Case Studies in Neuromuscular Disorders

Editor

AZIZ SHAIBANI

NEUROLOGIC CLINICS

www.neurologic.theclinics.com

Consulting Editor
RANDOLPH W. EVANS

August 2020 • Volume 38 • Number 3

ELSEVIER

1600 John F. Kennedy Boulevard • Suite 1800 • Philadelphia, Pennsylvania, 19103-2899

http://www.theclinics.com

NEUROLOGIC CLINICS Volume 38, Number 3
August 2020 ISSN 0733-8619, ISBN-13: 978-0-323-69771-2

Editor: Stacy Eastman
Developmental Editor: Donald Mumford

Neurologic Clinics (ISSN 0733-8619) is published quarterly by Elsevier Inc., 360 Park Avenue South, New York, NY 10010–1710. Months of issue are February, May, August, and November. Periodicals postage paid at New York, NY, and additional mailing offices. Subscription prices are $326.00 per year for US individuals, $696.00 per year for US institutions, $100.00 per year for US students, $408.00 per year for Canadian individuals, $843.00 per year for Canadian institutions, $427.00 per year for international individuals, $843.00 per year for international institutions, $210.00 for foreign students/residents, and $100.00 for Canadian students/residents. To receive student/resident rate, orders must be accompanied by name of affiliated institution, date of term, and the *signature* of program/residency coordinator on institution letterhead. Orders will be billed at individual rate until proof of status is received. Foreign air speed delivery is included in all *Clinics* subscription prices. All prices are subject to change without notice. **POSTMASTER:** Send address changes to *Neurologic Clinics*, Elsevier Health Sciences Division, Subscription Customer Service, 3251 Riverport Lane, Maryland Heights, MO 63043. **Customer Service: Telephone: 1-800-654-2452 (U.S. and Canada); 314-447-8871 (outside U.S. and Canada). Fax: 314-447-8029. E-mail: journalscustomerservice-usa@elsevier.com (for print support); journalsonlinesupport-usa@elsevier.com (for online support).**

Reprints. For copies of 100 or more of articles in this publication, please contact the Commercial Reprints Department, Elsevier Inc., 360 Park Avenue South, New York, New York, 10010-1710; Tel.: +1-212-633-3874; Fax: +1-212-633-3820, and E-mail: reprints@elsevier.com.

Neurologic Clinics is also published in Spanish by Nueva Editorial Interamericana S.A., Mexico City, Mexico.

Neurologic Clinics is covered in *Current Contents/Clinical Medicine, MEDLINE/PubMed (Index Medicus), EMBASE/Excerpta Medica, and PsycINFO, and ISI/BIOMED.*

Contributors

CONSULTING EDITOR

RANDOLPH W. EVANS, MD
Clinical Professor, Department of Neurology, Baylor College of Medicine, Houston, Texas, USA

EDITOR

AZIZ SHAIBANI, MD, FACP, FAAN, FANA
Director, Nerve and Muscle Center of Texas, Clinical Professor of Medicine, Baylor College of Medicine, Houston, Texas, USA

AUTHORS

EMILIO SUPSUPIN, Jr, MD
Assistant Professor, Neuroradiology, Department of Diagnostic and Interventional Imaging, McGovern Medical School, The University of Texas Houston Health Science Center, Houston, Texas, USA

JOHN M COLEMAN III, MD
Division of Pulmonary and Critical Care, Feinberg School of Medicine, Northwestern University, Chicago, Illinois, USA

SENDA AJROUD-DRISS, MD
Department of Neurology, Feinberg School of Medicine, Northwestern University, Chicago, Illinois, USA

HUSAM AL SULTANI, MD
Nerve and Muscle Center of Texas, Houston, Texas, USA

SUUR BILICILER, MD
Associate Professor of Neurology, UT Health Science Center in Houston, McGovern Medical School, Houston, Texas, USA

JACOB BOCKHORST, BA
University of Colorado, Anschutz Medical Campus, Aurora, Colorado, USA

JONATHAN R. BRENT, MD, PhD
Instructor, Department of Neurology, Feinberg School of Medicine, Northwestern University, Chicago, Illinois, USA

ENRICO BUGIARDINI, MD
Department of Neuromuscular Diseases, Queen Square Centre for Neuromuscular Diseases, University College London, London, United Kingdom

BAKRI H. ELSHEIKH, MBBS, MRCP
Associate Professor, Department of Neurology, The Ohio State University Wexner Medical Center, Columbus, Ohio, USA

KEVIN J. FELICE, DO
The Charles H. Kaman Foundation Neuromuscular and Muscular Dystrophy Association Care Center, Hospital for Special Care, New Britain, Connecticut, USA; Professor of Neurology, University of Connecticut School of Medicine, Farmington, Connecticut, USA

COLIN K. FRANZ, MD, PhD
Departments of Physical Medicine and Rehabilitation, and Neurology, Feinberg School of Medicine, Northwestern University, Shirley Ryan AbilityLab, Chicago, Illinois, USA

MELANIE D. GLENN, MD
Neuromuscular Medicine, Auckland, New Zealand

KELLY G. GWATHMEY, MD
Assistant Professor, Department of Neurology, Virginia Commonwealth University, Richmond, Virginia, USA

JOHANNA HAMEL, MD
Department of Neurology, University of Rochester Medical Center, Rochester, New York, USA

MICHAEL G. HANNA, FRCP, FMedSci
Department of Neuromuscular Diseases, Queen Square Centre for Neuromuscular Diseases, UCL Queen Square Institute of Neurology, National Hospital for Neurology and Neurosurgery, London, United Kingdom

YESSAR HUSSAIN, MD
Assistant Professor, The University of Texas at Austin, Dell Medical School, Director, Austin Neuromuscular Center, Austin, Texas, USA

STANLEY JONES P. IYADURAI, MSc, PhD, MD, FAAN
Neuromuscular Specialist, Department of Neurology, Johns Hopkins All Children's Hospital, St Petersburg, Florida, USA

DUAA JABARI, MD
Neuromuscular Medicine, University of Kansas Medical Center, Kansas City, Kansas, USA

HANS D. KATZBERG, MD, MSc, FRCPC
Associate Professor of Medicine (Neurology), Toronto General Hospital/University Health Network, Krembil Brain Institute, University of Toronto, Toronto, Ontario, Canada

JUSTIN KWAN, MD
Associate Professor of Neurology, Temple University, Lewis Katz School of Medicine, Philadelphia, Pennsylvania, USA

PEDRO M. MACHADO, MD, PhD
Department of Neuromuscular Diseases, Queen Square Centre for Neuromuscular Diseases, Division of Medicine, Centre for Rheumatology, University College London, London, United Kingdom

EMMA MATTHEWS, MRCP
Department of Neuromuscular Diseases, Queen Square Centre for Neuromuscular Diseases, UCL Queen Square Institute of Neurology, National Hospital for Neurology and Neurosurgery, London, United Kingdom

ASHIRWAD MERVE, FRCPath
Department of Neuropathology, UCL Queen Square Institute of Neurology, London, United Kingdom

SAMANTHA MILLER, MD
Neurology Resident, The University of Texas at Austin, Dell Medical School, Austin, Texas, USA

JASPER M. MORROW, FRACP
Department of Neuromuscular Diseases, Queen Square Centre for Neuromuscular Diseases, University College London, London, United Kingdom

PINKI MUNOT, MRCPCH
Dubowitz Neuromuscular Centre, Great Ormond Street Hospital for Children, London, United Kingdom

THY NGUYEN, MD
Associate Professor, Department of Neurology, McGovern Medical School, The University of Texas Houston Health Science Center, Houston, Texas, USA

MATTHEW PARTON, MD
Department of Neuromuscular Diseases, Queen Square Centre for Neuromuscular Diseases, University College London, London, United Kingdom

CECILE L. PHAN, MD
Associate Clinical Professor, Division of Neurology, Department of Medicine, University of Alberta, Edmonton, Alberta, Canada

DAVID S. SAPERSTEIN, MD
Director, Center for Complex Neurology, EDS & POTS, Clinical Associate Professor of Neurology, University of Arizona College of Medicine, Phoenix, Arizona, USA

AZIZ SHAIBANI, MD, FACP, FAAN, FANA
Director, Nerve and Muscle Center of Texas, Clinical Professor of Medicine, Baylor College of Medicine, Houston, Texas, USA

KAZIM SHEIKH, MD
Professor, Department of Neurology, McGovern Medical School, The University of Texas Houston Health Science Center, Houston, Texas, USA

PERRY B. SHIEH, MD, PhD, FAAN
Professor, Department of Neurology, University of California, Los Angeles, Los Angeles, California, USA

A. GORDON SMITH, MD
Professor and Chair, Department of Neurology, Virginia Commonwealth University, Richmond, Virginia, USA

RABI TAWIL, MD
Department of Neurology, University of Rochester Medical Center, Rochester, New York, USA

VINOJINI VIVEKANANDAM, MBBS, FRACP
Department of Neuromuscular Diseases, Queen Square Centre for Neuromuscular Diseases, UCL Queen Square Institute of Neurology, National Hospital for Neurology and Neurosurgery, London, United Kingdom

MEGAN A. WALDROP, MD
Assistant Professor, Center for Gene Therapy, Nationwide Children's Hospital, Department of Neurology, The Ohio State University Wexner Medical Center, Columbus, Ohio, USA

MATTHEW WICKLUND, MD
University of Colorado, Anschutz Medical Campus, Aurora, Colorado, USA

Contents

Preface xv

Aziz Shaibani

Skeletal Muscle Channelopathies 481

Vinojini Vivekanandam, Pinki Munot, Michael G. Hanna, and Emma Matthews

 Video content accompanies this article at http://www.neurologic.theclinics.com.

Skeletal muscle channelopathies are rare genetic neuromuscular conditions that include the nondystrophic myotonias and periodic paralyses. They cause disabling muscle symptoms and can limit educational potential, work opportunities, socialization, and quality of life. Effective therapy is available, making it essential to recognize and treat this group of disorders. Here, the authors highlight important aspects regarding diagnosis and management using illustrative case reports.

Limb Girdle Muscular Dystrophies 493

Jacob Bockhorst and Matthew Wicklund

 Video content accompanies this article at http://www.neurologic.theclinics.com.

The limb girdle muscular dystrophies (LGMDs) are genetic muscle diseases with primary skeletal muscle involvement in persons with the ability to walk independently at some point in the disease course. They usually have increased creatine kinase levels along with patterns of fatty and fibrous deposition on muscle imaging and/or dystrophic features on muscle biopsy. Distinctive clinical features provide valuable diagnostic clues to the diagnosis, and sometimes treatment, of these disorders. The advent of gene and cell-based therapies; gene replacement, editing, and modulation; along with stem cell and small molecule therapies may significantly ameliorate clinical severity in the LGMDs.

Spinal Muscular Atrophy in the Treatment Era 505

Megan A. Waldrop and Bakri H. Elsheikh

 Video content accompanies this article at http://www.neurologic.theclinics.com.

Spinal muscular atrophy is an autosomal-recessive degenerative neuromuscular disease that has historically been categorized into 5 types based on the individual's best functional ability. Two rather remarkable treatments have recently been approved for commercial use, and both have markedly changed the natural history of this disease. Here the authors report several cases of individuals, ranging from infants to adults, to highlight diagnostic considerations, along with initial and long-term treatment

Mutations in about 30 genes have been implicated. Diagnosis can be difficult. Treatment options vary depending on the specific genetic type.

Video content accompanies this article at http://www.neurologic.theclinics.com.

Diabetic lumbosacral radiculoplexus neuropathy, also known as diabetic amyotrophy, has a characteristic course of sudden onset of unilateral pain in the thigh and hip, which may spread to the other side in weeks to months and proceeds with progressive lower extremity weakness, often resulting in the inability to walk unassisted. The syndrome is typically monophasic, and most patients will recover at least to some degree. Less typical features include lack of pain, distal predominant weakness, absence of diabetes, and upper extremity involvement. This article provides a series of cases to highlight the diagnostic challenges and discusses management decision making.

Video content accompanies this article at http://www.neurologic.theclinics.com.

Amyotrophic lateral sclerosis (ALS) is a fatal disease with no cure; however, symptomatic management has an impact on quality of life and survival. Symptom management is best performed in a multidisciplinary care setting, where patients are evaluated by multiple health care professionals. Respiratory failure is a significant cause of morbidity and mortality in patients with ALS. Early initiation of noninvasive ventilation can prolong survival, and adequate use of airway clearance techniques can prevent respiratory infections. Preventing and treating weight loss caused by dysphagia may slow down disease progression, and expert management of spasticity from upper motor neuron dysfunction enhances patient well-being.

"Myasthenia gravis (MG) is the most common autoimmune neuromuscular disorder. This article highlights several cases that the practicing neurologist may encounter in the treatment of MG. Diagnostic uncertainty continues to be an issue in patients who are seronegative to the 2 most common antibodies, acetylcholine receptor and muscle-specific tyrosine kinase (MuSK). Specific populations of patients with MG including MuSK MG, thymomatous MG, refractory MG, and pregnant women also require special consideration. This article reviews specific cases and an update on current management."

Refractory Chronic Immune-mediated Demyelinating Polyneuropathy **591**

Aziz Shaibani and Husam Al Sultani

 Video content accompanies this article at http://www.neurologic.theclinics.com.

Please verify term, "alternative". Chronic immune-mediated demyelinating polyneuropathy (CIDP) is a treatable immune-related demyelinating polyneuropathy. Approximately 20% of cases do not respond to first-line therapies; most of these cases are due to alternative diagnoses, although some of them are due to severe CIDP. Unfortunately, a lack of universally accepted diagnostic criteria complicates the course of diagnosis and treatment. This article discusses videos of cases referred to a tertiary medical center for "refractory CIDP" and pitfalls in the diagnosis and management of this condition.

Small Fiber Neuropathy **607**

David S. Saperstein

Small fiber neuropathy has a broad array of presentations. Length-dependent symptoms and findings present little diagnostic difficulty, but non–length-dependent or multifocal symptoms can be challenging. Intraepidermal nerve fiber density (IENFD) testing in apparent fibromyalgia warrants further study, but skin biopsy testing of this patient population is reasonable. Avoidance of IENFD testing in situations where diagnosis of neuropathy is already clear or where neuropathy is not the cause of symptoms helps to prevent incorrect conclusions. Careful history and physical examination plus pretest probability are important factors to consider when assessing the results of an IENFD test report.

Other Myopathies **619**

Yessar Hussain and Samantha Miller

 Video content accompanies this article at http://www.neurologic.theclinics.com.

Healthy muscle relies on a complex and interdependent network that includes, but is not limited to, proteins, ion channels, and the production and utilization of ATP. Disruptions to the system can occur for a number of reasons (genetic mutations, toxins, systemic disease, inflammation), yet they clinically present with symptoms that are nonspecific and common to myopathies: weakness, muscle pain, cramping, hypotonia. This article uses a case-based format to review the clinical reasoning and diagnostic tools that guide the accurate diagnosis of myopathies. We specifically focus on toxic, metabolic, mitochondrial, and late-onset congenital myopathies.

Distal Myopathies **637**

Kevin J. Felice

The distal myopathies are a rare and heterogeneous group of neuromuscular disorders. Patients present with weakness of the hands, distal lower extremities, or both. Age of onset varies from early childhood to late

inflammatory and hereditary etiologies. This article discusses atypical cases and differential diagnoses and considers the role of imaging and histopathology in differentiating inclusion body myositis.

Immune-Mediated Neuropathies **711**

Kelly G. Gwathmey and A. Gordon Smith

 Video content accompanies this article at http://www.neurologic.theclinics.com.

The immune-mediated neuropathies are a broad category of diseases differentiated by time course, affected nerve fibers, and disease associations. This article spans the common, well-defined inflammatory demyelinating polyradiculoneuropathies (Guillain-Barré syndrome and chronic inflammatory demyelinating polyradiculoneuropathy) to the rarer, acquired demyelinating neuropathy variants (Miller-Fisher syndrome and multifocal motor neuropathy), vasculitic neuropathies, and sensory neuronopathies (dorsal root ganglionopathies). These case studies illustrate the characteristic clinical patterns of the immune-mediated neuropathies encountered in neurologic practice. Recommendations for diagnostic evaluation and treatment approach accompany each case. Prompt recognition of these disorders is imperative; delays in treatment may result in prolonged morbidity and permanent disability.

NEUROLOGIC CLINICS

FORTHCOMING ISSUES

November 2020
Applied Neurotoxicology
Michael R. Dobbs and Mam I. Ibraheem, *Editors*

February 2021
Therapy in Neurology
José Biller, *Editor*

May 2021
Neurologic Emergencies
Joseph D. Burns and Anna M. Cervantes-Arslanian, *Editors*

RECENT ISSUES

May 2020
Treatment of Movement Disorders
Joseph Jankovic, *Editor*

February 2020
Neuroimaging
Laszlo L. Mechtler, *Editor*

November 2019
Migraine and other Primary Headaches
Randolph W. Evans, *Editor*

RELATED SERIES

Neurosurgery Clinics
https://www.neurosurgery.theclinics.com/
Neuroimaging Clinics
www.neuroimaging.theclinics.com
Psychiatric Clinics
https://www.psych.theclinics.com/
Child and Adolescent Psychiatric Clinics
https://www.childpsych.theclinics.com/

Preface

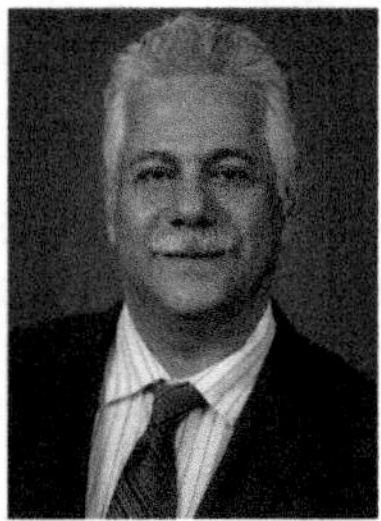

Aziz Shaibani, MD, FACP, FAAN, FANA
Editor

Neuromuscular disorders (NMD) is probably the most dynamic neurology subspecialty. The incidence of NMD as a group (160/100,000) is comparable to that of Parkinson disease and is increasing due to improved diagnosis and management. NMD carry high mortality and morbidity and economic burden.

Neuromuscular symptoms, such as muscle cramps, pain, muscle weakness, numbness, and fatigue, comprise approximately 50% of the presenting symptoms to the general neurology practice. Over the last 5 years, at least 7 new agents were approved by the Food and Drug Administration to treat NMD (Duchenne muscular dystrophy, spinal muscular atrophy [SMA], amyloidosis, amyotrophic lateral sclerosis [ALS], Lambert-Eaton syndrome, and myasthenia gravis [MG]). The current decade can be rightly labeled as the decade of biologics (in particular, monoclonal antibodies) and genetics when it comes to the diagnosis and treatment of NMD.

This issue of *Neurologic Clinics* is aimed at the general neurologist, NMD trainee, and general practitioner, who are eager to learn about new developments in the diagnosis and treatment of NMD.

I am honored to be the editor of this issue of *Neurologic Clinics*. I invited experts from different fields to update the readers about the diagnosis and management of a spectrum of NMD. The world of neuromuscular genetics has not stopped evolving. While genetic panels and whole-exome and -genome sequencing have become much more affordable, some cases remain challenging. A practical approach to the diagnosis of atypical genetic NMD is a needed update that is covered well by Shieh in this issue. Seeing children who were not expected to live beyond the first year of their life, crawling and walking, was not conceivable 10 years ago. New treatments for spinal muscular atrophy (SMA) have made that possible. Waldrop and Elsheikh cover these new and exciting developments. New therapies, albeit modest, are emerging for ALS. Brent and colleagues discuss the present and future of ALS management. Monoclonal antibodies have changed the therapeutic landscape of the refractory MG; this is addressed by Nguyen and colleagues. Epidermal nerve fiber density estimation for the diagnosis of small-fiber neuropathy has become very popular. The value and limitations are discussed by Saperstein. Muscle cramps are common, and their approach

Neurol Clin 38 (2020) xv–xvi
https://doi.org/10.1016/j.ncl.2020.05.002

lacks quantitative and objective measurements to guide treatment and clinical trials. Katzberg and Sadeghian discuss these issues. Inclusion body myositis, the most common myopathy after age 50 years, still has mimics. Machado and colleagues discuss the differential diagnosis. Immune-mediated neuropathies and myopathies are discussed by the Smith, Biliciler, and Shaibani groups. Genetic advances in facioscapulohumeral muscular dystrophy are discussed by Tawil, and congenital myasthenic syndromes are discussed by Iyadurai. Glenn and Jabari discuss the interesting syndrome of diabetic amyotrophy and its spectrum. Felice and Hussain discuss other myopathies. Increasingly reported mutations and changing classifications of chanelopathies are visited by Matthews and colleagues.

Throughout the issue, we use a similar style and emphasis on illustrations, algorithms, and videos to soften the stiff scientific material and enhance learning. I would like to thank the authors, for their contributions, and Mr Don Mumford, for the editorial support.

More articles on muscle than nerve disease may reflect my own prejudices as well the limitation of space.

I hope that the readers will be satisfied and happy.

Aziz Shaibani, MD, FACP, FAAN, FANA
Nerve and Muscle Center of Texas
Baylor College of Medicine
6624 Fannin Street, Suite 1670
Houston, TX 77030, USA

E-mail address:
ather@aol.com

Skeletal Muscle Channelopathies

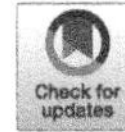

Vinojini Vivekanandam, MBBS, FRACP[a], Pinki Munot, MRCPCH[b], Michael G. Hanna, FRCP, FMedSci[a], Emma Matthews, MRCP[a,*]

KEYWORDS

- Myotonia • Myotonia congenita • Paramyotonia congenita • Periodic paralysis
- Channelopathies

KEY POINTS

- There are several conditions to consider in patients displaying myotonia on electromyography. Myotonic dystrophy type 1 is the most common differential diagnosis.
- Hypokalemic periodic paralysis can be more severe in men and require polypharmacy to control symptoms.
- Accurate diagnosis is important to inform effective treatment options available for skeletal muscle channelopathies.
- Cardiac conduction defects seen in Andersen-Tawil syndrome require monitoring and involvement from cardiac colleagues, even if asymptomatic.
- The skeletal muscle channelopathies can have significant impact on quality of life. Beyond myotonia and paralysis, pain and fatigue are important aspects to consider in management.

 **Video content accompanies this article at http://www.neurologic.theclinics.com.**

INTRODUCTION

Skeletal muscle channelopathies are a group of rare heterogeneous neuromuscular disorders characterized by episodic disabling symptoms of either myotonia or paralysis. They are genetic disorders, and onset is predominantly in childhood. Symptoms can have a significant impact on quality of life and influence educational opportunities, employment choice, and pregnancy. A subset develops fixed myopathy with progressive disability. They are important disorders to recognize and diagnose because

[a] Department of Neuromuscular Diseases, Queen Square Centre for Neuromuscular Diseases, UCL Queen Square Institute of Neurology and National Hospital for Neurology and Neurosurgery, London WC1N 3BG, UK; [b] Dubowitz Neuromuscular Centre, Great Ormond Street Hospital for Children, London, UK
* Corresponding author.
E-mail address: emma.matthews@ucl.ac.uk

Neurol Clin 38 (2020) 481–491
https://doi.org/10.1016/j.ncl.2020.04.003

symptomatic treatment is available and can make a significant difference to quality of life and morbidity.

Estimated minimum point prevalence of the skeletal muscle channelopathies is approximately 1.12 per 100,000.[1] With increased awareness, and the advent of next-generation sequencing, prevalence is now likely to be higher. The skeletal muscle channelopathies are broadly divided into the nondystrophic myotonias and the periodic paralyses. The nondystrophic myotonias include myotonia congenita (MC), paramyotonia congenita (PMC), and sodium channel myotonia. Myotonia is often experienced by patients as stiffness, cramps, and locking, which may be painful. MC, owing to mutations in the CLCN1 gene, is the most common of all the skeletal muscle channelopathies.[1] Myotonia predominantly affects the legs, and falls can be common. The hallmark of this condition is the warm-up phenomenon (improved myotonia with repetition). PMC owing to mutations in the SCN4A gene typically affects the hands and eye/facial muscle more than the legs. Paradoxic myotonia is demonstrated (worsening of myotonia with repetition). Episodes of weakness or even frank paralysis may occur in PMC. Sodium channel myotonia, also due to mutations in the SCN4A gene, has a similar distribution of muscle involvement to PMC but both warm-up and paradoxic myotonia may be found. Sodium channel myotonias are purely myotonic phenotypes without any episodic weakness. All of the non-dystrophic myotonias (NDMs) can be exacerbated by cold, but it is most striking in PMC, exercise, or prolonged rest. Muscle hypertrophy can also present in any NDM, although is typically highlighted in MC.

The periodic paralyses include hyperkalemic periodic paralysis caused by mutations in the SCN4A gene,[2,3] hypokalemic periodic paralysis caused by mutations in the CACNA1S gene (up to 80%) and the SCN4A gene,[4] and Andersen-Tawil syndrome (ATS) caused by mutations in the KCNJ2 gene.[5] ATS is the only skeletal muscle channelopathy to involve tissues other than skeletal muscle, namely the heart (cardiac conduction defects) and bone development (dysmorphic features).[6] During an attack of paralysis, patients experience disabling weakness and areflexia. Between attacks, muscle strength is often normal. Triggers can include exertion, carbohydrate-rich meals, cold, and stress.

The authors illustrate important clinical aspects regarding diagnosis and management of the skeletal muscle channelopathies with the use of 5 clinical cases.

CASE A: AN ALTERNATIVE

A 62-year-old woman presented with a history of muscle stiffness and myalgia since childhood. Past medical history included a previous hysterectomy for menorrhagia, hypercholesterolemia, and fatty liver.

Early history and development were normal, but at the age of 8 she recalls that her feet would often be "stuck" when skating on ice. At age 21, when playing rounders, she fell over when trying to run after hitting the ball. Symptoms worsened during each of her pregnancies, and climbing stairs became difficult. Her symptoms could be exacerbated in cold environments, and her condition deteriorated when she was prescribed a statin.

In her fifties, she noted the development of other symptoms. She felt unbalanced if standing unaided for long periods. Significant exercise left her fatigued the following day. She enjoyed hiking but found stepping over boulders very difficult even with walking poles. She lost the ability to jump.

In terms of family history, her 2 daughters reported difficulty opening jars and similar muscle stiffness during pregnancy. Her mother and sister had apparently reported "difficulty with cold hands and feet" but were not evaluated in the authors' clinic.

On examination at the time of referral in her fifties, she had hand grip myotonia (Video 1). Some mild proximal weakness was detected: medical research council grade 4+ in the shoulder abductors and hip flexors. Creatine kinase level was 418 IU/L. Electromyography (EMG) demonstrated myotonia and a positive short exercise test with Fournier type III pattern. This pattern of short exercise test is nonspecific and can be present in sodium channel myotonia, autosomal dominant MC, and myotonic dystrophy type 2 (DM2). Given the lack of systemic features, she was diagnosed with a nondystrophic myotonia on clinical grounds. There was no history of cardiac disease or symptoms; electrocardiogram (ECG) was normal, and she started mexiletine with significant symptomatic improvement.

Genetic testing identified a novel variant in the SCN4A gene (c.4805 A > G, p.Asn1602Ser) that was present in the proband and in one of her affected daughters who the authors had also assessed and confirmed to have a myotonic disorder. Her second daughter, who also reported symptoms, tested negative for this mutation. This discrepancy raised doubt as to the pathogenicity of the SCN4A variant. The authors recommended she be assessed in her local center because she lived abroad, and undergo an EMG. In parallel with this, additional laboratory-based functional testing to determine electrophysiological evidence of pathogenicity of this novel gene variant was started.

Laboratory-based assessment showed the variant had no significant effect on channel function, indicating it was a benign variant. The daughter's EMG demonstrated she had myotonia, confirming that she was affected, and therefore, the SCN4A variant did not segregate with disease in the family. Genetic testing for DM2 was requested in the proband and was positive with a CCTG repeat in intron 1 of the CNBP gene. This diagnosis was subsequently confirmed in both her daughters.

On the day of the proband's clinic appointment to discuss the new genetic results, she attended clinic and reported she had remained generally well but had just been diagnosed with cataracts.

What is the most common diagnosis in a patient presenting with myotonia?

1. Myotonia congenita
2. Paramyotonia congenita
3. Myotonic dystrophy type 2
4. Pompe disease
5. Myotonic dystrophy type 1

Correct answer: 5

Discussion

Differential diagnosis of myotonia

Myotonia is delayed relaxation of skeletal muscle after voluntary contraction. It is often described by patients as muscle stiffness, cramp, or "locking." Symptoms commonly affect the hands and legs but can involve any skeletal muscle, including those of the face, jaw, tongue, and trunk. In some patients, it can even affect intercostal muscles causing dyspnea. Myotonia is best examined with initiation of gait, in the hands and eyes (Video 2). In MC, myotonia lessens with repetition, whereas in paramyotonia, myotonia worsens with repetition (Video 3).

Myotonia can be present in several conditions, including the nondystrophic myotonias and myotonic dystrophy type 1 and 2. Myotonic dystrophy 1 (DM1) is the most common myotonic disorder with an incidence of 1 in 8000, and although typically accompanied by a degree of distal weakness and/or extramuscular manifestations, such as cataracts, diabetes, frontal balding, and testosterone deficiency, these features may not yet be evident early in the disease course (or at the age when NDM typically presents).[7] Extramuscular features are likewise reported in DM2 along with proximal weakness but may be mild. It is always important to consider a differential diagnosis of DM in patients with myotonia because the systemic and cardiac features require a different monitoring and management approach to the skeletal muscle exclusive of nondystrophic myotonias.

Electrical myotonia, often without overt clinical myotonia, can also be seen in other neuromuscular disorders, including acid maltase deficiency (Pompe disease), myopathies, including myofibrillar myopathies, denervation, drug-induced hypothyroidism, and colchicine-induced myopathy.[8]

Differentiating Nondystrophic Myotonia from myotonic dystrophy

Obvious systemic features associated with DM versus an isolated myotonic disorder generally assist in differentiating these diseases, although the caveats above of early disease course in DM1 and milder symptoms in DM2 can cause confusion (as in the described family). Myalgia is often suggested as a pointer toward DM2, but it is not specific and can be significant among the NDMs as well. The short exercise test with variable patterns as described by Fournier can be indicative if characteristic (patterns 1 and 2), but as in this case, pattern 3 is noninformative.[9] Genetic testing is ultimately diagnostic, although the possibility of polymorphisms in a candidate gene can be misleading (as in this case). It is also notable that single heterozygous CLCN1 gene mutations and DM2 can coexist[10] or can modify a sodium channel phenotype.[11]

Is it safe to use mexiletine to treat myotonia in myotonic dystrophy?

The proband derived significant benefit from taking the class I antiarrhythmic sodium channel blocker mexiletine. In the NDMs, that is, those without preexisting heart disease, it has a good safety profile, and this is largely considered to be first-line therapy. It can be arrhythmogenic however, and this raises greater concern in DM because of the risk of preexisting cardiac disease. Atrioventricular and interventricular conduction defects are common.[12] In addition, approximately 14% have left ventricular systolic dysfunction. In a trial of mexiletine in patients with DM, no significant difference was seen in ECGs and cardiac events between mexiletine and placebo groups.[13] However, patients with significant cardiac arrhythmias were excluded from this study. Given the theoretic arrhythmogenic risk with mexiletine, caution should be taken when using it in patients with DM and associated cardiac disease.

The authors' patients had normal ECGs performed as part of routine monitoring while on mexiletine and reported no symptoms suggestive of cardiac disease. Following the diagnosis of DM2, they were additionally reviewed by cardiologists who recommended they could continue to take the medicine with a yearly cardiac review.

CASE B: RUNS IN THE FAMILY

A 32-year-old man was referred to clinic with a history of muscle stiffness. Early childhood development was normal. He was active in primary school. Symptom onset was at age 12. He noticed stiffness and locking in his legs, hands, and occasionally jaw and tongue. He enjoyed hockey, but was unable to keep playing because stiffness predominantly affected his legs (especially initiation of movement or sudden movement) and was particularly troublesome in the cold. Muscle symptoms had a tendency to improve as he warmed up.

Examination was notable for calf hypertrophy and gait and grip myotonia.

In terms of family history, his brother described similar symptoms, but his parents and sister were unaffected.

Clinical history and examination were indicative of MC, and genetic testing identified a heterozygous c.654 G > A, p. Gly285Glu mutation in the chloride channel gene CLCN1, confirming the diagnosis. This mutation is pathogenic and described in numerous unrelated families with MC. The inheritance pattern in some, however, is autosomal dominant and in others is autosomal recessive. Segregation testing was undertaken in the family. His asymptomatic mother and sister did not carry the mutation, whereas his symptomatic brother did. His father, although asymptomatic and without any EMG evidence for myotonia, was also found to be heterozygous for the mutation.

All coding regions of the CLCN1 gene were sequenced, and multiplex ligation-dependent probe amplification (MLPA) was performed to exclude any gene rearrangements. Genetic analysis of the SCN4A gene and testing for DM1 and DM2 was also negative.

What can be the inheritance pattern in myotonia congenita?

1. Autosomal dominant
2. Autosomal recessive
3. De novo dominant
4. Autosomal dominant with reduced penetrance
5. Any of the above

Correct answer: 5

Discussion

What is the inheritance pattern in the family?

To further assess the effect of the Gly285Glu CLCN1 mutation, cell-based electrophysiological characterization of the effects of the mutation in an oocyte model was undertaken. The mutation had definite effects on chloride channel function, and these effects are similar to those seen in other dominantly inherited CLCN1 mutations. In this family, 2 individuals who were heterozygous for the mutation displayed clinical symptoms, whereas their father was asymptomatic. In the authors' diagnostic service, the inheritance pattern seen in families with this variant is variable, reflecting what is reported in the literature, that is, some appear dominant and others appear recessive. The authors excluded other scenarios, for example, concomitant DM2.

Overall, given 2 symptomatic family members who were both heterozygous for the mutation, previous descriptions of the CLCN1 Gly285Glu mutation in multiple dominant pedigrees, the cell electrophysiology compatible with dominant inheritance, and the lack of any confounding genetic variants in other genes, the inheritance pattern in this family was thought to be most consistent with dominant inheritance with reduced penetrance.

CASE C: A TREATMENT CHALLENGE

A 15-year-old boy was transitioned from pediatric services. He was born premature but reached developmental milestones well. At age 8, following a viral gastroenteritis, he developed weakness of arms and legs lasting 24 hours. In subsequent years, he had a similar episode once or twice per year, but in the few years before transition, this had escalated to 2 to 3 episodes per week. At the age of 14, he was admitted to hospital with quadriparesis. Serum potassium level was 2.5 mmol/L. A diagnosis of hypokalemic periodic paralysis was confirmed with a genetic mutation in CACNA1S (p.Arg528His). He was started on acetazolamide, and attack frequency reduced to 2 to 3 per month.

His attacks of paralysis typically occur in the morning, on waking. They can be triggered by high carbohydrate intake. Occasionally, his hands become weak in the cold, or he may have some weakness if exercising after a significant break.

At review on transition to the adult clinic, his symptoms had deteriorated again to 2 to 3 attacks per week, despite being prescribed acetazolamide 250 mg 3 times daily. He reported however that because of commitments at school he would often forget the midday dose. At this stage, his acetazolamide dose was changed to a twice daily dose of 500 mg, allowing for easier administration and a slight dose increase. He additionally started daily Sando-K (potassium supplementation) 2 tablets in the morning.

He enrolled in college, but on average would miss 2 days per week because of attacks. If he woke with weakness, he could not get out of bed until 2 PM Amiloride 5 mg daily, increasing to 5 mg twice daily, was added to acetazolamide and Sando-K. This regimen improved some severity of symptoms but not to a degree sufficient to prevent days off.

Amiloride was changed to spironolactone 50 mg daily in an attempt to gain better control of the attacks, but this was not tolerated because of side effects and was changed to eplerenone. A combination of eplerenone, acetazolamide, and daily Sando-K reduced the duration and frequency of attacks, although did not abolish them entirely.

His mother carries the same CACNA1S mutation and has reported symptoms since age 17. However, she has mild, infrequent episodes of weakness that do not significantly impair function or prevent work attendance and have not required treatment.

Which of the following is not a treatment for hypokalemic periodic paralysis?

1. Spirinolactone
2. Acetazolamide
3. Bendroflumethiazide
4. Amiloride
5. Potassium supplements

Correct answer: 3

Discussion

Why was the proband more severely affected than his mother when they both have the same genetic mutation?

Reduced penetrance and variable severity of phenotype with the same mutation are relatively common in skeletal muscle channelopathies.[14] The same mutation can even cause different phenotypes within the same family (see also case 2). Phenotypic variability may be influenced by epigenetic factors and differential allelic expression.[15] In addition, it is reported that men are more severely affected by the periodic paralyses than women.[14] A gender difference was illustrated in the proband with severe, treatment-resistant symptoms, whereas his mother with the same CACNA1S mutation is mildly affected, not requiring any pharmacologic treatment.

What should the approach to treatment in hypokalemic periodic paralysis consider?

Because of the episodic nature of symptoms in the channelopathies with return to baseline, they are sometimes regarded as relatively benign. Frequent, prolonged, and severe episodes however are severely limiting with additional disability or disadvantages accrued if unable to participate in education, socialization (especially in teenage years), and work.[16] Frequency and severity of symptoms, detrimental effect on daily life/activities, and any obvious triggers to symptoms are all factors to consider in the approach to management.

Identification and minimization of triggers, for example, consumption of large carbohydrate loads, is useful in all cases, regardless of overall severity. Keeping a food diary can be a useful way to highlight foods that may be especially detrimental to an individual. Including the timing of meals is also helpful because many patients report the influence of carbohydrates in the evening is worse the less time they are taken before going to sleep.

Those with mild and infrequent episodes may prefer not to take daily medication. Most patients in the authors' clinical experience require management with at least 1 agent, although they may be more severely affected individuals by the nature of their referral to clinic. If pharmacologic agents are considered, Acetazolamide, a carbonic anhydrase inhibitor, is often used as first-line treatment and can be effective in any form of periodic paralysis. In hypokalemic periodic paralysis specifically, other agents aim to prevent low serum potassium, for example, potassium-sparing diuretics, such as amiloride or spironolactone, which are taken daily as a prophylactic attempt to prevent attacks or reduce their frequency. Potassium supplementation is more rapid acting and frequently taken at the onset of an attack to try and reduce its duration and/or severity. A small regular daily adjunctive dose in conjunction with other prophylactic medications can also sometimes be beneficial. In difficult-to-treat cases, a combination of agents may be required.

The aim of therapy is ultimately to reduce the frequency, duration, and severity of episodic symptoms. A subset of patients develop progressive fixed weakness, but it is unclear as yet the extent that this relates to frequency of attacks and whether aggressive symptomatic treatment would prevent or reduce this.

More recently, MRI has been used to identify patients with significant short T1 inversion recovery (STIR) signal change in muscles. STIR signal suggests edema related to an attack in these patients and may be a potential biomarker for treatment efficacy, although this requires further exploration.

Other factors to consider in management include providing an emergency plan to the local team with instructions for administering intravenous potassium and cardiac monitoring in the event of a profound quadriparesis and significantly low serum potassium. Education regarding the condition and suitable adjustments should also be provided to school and work.

CASE D: ALL MUSCLE

An 18-year-old boy was born at term with no perinatal complications. He was smaller than average at birth, but well, and subsequent development was normal. He was sporty in primary school, with comparable abilities to his peers and enjoyed playing football. He had some dental abnormalities requiring an orthodontist's input for overcrowding and misalignment.

There was no significant family history. His parents and older sister were well.

At age 11, he collapsed at school. Bystanders described sudden loss of consciousness and thought he had a fit. When an ambulance arrived, an unspecified cardiac ventricular arrhythmia was detected. On arrival to hospital, nodalol was started but did not control the rhythm. He was subsequently started on Flecainide and Verapamil with control of the rhythm achieved. Subsequent cardiac monitoring in childhood recorded transient ventricular tachycardias. At age 14, a Reveal device was implanted to aid monitoring.

Despite intermittent cardiac conduction abnormalities, he did not report any palpitations or other cardiac symptoms. On specific questioning, he did notice a little weakness in his legs after exercise but had thought this was normal. He had no episodes of paralysis. On examination, he was of short stature with evidence of micrognathia, hypertelorism, and clinodactyly. Neurophysiology testing demonstrated a positive long exercise test. Genetic testing revealed a KCNJ2 mutation (c.368 T > G, p.Val123Gly) consistent with a diagnosis of ATS.

In a patient presenting with suspected periodic paralysis, which test is most helpful in indicating a diagnosis of Andersen-Tawil syndrome?

1. Creatine kinase
2. An ECG
3. A muscle biopsy
4. Their height
5. Clinodactyly

Correct answer: 2

Discussion

What is the cardiac spectrum of disease in Andersen-Tawil syndrome?

ATS has historically been thought to have a generally benign cardiac phenotype with life-threatening arrhythmias occurring only rarely. The key features reported include presence of U waves on the ECG (**Fig. 1**) and ventricular ectopics.[17] However, there is increasing literature on the occurrence of more severe arrhythmias and the need for implantable cardiac defibrillators. In the authors' cohort of 62 patients at the National Hospital for Neurology and Neurosurgery, 8% of those with genetically confirmed ATS have required an implantable cardiac defibrillator for sustained ventricular tachycardia or cardiac arrest. In addition, 12.5% have cardiogenic syncope. Patients typically complain of few cardiac symptoms or only palpitations, and without regular monitoring, there is a risk serious arrhythmia will be undetected. The authors

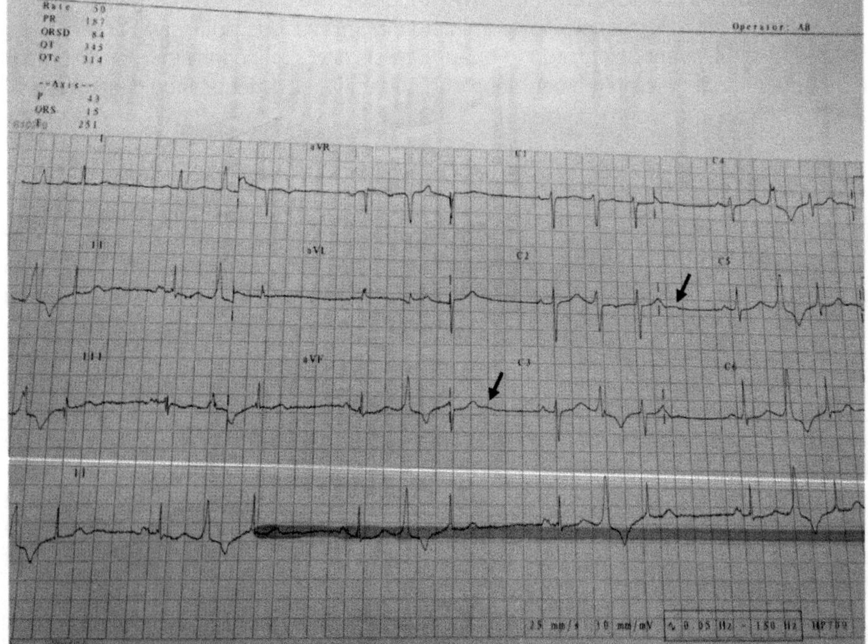

Fig. 1. Ventricular ectopics and U waves (*black arrows*) seen on a resting ECG in patients with ATS.

recommend all ATS patients (with or without cardiac symptoms) have at least yearly cardiac review, including a minimum of 24-hour Holter monitoring.

What characteristic features are seen in Andersen-Tawil syndrome, and can they aid diagnosis?
ATS is described as a triad of periodic paralysis, cardiac conduction defects, and dysmorphic features, but only 2 out of 3 are required for diagnosis. It is notable that the episodic muscle weakness in ATS is also often not profound or does not result in quadriparesis (as in the authors' case), meaning this feature can be present but its significance overlooked. Similarly, not all patients complain of cardiac symptoms or may only report occasional palpitations. An ECG is often abnormal however (see **Fig. 1**) and can be a useful investigation in anyone presenting with periodic paralysis, even if they do not appear dysmorphic.

Classically described dysmorphic features include short stature, hypertelorism, low-set ears, micrognathia, small hands and feet, clinodactyly, and syndodactyly.[5,6] However, in some patients, these features may be subtle, and certainly not all aspects are present in everyone. Some patients may be of normal height or even tall for their gender and age. In the authors' practice, the most consistently present feature appears to be clinodactyly, but this is a relatively common dysmorphic feature and not specific to ATS. This broad range of distinctive features and even the complete absence (or subtlety) of distinctive features is important to be aware of. The absence of these features should not dissuade clinicians from pursuing genetic testing for KCNJ2 mutations.

CASE E: FATIGUE

A 13-year-old boy presented with lethargy. He was born at term, and development was normal. At age 9, he noticed myalgia and limb pain, which was exacerbated during an intercurrent illness. Despite recovering from the upper respiratory tract infection, he had persistent although variable lethargy and pain and slept and ate poorly. He missed a substantial amount of school. At this stage, routine investigations were normal with the exception of a slightly elevated for age creatinine kinase level of 305 IU/L. He was diagnosed with chronic fatigue syndrome, and symptoms persisted. There was no significant family history or other past medical history.

Two years later, he woke with heaviness and weakness in his legs, which progressed over the course of the day. He went on a school trip, but by that evening, he was unable to walk or sit upright, had paralysis of all limbs, and poor head control. He was taken to the emergency department where a serum potassium level of 2 mmol/L was recorded. This serum potassium level was corrected with oral potassium supplementation, and the weakness subsequently improved over the following 48 hours. He had 3 further similar episodes over the next 3 months. The weakness was always worse in the mornings, with some improvement in strength over the day. There were no identifiable triggers. Daily episodes of myalgia and heaviness in the legs continued. School attendance remained poor.

On examination, there was no fixed muscle weakness, atrophy, or hypertrophy. A long exercise test was normal. Creatine kinase level was mildly elevated at 495 IU/L. Genetic testing identified a pathogenic de novo CACNA1S mutation, confirming a diagnosis of hypokalemic periodic paralysis.

Subsequent treatment with potassium supplementation, acetazolamide, and amiloride was effective in reducing the severity and frequency of weakness and fatigue as well as episodes of full paralysis. School attendance significantly improved.

Which of the following are not symptoms of hypokalemic periodic paralysis?

1. Episodic muscle weakness
2. Fatigue
3. Syncope
4. Myalgia
5. Progressive muscle weakness

Correct answer: 3

Discussion

Are the symptoms of fatigue and myalgia relevant?

Fatigue and myalgia as the presenting symptom of periodic paralysis are rare; however, a significant proportion of patients do describe fatigue and report that lack of energy is a significant aspect to the impact on quality of life.[18] The Independent Quality of Life questionnaire and 36-Item Short Form Health Survey were administered to 66 patients with skeletal muscle channelopathies. Patients with MC and hypokalemic periodic paralysis had the worst perception of the quality of their life. Muscle weakness and fatigue were important contributors to this perception.

When this patient was referred to the authors, the authors in retrospect some of his fatigue and myalgia were accompanied by weakness and probably did reflect the onset of periodic paralysis symptoms, but it was not until his presentation with quadriparesis that this became evident.

This case also highlights the impact of hypokalemic periodic paralysis on educational potential. Because attacks often occur first thing in the morning but can resolve by the afternoon, they can also be misinterpreted as school avoidance. Liaising with the school to ensure adequate understanding of the condition, allowing pupils to attend in the afternoon even if they have missed the morning, and sending school work to be done at home are all useful avenues that can be deployed to limit the impact on learning and achievement.

DISCLOSURES

Part of this work was undertaken at University College London Hospitals/University College London, which received a proportion of funding from the Department of Health's National Institute for Health Research Biomedical Research Centres funding scheme. M.G. Hanna receives research funds from the Medical Research Council and the UCLH Biomedical Research Centre. E. Matthews receives research funds from Wellcome.

SUPPLEMENTARY DATA

Supplementary data related to this article can be found online at https://doi.org/10.1016/j.ncl.2020.04.003.

REFERENCES

1. Horga A, Raja Rayan DL, Matthews E, et al. Prevalence study of genetically defined skeletal muscle channelopathies in England. Neurology 2013;80(16):1472–5.
2. Fontaine B, Khurana TS, Hoffman EP, et al. Hyperkalemic periodic paralysis and the adult muscle sodium channel alpha-subunit gene. Science 1990;250(4983):1000–2.
3. Ptacek LJ, George AL Jr, Griggs RC, et al. Identification of a mutation in the gene causing hyperkalemic periodic paralysis. Cell 1991;67(5):1021–7.

4. Bulman DE, Scoggan KA, van Oene MD, et al. A novel sodium channel mutation in a family with hypokalemic periodic paralysis. Neurology 1999;53(9):1932–6.
5. Tawil R, Ptacek LJ, Pavlakis SG, et al. Andersen's syndrome: potassium-sensitive periodic paralysis, ventricular ectopy, and dysmorphic features. Ann Neurol 1994;35(3):326–30.
6. Andersen ED, Krasilnikoff PA, Overvad H. Intermittent muscular weakness, extrasystoles, and multiple developmental anomalies. A new syndrome? Acta Paediatr Scand 1971;60(5):559–64.
7. Matthews E, Fialho D, Tan SV, et al. The non-dystrophic myotonias: molecular pathogenesis, diagnosis and treatment. Brain 2010;133(Pt 1):9–22.
8. Miller TM. Differential diagnosis of myotonic disorders. Muscle Nerve 2008;37(3): 293–9.
9. Fournier E, Arzel M, Sternberg D, et al. Electromyography guides toward subgroups of mutations in muscle channelopathies. Ann Neurol 2004;56(5):650–61.
10. Suominen T, Schoser B, Raheem O, et al. High frequency of co-segregating CLCN1 mutations among myotonic dystrophy type 2 patients from Finland and Germany. J Neurol 2008;255(11):1731–6.
11. Furby A, Vicart S, Camdessanche JP, et al. Heterozygous CLCN1 mutations can modulate phenotype in sodium channel myotonia. Neuromuscul Disord 2014; 24(11):953–9.
12. Smith CA, Gutmann L. Myotonic dystrophy type 1 management and therapeutics. Curr Treat Options Neurol 2016;18(12):52.
13. Groh WJ. Mexiletine is an effective antimyotonia treatment in myotonic dystrophy type 1. Neurology 2011;76(4):409 [author reply: 409].
14. Venance SL, Cannon SC, Fialho D, et al. The primary periodic paralyses: diagnosis, pathogenesis and treatment. Brain 2006;129(Pt 1):8–17.
15. Duno M, Colding-Jorgensen E, Grunnet M, et al. Difference in allelic expression of the CLCN1 gene and the possible influence on the myotonia congenita phenotype. Eur J Hum Genet 2004;12(9):738–43.
16. Matthews E, Silwal A, Sud R, et al. Skeletal muscle channelopathies: rare disorders with common pediatric symptoms. J Pediatr 2017;188:181–5.e6.
17. Zhang L, Benson DW, Tristani-Firouzi M, et al. Electrocardiographic features in Andersen-Tawil syndrome patients with KCNJ2 mutations: characteristic T-U-wave patterns predict the KCNJ2 genotype. Circulation 2005;111(21):2720–6.
18. Sansone VA, Ricci C, Montanari M, et al. Measuring quality of life impairment in skeletal muscle channelopathies. Eur J Neurol 2012;19(11):1470–6.

Limb Girdle Muscular Dystrophies

Jacob Bockhorst, BA[a], Matthew Wicklund, MD[b,*]

KEYWORDS

- Limb girdle muscular dystrophies • Anoctamin 5 • Calpain 3 • Caveolin 3
- Lamin A/C

KEY POINTS

- As a group, the limb girdle muscular dystrophies are the fourth most common of the genetic muscle diseases.
- Distinctive clinical features can facilitate diagnosis and/or treatment in some of the limb girdle muscular dystrophy genetic subtypes.
- A definitive genetic diagnosis in the limb girdle muscular dystrophies spurs appreciation for possible other organ system involvement in each genetic subtype.
- The advent of gene-based therapies and systemic viral vector gene replacement, editing, and modulation may significantly ameliorate clinical severity in the limb girdle muscular dystrophies.

 **Video content accompanies this article at http://www.neurologic.theclinics.com.**

As a collective whole, the limb girdle muscular dystrophies (LGMDs) are the fourth most common of the genetic muscle diseases behind facioscapulohumeral muscular dystrophy, the dystrophinopathies (Duchenne, Becker, manifesting carriers with pathogenic variants in *DMD*), and the myotonic dystrophies. LGMDs are currently defined by 7 features: a (1) genetically inherited condition that (2) primarily affects skeletal muscle because of loss of muscle fibers, leading to (3) progressive, predominantly proximal weakness in persons who (4) achieve independent walking at some point in their lives and have (5) increased serum muscle enzyme levels, show (6) degenerative changes on muscle imaging, and can have (7) dystrophic features on muscle histology.[1]

[a] University of Colorado School of Medicine, Anschutz Medical Campus, Mail Stop B185, Academic Office 1, 12631 East 17th Avenue, Aurora, CO 80045, USA; [b] University of Colorado School of Medicine, Anschutz Medical Campus, Mail Stop B185, Academic Office 1, 12631 East 17th Avenue, Aurora, CO 80045, USA
* Corresponding author.
E-mail address: Matthew.Wicklund@CUAnschutz.edu

Neurol Clin 38 (2020) 493–504
https://doi.org/10.1016/j.ncl.2020.03.009
0733-8619/20/

The nomenclature of the LGMDs is in transition. Formerly, LGMDs were labeled with a number (1 for dominant and 2 for recessive) followed by a letter (which designated the order in which that disorder's chromosomal locus was delineated). Thus, the most common of the LGMDs, caused by mutations in *CAPN3* (the gene for calpain 3), was designated as LGMD 2A (because it was the first recessive LGMD discovered). A major problem occurred in 2016 when the letter Z was used in a recessive LGMD. The entire alphabet had been consumed, presenting a problem for the next recessive LGMD discovered. Therefore, the new nomenclature includes a letter (D for dominant and R for recessive) followed by a number (delineating the order in which that disorder's chromosomal locus was delineated), followed by the protein product of that disorder. One advantage of this new nomenclature is that the use of numbers precludes the problem of running out of letters. Now, disorders related to *CAPN3* are referred to as LGMD R1 calpain3- related.[1] Throughout this article, both nomenclatures are used for clarity and to facilitate access to the older literature. Because future therapies are likely to be genetically based, future nomenclatures would most reasonably include the gene of the affected LGMD. **Box 1** lists genes associated with an LGMD phenotype.

The overall prevalence of the LGMDs is 2 to 10 per 100,000 persons.[2,3] Among the different LGMD subtypes, in the United States, LGMD 2A/R1, calpain 3 related is the most common.[4] However, when evaluating pathogenic variants in a large DNA database with roughly one-third of a million people, LGMD 2L/R12, anoctamin 5 related ranked highest in lifetime prevalence.[3]

The diagnostic algorithm for the LGMDs has changed. At present, once there is clinical suspicion after the history and physical examination for a disorder of muscle with progressively worsening weakness over years or decades, genetic testing through panel, exome, or genome sequencing should be used. This approach is different from the past when patient evaluation flowed through history, examination, laboratory testing, electrodiagnostic studies, muscle imaging, and on to muscle biopsy. In modern times, ancillary tests are useful in adjudicating variants of uncertain significance. Anti–3-hydroxy-3-methylglutaryl coenzyme A reductase (HMGCR) antibodies have been found in persons with many years of a progressive LGMD phenotype.[5] Therefore, it is important to exclude acquired disorders of muscle, which may be responsive to immune-based or other therapies, in patients with chronic, progressive muscle disorders.

The LGMDs are discussed next through a case-based approach. This article presents 5 patient stories illustrative of the breadth of distinct differences among a common phenotype.

CASE 1

A 42-year-old man presented to the neuromuscular center for leg weakness and a family history of muscular dystrophy. He did not walk until nearly 2 years of age. In

Box 1
Genes commonly associated with a limb girdle muscular dystrophy phenotype

Dominant: *CAPN3, CAV3, COL6Ax, DES, DNAJB6, HNRNPDL, LMNA, MYH2, MYH7, MYOT, RYR1, TNPO3, VCP, ZNF9*

Recessive: *ANO5, BVES, CAPN3, COL6Ax, CRPPA, DAG1, DES, DYSF, FCMD, FKRP, GAA, GNE, GMPPB, LAMA2, LIMS2, PLEC1, POGLUT1, POMGnT1, POMGnT2, POMT1, POMT2, PRTF, RYR1, SGCA, SGCB, SGCD, SGCG, TCAP, TOR1AIP1, TRAPPC11, TRIM32, TTN*

X linked: *DMD, FHL1, TAZ*

high school, he was slower than the other children, but participated in varsity sports (football as an offensive guard and wrestling in the heavyweight class) because of his size (1.9 m [6 feet 4 inches] tall and 116 kg [255 pounds]). As a teen, he was able to bench press more than 135 kg [300 pounds], but could only lift perhaps 55 kg [120 pounds] when doing squats. By his 30s, he was having trouble ascending stairs and started to note episodes of his heart racing. At present, he has a cardiac pacer-defibrillator and remains able to traverse stairs (except when tired at the end of the day). His father also had a muscular dystrophy requiring use of a wheelchair at around 41 years of age. His father had a pacemaker for an arrhythmia and died at age 52 years from sudden cardiac arrest.

On examination, the patient had a paced heart rate. Interestingly, his body habitus was of relative truncal adiposity with a relative paucity of subcutaneous fat in his lower extremities. His strength (MRC [Medical Research Council] scale) was 4 to 4+ in a humeroperoneal pattern. There were mild contractures of the ankles, elbows, and neck extensors. His gait was mostly normal, but he was not able to walk well on his heels.

Evaluation revealed a creatine kinase level of 475 U/L. His nerve conduction studies (NCS)/electromyogram (EMG) showed normal motor and sensory responses, no decrement on repetitive stimulation, and a proximal myopathy with minimal muscle membrane instability, but no myotonic discharges. The next step in the evaluation was genetic testing (Video 1).

The diagnosis in this patient is:

1. LGMD 1A caused by a pathogenic variant in the gene for myotilin, *MYOT*.
2. LGMD 1B caused by a pathogenic variant in the gene for lamin A/C, *LMNA*.
3. LGMD 1C caused by a pathogenic variant in the gene for caveolin 3, *CAV3*.
4. LGMD 1D caused by a pathogenic variant in the gene for DNAJB6-related protein, DNAJB6.
5. LGMD 1E caused by a pathogenic variant in the gene for desmin, *DES*.

As expected from his history, phenotype, and examination, genetic testing revealed a pathogenic variant in *LMNA*, c.1130G>A (p.Arg377His). This variant has been reported to segregate in families with LGMD with atrioventricular conduction disturbances and in families with dilated cardiomyopathy with quadriceps weakness. Through alternate splicing of the gene, LMNA produces the proteins lamin A and lamin C, integral proteins of the inner nuclear envelop. LMNA-related disease involves a myriad of phenotypes (often overlapping), including limb girdle and Emery-Dreifuss muscular dystrophies, axonal polyneuropathy, arrhythmogenic and dilated cardiomyopathies, lipodystrophy, progeria, restrictive dermopathy, mandibuloacral dysplasia, and others.[6] This patient had muscular dystrophy, cardiac conduction disease, mild lipodystrophy, and contractures of the neck extensor, biceps, and Achilles tendons.

Patients with LGMD 1B often have symptoms in the first decade, but weakness can progress at variable rates. Some infants have early and progressive weakness requiring wheelchair use. Others, like the patient in case 1, may remain ambulatory and active through the later decades of life. Although age of onset of weakness is broad, the median age in a large cohort was in the third decade.[7] Weakness tends to be in a humeroperoneal pattern but may also involve the quadriceps. Contractures of the ankle plantar flexors, elbow flexors, and neck extensors are common. Scoliosis can occur with onset of weakness at an early age. Although respiratory insufficiency is not common, up to 10% of patients require noninvasive ventilation in their lifetimes. Creatine kinase levels may be normal and up to 10-fold the upper limit of normal.

Cardiac involvement in LGMD 1B is not universal, but is nearly so in a lifetime. There is a family history of heart disease in most patients with LGMD 1B. Motor weakness generally precedes cardiac symptoms by around a decade, but cardiac symptoms may be the first symptom bringing the patient to medical attention. The incidence of cardiac manifestations increases with age, being uncommon in the first decade and nearly uniform by the sixth decade. Sudden cardiac death may account for more than 25% of mortality in LGMD 1B,[7] which underscores the importance of routine cardiac surveillance (electrocardiogram, Holter/Zio monitor, and echocardiogram) starting no later than the second decade of life in patients with LGMD 1B.[8] Placement of cardiac pacer-defibrillators for arrhythmogenic disease and cardiac transplant for cardiomyopathies with heart failure are both indicated for LGMD 1B.

CASE 2

A 32-year-old man presented for evaluation for muscle pain and cramping since his early teenage years. From age 20 years onward, he has noted increased weakness with trouble arising from the floor or ascending steps. In his job as a heavy equipment mechanic, he needs assistance for tasks above his head and for twisting or unscrewing pipes, screws, or bolts. With physical activity, he notes his muscles wear out more rapidly, hurt more after use, and cramp with less and less exertion. Now, his muscles feel tight and sore nearly all the time, even interfering with sleep. Interestingly, he describes that sometimes he feels and sees a rolling of the muscles of his calves or quadriceps before cramping, when contracting a muscle, or when he bumps a muscle. He recalls dark urine on 2 occasions after sporting activities. He does not have shortness of breath, palpitations, chest pain, or episodes of syncope. Noteworthy, his mother and maternal grandfather have a similar disorder. His mother now uses a wheelchair for distances, and his maternal grandfather was wheelchair dependent late in life.

On examination, his strength was fairly well preserved with normal strength except as follows (MRC scores, right/left): shoulder abductors, 4+/4+; elbow flexors, 4+/4+; finger flexors, 4+/4+; finger abductors, 4+/4+; hip abductors, 4+/4+; hip adductors,4+/4+; knee flexors, 4+/4+; ankle dorsiflexors, 5−/5−; toe flexors, 4/4. Sensation, coordination, and reflexes were normal. His gait was initially stiff legged, then transitioned to normal after 8 to 10 steps. Interesting features on his examination included male pattern baldness, mild percussion myotonia at the thenar eminences, and a rippling of his muscles when struck by the reflex hammer. His only evaluation before genetic testing was a creatine kinase level of 544 U/L (Video 2).

The diagnosis in this patient is:

1. LGMD 1A caused by pathogenic variants in *MYOT*, the gene for myotilin.
2. LGMD 1C caused by pathogenic variants in *CAV3*, the gene for caveolin 3.
3. Myotonic dystrophy type 1.
4. Myotonic dystrophy type 2.
5. A thymoma.

Genetic testing in this patient confirmed the diagnosis of LGMD 1C with the known pathogenic variant, *CAV3*, c.80G>A (p.Arg27Gln). This variant has been reported in families with a proximal, LGMD pattern of weakness, distal weakness, autosomal dominant rippling muscle disease, and asymptomatic hyperCKemia. One of the unique clinical examination findings in LGMD 1C is increased muscle membrane irritability, which manifests as percussion-induced rapid contractions, muscle mounding when struck or bumped, and muscle rolling or rippling. Remarkably, when muscles ripple, they roll perpendicularly to the long axis of a muscle. Muscle pain, cramps, and stiffness are common concerns of patients. Weakness in LGMD 1C ranges from asymptomatic to wheelchair dependence. Because pathogenic variants in *CAV3* have been reported in families with hypertrophic cardiomyopathy, patients with LGMD 1C should undergo cardiac evaluation at diagnosis and intermittently thereafter. Creatine kinase levels range from 3 to 30 times the upper limit of normal.[9] MRI of the thigh often reveals preferential involvement of the rectus femoris and semitendinosus, often with a peripheral predilection for fatty and fibrous replacement in a ringlike pattern.[10] In the diagnostic evaluation of a person with an autosomal dominant family history of weakness along with rippling and rolling of muscles, the first step should be to check a muscle enzyme level and then move directly to genetic testing.

CASE 3

A woman presented for further evaluation at 52 years of age. In her teenage years, friends commented that her walk was unusual. By 17 years of age, she was noted to have a waddling gait, walking erect and with her arms somewhat hyperextended behind her. She noted difficulty with stairs. During an evaluation at age 27 years, her creatine kinase level was found to be 2616 U/L, with several subsequent, contemporaneous levels in the 1200 to 5300 U/L range. Subsequently an EMG revealed myopathic motor units with fibrillation potentials and positive sharp waves in proximal muscles, and a quadriceps muscle biopsy revealed so-called moth-eaten muscle fibers. Over the next 2 decades, she had greater difficulties in walking independently, and by age 45 years began to use a Rollator walker regularly. Around age 50 years, she used a power wheelchair most of the time and anytime outside her home. Once using the wheelchair regularly, she gained a substantial amount of weight, with her body mass index exceeding 40 kg/m^2. Around this time, she was started on nocturnal bilevel positive airway pressure at night because of a forced vital capacity (FVC) of 72% predicted in the upright position, an FVC of 58% in the supine position, and an overnight polysomnogram with an apnea-hypopnea index at 99 events per hour and with oxygen saturation less than 89% for 35% of her sleep time. There is no family history of a similar disorder.

On examination, her general and mental status examinations were normal except for obesity. Cranial nerves were normal with normal extraocular and perioral strength and the ability to whistle normally. Strength was graded as follows (MRC scale, right/left): shoulder abductors, 3−/3−; elbow flexors, 2/3−; elbow extensors, 3−/3−; wrists/fingers, 5/5; hip flexors, 3−/3−; hip extensors, 2/2; hip abductors, 5/5; hip adductors, 2/2; knee extensors, 5/5; knee flexors, 2/2; ankles/toes, 5/5. There was prominent scapular winging, bilaterally. Sensation and coordination were normal. She was able to arise from a chair without the use of her arms. Her gait was hyperlordotic with her arms held behind her and her legs splayed apart, and she was able to walk without an ambulatory aid for 6 to 15 m (20–50 feet). At age 52 years, genetic testing confirmed the diagnosis suspected in this woman (Video 3).

The diagnosis in this woman is:

1. LGMD 2A/R1 caused by pathogenic variants in *CAPN3*, the gene for calpain 3.
2. LGMD 2B/R2 caused by pathogenic variants in *DYSF*, the gene for dysferlin.
3. LGMD 2L/R12 caused by pathogenic variants in *ANO5*, the gene for anoctamin 5.
4. Manifesting dystrophinopathy carrier caused by a pathogenic variant in *DMD*.
5. Facioscapulohumeral muscular dystrophy caused by a truncation in the number of D4Z4 repeats on chromosome 4.

This patient has LGMD 2A/R1 caused by compound heterozygous pathogenic variants in *CAPN3*, c.550delA and c.1250C>T. Calpainopathies are the most prevalent LGMD in the United States. Symptoms generally begin in LGMD 2A/R1 between 5 and 15 years of age. Weakness has a distinct pattern with marked disparities in strength in antagonist muscles across the hip and knee joints. Thus, the hip adductors, hip extensors, and knee flexors are substantially weaker than the hip abductors, hip flexors, and knee extensors. Retained quadriceps strength allows patients to walk much longer. Nearly half of patients have scapular winging, sometimes prominent. In general, cardiopulmonary function is not affected early in the disease course.[11] Later, respiratory insufficiency requiring nocturnal noninvasive ventilation occurs in around 20%. Although most patients with calpainopathy inherit their disease in an autosomal recessive fashion, up to one-third of patients may have disease with only 1 pathogenic variant in *CAPN3*.[12] In autosomal dominant calpainopathy, onset of disease tends to be 10 to 20 years later than in LGMD 2A/R1.

In LGMD 2A/R1, creatine kinase levels range from normal late in disease to in excess of 20,000 U/L. Muscle biopsies often reveal lobulated fibers on oxidative enzyme stains. In this patient with obesity, the question arose as to whether bariatric surgery would be appropriate. There is mounting evidence that bariatric surgery is safe in the LGMDs, and that subsequent weight loss may improve function without worsening the disease course.[13,14]

CASE 4

A man initially presented at 48 years of age for evaluation of a 3-year history of progressive weakness of his bilateral biceps and left leg. As a youth, he was athletically gifted, winning the state wrestling championship in his weight class. Through his 20s and 30s, he remained physically active and was able to bench press 135 kg (300 pounds), squat 180 kg (400 pounds), and bicycle 4830 km (3000 miles) per year. Around 47 years of age, he noted left calf hypertrophy, but, ironically, noted greater difficulty standing on his toes, bilaterally. Over the ensuing decade, his strength declined such that he could not traverse stairs, arise from the floor, and now uses a walking stick regularly. His past history is significant for gynecomastia surgery when younger. He also experiences frequent premature ventricular contractions (>10,000 on 48-hour Holter monitor) since his early 30s. Noteworthy, his unaffected parents are first cousins. Of 6 siblings, 2 younger brothers also have milder weakness; 1 younger sister has persistently increased aspartate transaminase, alanine transaminase, and creatine kinase levels, but no weakness, and 2 sisters have multiple sclerosis. No aunts, uncles, or grandparents have neurologic disease.

On examination at 58 years of age, his motor examination revealed the following strengths (MRC scale, right/left): deltoid, 5/5; biceps, 2/4−; triceps, 3/4; wrist and finger muscles, 5/5; hip flexors, 4−/4−; hip extensors, 2/2; hip abductors, 5/4+; hip adductors, 2−/2−; knee extensors, 4/3; knee flexors, 2/2; ankle dorsiflexion, 5/5; and ankle plantar flexion, 4/4−. He was able to walk on his heels bilaterally, but unable to stand on his toes bilaterally.

In terms of evaluation, at 48 years of age, his creatine kinase level was 4852 U/L, and, at age 58 years, his creatine kinase level was 1374 U/L. NCS/EMG revealed a nonirritable, proximal myopathy both at age 48 years and again at age 58 years. His MRI of the thighs and calves at age 58 years revealed bilateral marked fatty and fibrous replacement of his hamstring, adductor, and vasti muscles with sparing of the rectus femoris muscle in the thighs, and marked fatty and fibrous replacement of the bilateral gastrocnemius muscles and left soleus muscle with sparing of the anterior compartment of the calves (**Fig. 1**). A right biceps muscle biopsy at age 53 years revealed end-stage muscle with a few muscle fibers among fatty and fibrous tissue. A deltoid muscle biopsy at age 58 years revealed nonspecific myopathic changes (**Fig. 2**, Video 4).

The diagnosis in this patient is:

1. LGMD 2A/R1 caused by pathogenic variants in *CAPN3*, the gene for calpain 3.
2. LGMD 2B/R2 caused by pathogenic variants in *DYSF*, the gene for dysferlin.
3. LGMD 2L/R12 caused by pathogenic variants in *ANO5*, the gene for anoctamin 5.

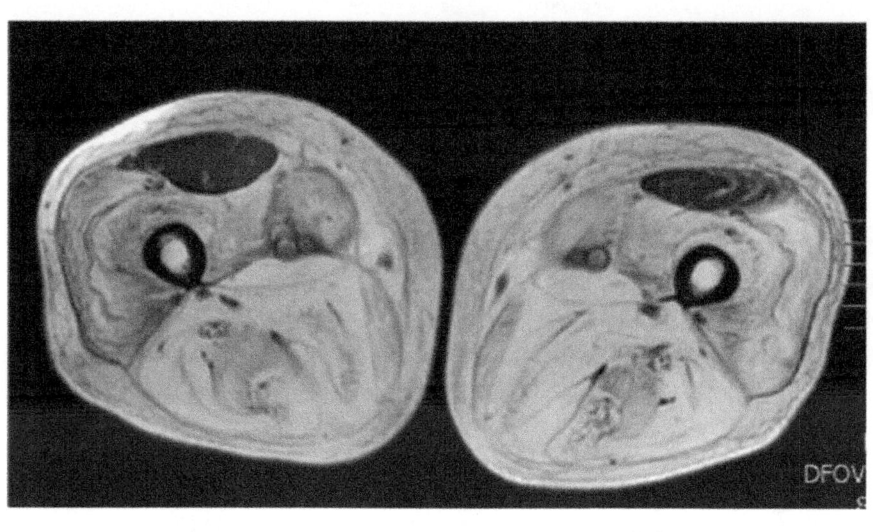

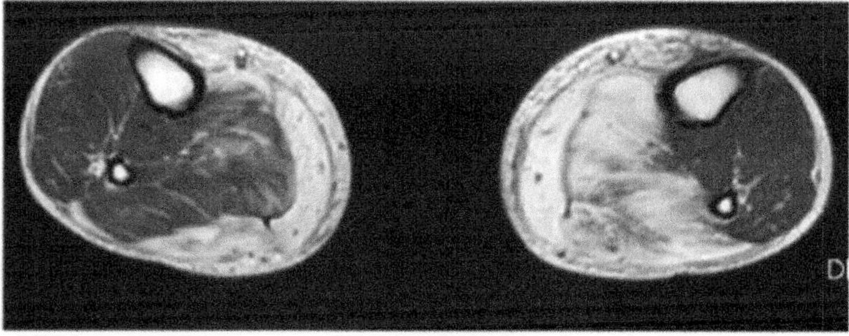

Fig. 1. MRI (T1-weighted, axial images) of the thigh and calf in a man with LGMD 2L/R12. In the thighs, note the nearly complete fatty atrophy of the hamstring muscles, severe fatty atrophy of the vasti muscles, and sparing of the rectus femoris muscles, bilaterally. In the calves, note the asymmetric involvement in the gastrosoleus complex, with greater fatty and fibrous replacement on the left.

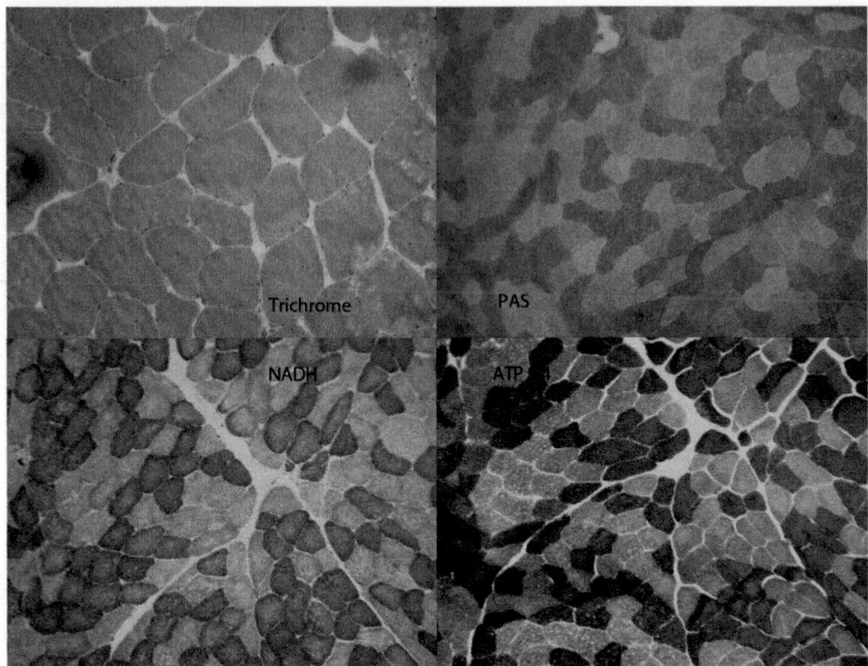

Fig. 2. Muscle biopsy of the barely affected deltoid muscle in this patient with LGMD 2L/R12. NADH, nicotinamide adenine dinucleotide plus hydrogen; PAS, periodic acid–Schiff. NADH magnification was 200x. Trichrome, PAS and ATP 9.4 magnifications were 100x.

4. Becker muscular dystrophy caused by a pathogenic variant in *DMD*.
5. Bulbospinal muscular atrophy or Kennedy disease caused by the gynecomastia with a CAG repeat in the gene for the androgen receptor.

This patient has LGMD 2L/R12 caused by homozygous pathogenic variants in *ANO5*, c.172C>T (p.R58 W). LGMD 2L/R12 is highly prevalent in persons of northern European ancestry. Patients with 2 pathogenic variants in ANO5 can present with a proximal, limb girdle pattern or with a distal pattern (Miyoshi-like muscular dystrophy type 3). Onset of weakness is later than in most LGMDs, often in the third to fifth decades. In persons with the same pathogenic variants, women tend toward less weakness than men. The muscles most affected include the quadriceps and biceps muscles. Early inability to walk on the toes can occur, similar to LGMD 2B/R2. Cardiac arrhythmias are more prevalent than in the general population, but heart failure is less common. Muscle enzyme levels generally are 10-fold to 50-fold the upper limit of normal at diagnosis, but may exceed 30,000 U/L. MRI shows fatty and fibrous replacement in the posterior thigh muscles along with the biceps muscle. Muscle biopsies may be nearly normal early in disease, or in less affected muscles, but later show fatty and fibrous (dystrophic) changes.[15,16]

CASE 5

A 54-year-old woman initially noted greater fatigue in middle school and high school. At that time, she was never able to accelerate quickly, and had trouble running the 50-yard (46-m) dash with any speed. She could never jump very high. In her 20s, she noted greater difficulty running. In her 30s, she noted difficulty with ascending stairs, using her arms over her head, and some mild foot drop. At that time, she was diagnosed with LGMD. By her early 50s, she was unable to ride a bicycle, hike, play golf, or walk any significant distance. She was falling perhaps once a month. There was no family history of a similar disorder.

On general examination, she had enlarged calves, but did not have tongue hypertrophy. Mental status and cranial nerves were normal (specifically, she had no ptosis and no diplopia). Strength testing revealed symmetric weakness graded as follows (MRC scale) in the upper extremities: shoulders and elbows, 4 to 4+; wrists and fingers, 5. Her lower extremity strength was: hip flexors, 4−; knee extensors, 5; ankle dorsiflexors, 3; ankle plantar flexors, 5; hip extensors, adductors, and abductors, 2; knee flexors, 4+. Station and gait revealed a camptocormic thoracic spine with forward hip posture. She had trouble standing erectly.

Her evaluation extended over 3 decades. Creatine kinase levels ranged from 900 to 2700 U/L. EMGs in her 30s were consistent with a myopathy. Muscle biopsies in her 30s revealed myopathic changes and a mildly dystrophic pattern with fatty and fibrous replacement. At age 54 years, ultrasonography of her muscle was consistent with a generalized myopathy without a distinct pattern. MRI of her lumbar spine revealed complete fatty replacement of the lumbar paraspinal muscles with relative preservation of her iliopsoas muscles (**Fig. 3**). MRI of the brain was normal. Pulmonary function tests revealed an FVC at 74% of predicted in the upright position, but only 56% of predicted in the supine position. Echocardiogram was normal. Electrodiagnostic testing at age 54 years revealed a myopathic pattern, mostly in proximal muscles, but also repetitive stimulation at 3-Hz stimulation of the spinal accessory nerve to the trapezius muscle revealed a decrement of 23%. This decrement repaired with treatment with pyridostigmine. The patient was started on pyridostigmine and her strength and endurance improved and she no longer had falls (Video 5).

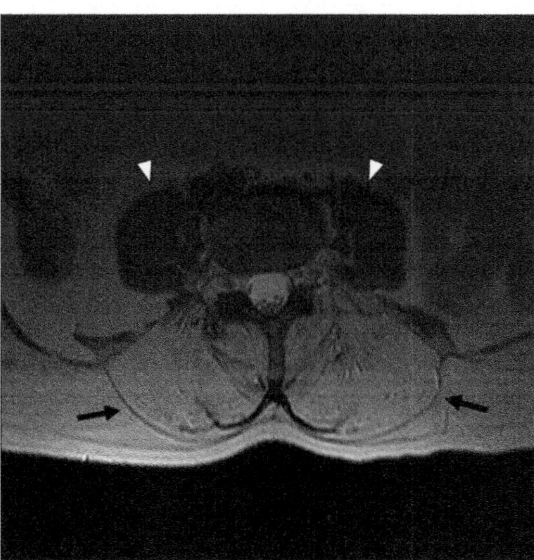

Fig. 3. MRI lumbar spine (T2-weighted, axial images) in a patient with LGMD 2T/R19. Note the nearly complete fatty replacement of the lumbar paraspinal muscles, bilaterally (*black arrows*), with nearly normal iliopsoas muscles, bilaterally (*white arrowheads*).

The diagnosis in this woman is:

1. Myasthenia gravis caused by antibodies to the acetylcholine receptor.
2. LGMD 2A/R1 caused by pathogenic variants in *CAPN3*, the gene for calpain 3.
3. LGMD 2I/R9 caused by pathogenic variants in *FKTN*, the gene for Fukutin-related protein.
4. LGMD 2T/R19 caused by mutations in *GMPPB*, the gene for guanosine diphosphate (GDP) mannose pyrophosphorylase B.
5. Congenital myasthenic syndrome caused by pathogenic variants in *DOK7*, the gene for DOK7-related protein.

Genetic testing in this patient revealed 2 pathogenic variants in *GMPPB*: c.79G>C (p.Asp27His) and c.1099G>A (p.Gly367Arg). *GMPPB* encodes the protein GDP-mannose pyrophosphorylase B, one of 18 genes associated with glycosylation of alpha-dystroglycan. Two pathogenic variants in *GMPPB* may lead to the spectrum of phenotypes including congenital muscular dystrophy with brain and eye involvement, congenital myasthenic syndrome, and a milder muscle phenotype (LGMD2T).[17] In some cases, there are components of more than 1 phenotype. This case had predominant limb girdle pattern muscular dystrophy with proximal weakness and fatty and fibrous replaced muscles but also had a partially reversible neuromuscular junction component. Progressive muscle weakness in the disease course with myopathic changes on muscle biopsy, along with evidence for abnormal transmission at the neuromuscular junction, may also be seen in other myopathies, such as *BIN1*, *DES*, *DNM2*, *MTM1*, and *PLEC*, as well as in other congenital myasthenic syndromes, such as *DOK7*, *ALG2*, *ALG14*, *COL13A1*, *DPAGT1*, and *GFPT1*.[18] For this reason, evaluation for abnormalities of the neuromuscular junction, either repetitive nerve stimulation or single-fiber EMG, should be performed in all patients presenting with weakness, even in the presence of myopathic motor units.

The age of onset in LGMD 2T/R19 ranges from congenital weakness to later adult life. Calf hypertrophy commonly occurs in LGMD 2T/R19. Lumbar paraspinal, adductor, hamstring, and medial gastrocnemius muscles is the pattern that tends to be most involved. Creatine kinase levels are increased, running from 300 to 10,000 U/L. Lumbar paraspinal muscles tend to be the most affected on total-body MRI of muscles.[19] In terms of genetics, there are genotype/phenotype correlations. The common c.79G>C pathogenic variant tends to be associated with milder weakness and more so with a myasthenic syndrome phenotype.[20] Treatment with pyridostigmine and/or salbutamol improves the strength and endurance in some patients with LGMD 2T/R19.

TREATMENT

Treatment of the LGMDs is transforming from supportive to disease-specific genetic correction strategies. The mainstay for patients with LGMD has always been therapy services. Physical, occupational, and speech therapists, along with nutrition specialists, significantly improve patients' daily lives. Involvement of cardiology, pulmonary, and bone health specialists also markedly reduces other organ system dysfunction.[21] Genetic therapies involving modulation, editing, skipping, and transfer of genes are in various stages of advancement in the LGMDs. Ongoing systemic viral vector gene therapies in humans for calpainopathies, dysferlinopathies, sarcoglycanopathies, anoctaminopathies, and fukutin-related protein (FKRP) syndromes promise bright futures for this group of disorders without previous disease-specific corrective therapies.[22]

DISCLOSURE

J. Bockhorst has nothing to disclose. M. Wicklund has served on advisory boards, consulted for, and received research funding from Sarepta Therapeutics. He has consulted for ML Bio Solutions.

SUPPLEMENTARY DATA

Supplementary data to this article can be found online at https://doi.org/10.1016/j.ncl.2020.03.009.

REFERENCES

1. Straub V, Murphy A, Udd B, et al. 229th ENMC international workshop: limb girdle muscular dystrophies nomenclature and reformed classification. Neuromuscul Disord 2018;28:702–10.
2. Norwood FL, Harling C, Chinnery PF, et al. Prevalence of genetic muscle disease in Northern England: in depth analysis of a muscle clinic population. Brain 2009; 132:3175–86.
3. Liu W, Pajusalu S, Lake N, et al. Estimating prevalence for limb-girdle muscular dystrophy based on public sequencing databases. Genet Med 2019;21: 2512–20.
4. Nallamilli BRR, Chakravorty S, Kesari A, et al. Genetic landscape and novel disease mechanisms from a large LGMD cohort of 4656 patients. Ann Clin Transl Neurol 2018;5:1574–87.
5. Mohassel P, Mammen AL. Anti HMGCR myopathy. J Neuromuscul Dis 2018;5: 11–20.
6. Maggi L, D'Amico A, Pini A, et al. *LMNA*-associated myopathies: the Italian experience in a large cohort of patients. Neurology 2014;83:1634–44.
7. Perretto G, Di Resta C, Perversi J, et al. Cardiac and neuromuscular features of patients with *LMNA*-related cardiomyopathy. Ann Intern Med 2019;171:458–63.
8. Choi SA, Cho A, Kim SY, et al. Importance of early diagnosis in *LMNA*-related muscular dystrophy for cardiac surveillance. Muscle Nerve 2019;60(6):668–72.
9. Bruno C, Sotgia F, Gazzerro E, et al. Caveolinopathies. In: Adam MP, Ardinger HH, Pagon RA, et al, editors. GeneReviews [Internet]. Seattle (WA): University of Washington, Seattle; 2012. p. 1993–2019.
10. Ishiguro K, Nakayama T, Yoshioka M, et al. Characteristic findings of skeletal muscle MRI in caveolinopathies. Neuromuscul Disord 2018;28:857–62.
11. Richard I, Hogrel JY, Stockholm D, et al. Natural history of LGMD2A for delineating outcome measures in clinical trials. Ann Clin Transl Neurol 2016;2(4):e89.
12. Vissing J, Barresi R, Witting N, et al. A heterozygous 21-bp deletion in *CAPN3* causes dominantly inherited limb girdle muscular dystrophy. Brain 2016;139: 2154–63.
13. Williams GJ, Georgiou DM, Cocker DM, et al. The safety and efficacy of bariatric surgery for obese, wheelchair bound patients. Ann R Coll Surg Engl 2014;96: 373–6.
14. Abel EEDH, Cup EHC, Lanser A, et al. Experiences with bariatric surgery in patients with facioscapulohumeral dystrophy and myotonic dystrophy type 1: a qualitative study. Neuromuscul Disord 2018;28:938–46.
15. Liewluck T, Winder TL, Dimberg EL, et al. *ANO5*-muscular dystrophy: clinical, pathological and molecular findings. Eur J Neurol 2013;20:1383–9.

16. Papadopoulos C, Laforet P, Nectoux J, et al. HyperCKemia and myalgia are common presentations of anoctamin-5-related myopathy in French patients. Muscle Nerve 2017;56:1096–100.
17. Balcin H, Palmio J, Penttilä S, et al. Late-onset limb-girdle muscular dystrophy caused by *GMPPB* mutations. Neuromuscul Disord 2017;27:627–30.
18. Nicolau S, Kao J, Liewluck T. Trouble at the junction: when myopathy and myasthenia overlap. Muscle Nerve 2019;60(6):648–57.
19. Oestergaard ST, Stojkovic T, Dahlqvist JR, et al. Muscle involvement in limb-girdle muscular dystrophy with *GMPPB* deficiency (LGMD2T). Neurol Genet 2016;2:e112.
20. Montagnese F, Klupp E, Karampinos DC, et al. Two patients with *GMPPB* mutation: the overlapping phenotypes of limb-girdle myasthenic syndrome and limb-girdle muscular dystrophy dystroglycanopathy. Muscle Nerve 2017;56:334–40.
21. Narayanaswami P, Weiss M, Selcen D, et al. Evidence-based guideline summary: diagnosis and treatment of limb-girdle and distal dystrophies. Neurology 2014;83:1453–63.
22. Crudele JM, Chamberlain JS. AAV-based gene therapies for the muscular dystrophies. Hum Mol Genet 2019;28:R102–7.

Spinal Muscular Atrophy in the Treatment Era

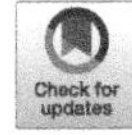

Megan A. Waldrop, MD[a,b], Bakri H. Elsheikh, MBBS, MRCP[b,*]

KEYWORDS

- Spinal muscular atrophy • Nusinersen • Onasemnogene abeparvovec-xioi
- Newborn screen • Multidisciplinary care

KEY POINTS

- Early/presymptomatic treatment in spinal muscular atrophy provides the most benefit, making newborn screening essential.
- Later treatment in infants and children with spinal muscular atrophy can still provide meaningful functional and quality-of-life improvements.
- Nusinersen treatment and related procedures are well tolerated in adults with spinal muscular atrophy with encouraging early efficacy data.
- More information is needed to help guide clinicians for those patients who are eligible for multiple treatments.
- Continued multidisciplinary care for individuals with spinal muscular atrophy is essential.

Video content accompanies this article at http://www.neurologic.theclinics.com.

INTRODUCTION

The term spinal muscular atrophy (SMA) is used to encompass a diverse group of hereditary disorders of the lower motor neuron. Most cases, ~95%, have a proximal predominant autosomal-recessive disease that was first described clinically in 1890 and is characterized by a progressive loss of motor neurons owing to the absence of the *SMN1* gene.[1] Disease severity is most often modified by the presence of a back-up gene, *SMN2*, although it is suspected that other modifiers exist as well.[2] Historically, 5 types have been described, and the natural history of type 1 has been well documented, with most of these individuals succumbing to the disease before age 2.[3,4] Most type 2 individuals live into adulthood, and those with type 3 and 4 have a normal lifespan.

[a] Center for Gene Therapy, Nationwide Children's Hospital, 700 Children's Drive, Columbus, OH 43205, USA; [b] Department of Neurology, The Ohio State University Wexner Medical Center, 395 West 12th Avenue, Columbus OH 43210, USA
* Corresponding author.
E-mail address: Bakri.Elsheikh@osumc.edu

Neurol Clin 38 (2020) 505–518
https://doi.org/10.1016/j.ncl.2020.03.002
0733-8619/20/

The first genetic therapy for SMA, using *SMN2* RNA transcript modification, was Food and Drug Administration (FDA) approved in December 2016 for all ages, and the second, *SMN1* gene replacement, was approved in May 2019 for children under the age of 2, both of which are markedly changing the natural history of this disease with minimal side effects.[5,6] Given the change in disease trajectory with these treatments, the limitations of the historic classifications based on age of onset and maximal function achieved became evident. A pragmatic approach using additional classifications based on genotype and the current functional status is being increasingly considered. The cases in later discussion highlight the diagnostic, treatment, and outcome considerations that are now relevant in the therapeutic era of SMA.

CASE: A DELAYED DIAGNOSIS

Case Presentation

This patient was born full term via cesarean section due to breech presentation. After birth, there were no complications, and she breast fed well. She seemed to be growing and developing normally, but at her 4-month well-child check, she could not lift her head when prone and was referred for therapy. Because she was not making progress, she was seen by neurology at ~5.5 months of age, where SMA genetic testing was sent and was positive (*SMN1* 0, *SMN2* 2). At 6 months of age, she was seen by neuromuscular and was unable to roll or sit (**Fig. 1**). She did move her arms, barely getting her elbows antigravity, and there was some distal leg movement. Her Children's Hospital of Philadelphia Infant Test of Neuromuscular Disorders (CHOP-INTEND) score was 25. She had a weak cough and a history of frequent and prolonged respiratory infections but no hospitalizations. She was continuing to grow with breast milk

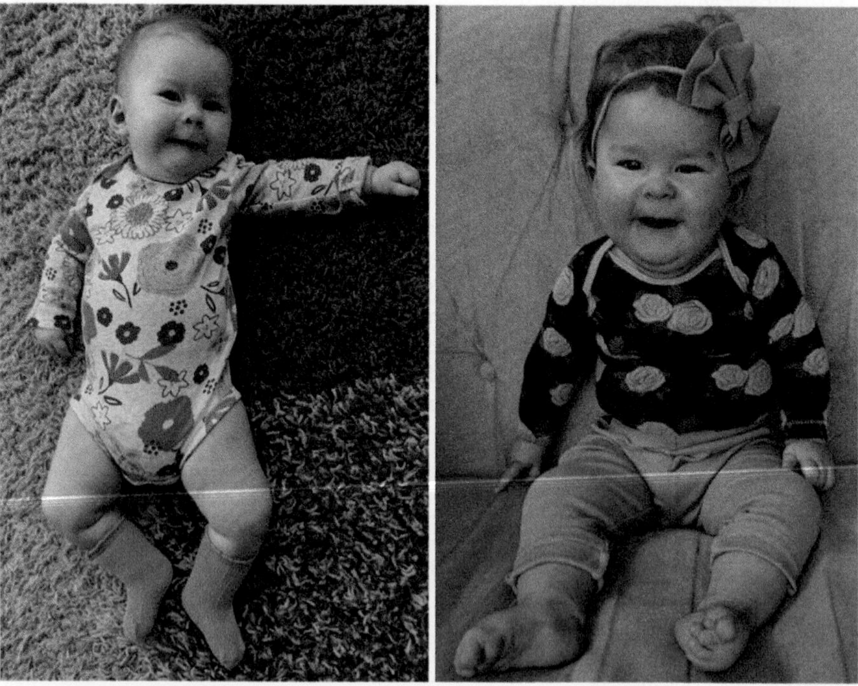

Fig. 1. (*left*) Patient just before diagnosis at 6 months of age. (*right*) Patient at 13 months of age.

as her only intake. Because of concerns about her safety in feeding, she was admitted, and a video swallow study (VSS) showed silent aspiration; Therefore, a gastrostomy tube was placed, and bilevel positive airway pressure (BiPAP) at night was initiated. She was started on nusinersen at 6.5 months of age and received 3 loading doses before transition to AVXS-101 via the expanded access program. Her CHOP-INTEND score before gene transfer was 26. She has experienced continued improvement and is now sitting with minimal support for ~10 seconds. Her CHOP-INTEND score is now 40* (*on a day when she was tired), 5.5 months after gene transfer (see **Fig. 1**).

Clinical Question

Which of the following is true regarding newborn screening for SMA?

a. Newborn screening is implemented in most states and will catch all cases of 5q SMA.
b. Newborn screening is implemented in some states and will catch all cases of 5q SMA.
c. Newborn screening is implemented in some states and will catch most cases of 5q SMA.
d. Newborn screening is implemented in all states and will catch most cases of 5q SMA.

Discussion

The evidence is clear that earlier treatment of these individuals is better. Although a federal advisory committee recommended that SMA be added to the Recommended Uniform Screening Panel on March 13, 2018, each state must then decide when and how to implement screening. As of the end of September 2019, newborn screening has been adopted and fully implemented in 10 states, adopted but not yet fully implemented in 18 states, and finally, 3 states are in a pilot phase (CureSMA, accessed October 21, 2019, https://www.curesma.org/newborn-screening-for-sma/). This patient was born when the pilot phase of the Ohio program was being rolled out and was, unfortunately, not tested. Her parents were following routine follow-up recommendations, and at 4 months of age, she was referred to Help Me Grow for therapy. With the current treatment options available for patients with SMA, earlier consideration of SMA in any infant with hypotonia, motor delay, and absent reflexes and urgent consultation with a pediatric neurologist or neuromuscular specialist should be completed. For most cases seen by pediatricians, referral to therapy can provide significant and sufficient benefit, but urgency on the part of the pediatrician can ensure that all infants with SMA are treated as soon as possible. Pediatrician vigilance is particularly important now because not all states have newborn screening, but will also remain important once it is implemented in all states because newborn screening will only pick up ~95% of patients with SMA. Newborn screening only detects the *SMN1* deletion. A patient who has only 1 copy of *SMN1* deleted and then a pathogenic point mutation on the second copy would be resulted as negative. If suspicion for SMA remains OR develops in a patient with a negative newborn screen, it is imperative for the pediatrician and/or neurologist to send further genetic testing (*SMN1* sequencing) (**Fig. 2**).

Although this patient was not diagnosed via newborn screening, she still had a rather remarkable benefit from treatment. Based on the initial gene replacement trial data,[6] one may assume that an 8 month old would experience no benefit from gene therapy. However, this patient clearly adds additional evidence to the literature that a patient treated at 8 months of age can experience significant benefit from treatment,

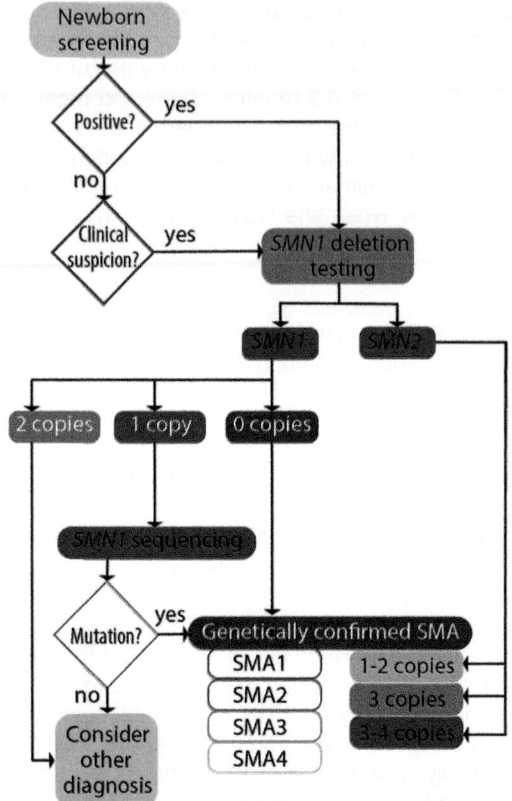

Fig. 2. Newborn screening diagnostic algorithm. (*Reproduced with permission from* Rai W and Elsheikh B. Spinal Muscular Atrophy. Practical Neurology. 2019; 18(6):61–66.)

as shown by her CHOP-INTEND score increase from 26 to 40. The CHOP-INTEND score ranges from 0 to 64, and in untreated individuals with SMA type 1, the score declines over time.[3,7] In the original gene replacement trial, treated individuals had a mean increase of 9.8 points at 1 month and 15.4 points at 3 months.[6]

CASE: AN "ASYMPTOMATIC" DIAGNOSIS

Case Presentation

This patient was born full term via repeat cesarean section without complication. He was immediately started on bottle feeds, which he tolerated well. On day of life 6, his newborn screen returned positive for SMA. He was seen in clinic on day of life 8, and his mother reported normal arm and leg movements, no concerns about breathing or feeding, and that he had a loud cry. On examination, he had normal reflexes and good antigravity movement of all extremities and age-appropriate head control. The only finding was very mild hip flexion weakness. His CHOP-INTEND score was 54. Confirmatory genetic testing was sent and was positive (*SMN1* 0, *SMN2* 4), and the modifier gene (c.859G > C in *SMN2*) was not present.[2] He was started on nusinersen at 4 weeks of age, which was well tolerated. He was followed regularly in the multidisciplinary SMA clinic, and at 4 months old his mother noted that he sometimes seemed like he was choking with feeds. A VSS was ordered and showed deep laryngeal penetration with thin liquids, so he was transitioned to nectar thick liquids. At 6 months of age, he received onasemnogene abeparvovec-xioi, and nusinersen was discontinued. His overall gross and fine motor development has progressed to be on time or even early, with him pushing onto all fours just after 6 months, starting to pull to stand at 7 months of age, and now starting to cruise at 8 months. His CHOP-INTEND score has plateaued at 64 ~2 months after gene transfer and 5 months since his last dose of nusinersen (Video 1). A follow-up VSS has been scheduled.

Clinical Questions

In a patient who was identified from newborn screening and was relatively asymptomatic, the following is true:

a. Continued follow-up care in a multidisciplinary clinic may or may not be indicated.
b. Continued follow-up care with the primary care physician is sufficient.
c. Continued follow-up care on a regular basis in a multidisciplinary SMA clinic is essential.
d. Continued follow-up care may be determined based on the comfort of the patient's primary care physician.

In a patient who has been treated with 1 SMA disease-modifying therapy, the following is true:

a. There is no indication for the addition of a second agent.
b. There is no reason not to add on a second agent.
c. There is no evidence to guide decision making at this time.
d. Parent preference should be the driving factor in the decision-making process.

Discussion

Although both available treatments have provided rather remarkable benefits in terms of functional outcomes, neither should be considered a "cure." Thus, all patients, treated or untreated, must still be considered patients with SMA and followed routinely in a multidisciplinary SMA or Muscular Dystrophy Association clinic. This point is highlighted in the patient above who developed mild bulbar weakness (requiring thickened feeds to avoid aspiration) despite treatment with nusinersen since 4 weeks of age. In several studies, nusinersen has been shown to have significant impact on motor function, but its impact on bulbar function is less well reported.[5,8,9] In the small cohort of patients treated with gene replacement, all patients had stable or improved swallow function.[10] Thus, the decision was made to transition this patient to onasemnogene abeparvovec-xioi. Further considerations that will be best addressed with continued care in a multidisciplinary clinic include the development of any potential adverse effects from these treatments and the persistence or waning of response to treatment. In addition, monitoring for any potential toxicity that may develop over time must be considered because in vivo models have shown an early peak of SMN protein levels and then a decline over time,[11] so the impact of high levels of SMN throughout an individual's lifetime is unknown. Finally, SMN, despite being of particular importance for motor neuron development, is also present systemically and may be important for the health of other organ systems,[12,13] and it will be necessary to thoughtfully monitor patients who have been treated with systemic therapy versus intrathecal therapy for any potential health issues that may arise because of differences in treatment.

With the approval of onasemnogene abeparvovec-xioi, nearly all families of a child with SMA less than the age of 2 were interested in receiving this treatment. Many patients had previously been receiving nusinersen and the addition of, or a switch to, gene replacement has not been studied. Several questions arise pertaining to the safety of switching or dual therapy. Is there an ideal time after last nusinersen dose to dose with gene replacement? Are there any additional safety concerns or monitoring that needs to be done? Can nusinersen safely be restarted? Is there even need to restart nusinersen? Could it be harmful to have too much SMN? Although a study is planned in patients who have previously received nusinersen, the current study design is to not dose with gene replacement until the patients are at least 4 months out from the last nusinersen dose. Thus, extensive conversation with the family about the known and unknown risks and benefits of switching and/or dual therapy is essential. It would be reasonable to switch to gene replacement if full benefit has not been obtained after use of nusinersen. In the patient above, despite treatment with nusinersen, it appeared that his swallow function was declining; thus, the hope would be with the addition of gene replacement, some additional motor improvements could be obtained. In a patient who had obtained normal or near normal function on nusinersen, a discussion is needed taking into account potential risks of gene therapy versus continued lumbar punctures (with or without sedation) every 4 months. The authors would encourage caution and ensuring that parents are making a well-informed decision if choosing to switch from nusinersen to gene replacement or resume treatment with nusinersen after receiving gene replacement.

CASE: TREATMENT OPTIONS

Case Presentation

This patient was born full term after induced vaginal delivery. She was breast fed and was doing well until 3.5 months of age when she stopped pushing her head up. At 4 months, she rolled front to back but was not really moving her legs. At 5 months of age, she was hospitalized for a respiratory illness and poor feeding, and further workup was done. Genetic testing for SMA was sent and returned positive for SMA (*SMN1* 0, *SMN2* 3). At 6.5 months of age, she was able to sit unsupported when placed into a seated position. Her parents were very interested in gene therapy and were aware of the intrathecal gene therapy trial. However, despite repeated evaluation, she was unable to meet the inclusion criteria of sitting unsupported without using her arms or hands to support herself for at least 10 seconds. Her CHOP-INTEND score was 37. She was then seen by the authors' clinical team to discuss both FDA-approved therapies, and the process was initiated to obtain approval for onasemnogene abeparvovec-xioi, which she received at 10 months of age. She has experienced benefit, now with a CHOP-INTEND score of 54 at 13 months (Video 2).

Clinical Question

In a patient who is eligible for both FDA-approved therapies, there is sufficient evidence to make counseling families easy.

a. True
b. False

Discussion

This conversation is difficult to have with families because there has been no direct comparison studied. First a physician and the family of a child under the age of 2 years must discuss nusinersen versus onasemnogene abeparvovec-xioi. Nusinersen performs very well in terms of improved outcomes with minimal side effects in several ages and SMA types,[5,8,9,14] but one may wonder about the extent of potential benefit in those with fewer *SMN2* copy numbers based on the mechanism of action. For those who require anesthesia, there is a concern about repeated sedation events. Onasemnogene abeparvovec-xioi also performs very well with minimal concern for liver toxicity, but the data are only in infants, and the sample size is much smaller.[6,10] An additional intravenous study is underway in presymptomatic infants with similar findings (NCT03505099), but the evidence for the safety and efficacy of onasemnogene abeparvovec-xioi in older individuals is lacking. Thus, several questions remain that cannot be answered when discussing options with families. Is one better for bulbar function? Is one better for limb function? Is one better in presymptomatic individuals? Is one better for symptomatic individuals? Which one is safer for my child? In this case, the family had a preference for gene replacement therapy and was aware of both the clinical trial opportunity and the commercial opportunity. When discussing intravenous versus intrathecal, one must consider if 1 mode is better than the other. The intravenous formulation is FDA approved for the patient above, but do we know if that is that the best option? The viral vector, AAV9, is known to have a high affinity for the central nervous system and does cross the blood-brain barrier, so we expect and have seen that it can transduce motor neurons. It also transduces other cells types and uses a promoter that works in all cell types,[15–17] meaning systemic administration may have effects throughout the body. However, without clinical evidence of safety and efficacy in this patient's specific age group and SMA type, the intrathecal clinical trial option was also considered. Intrathecal administration will result in the highest exposure of the motor neurons to the delivered *SMN1* and may perhaps be more efficacious for motor outcomes but will likely not have as much systemic exposure as intravenous administration. Importantly, it is still in the research phase, and clinical efficacy and safety have not yet been determined by the FDA.

CASE: NUSINERSEN IN ADOLESCENCE

Case Presentation

This patient was born full term without complication and breast fed, grew, and developed well, although his parents noted that he was an "army crawler." At 2.5 years of age, he was not walking well and was unable to climb stairs. Genetic testing was positive for SMA (*SMN1* 0, *SMN2* 4). He had some improvements in his motor function but then started to decline at around age 5, when he was only able to safely walk around the house. At 9 years of age, he lost the ability to walk independently. He was started on nusinersen just after turning 12 years old. A baseline Hammersmith Functional Motor Scale Expanded (HFMSE) score was 20 and is now 30 at 14 years of age. Both he and his parents are impressed with the skills he has regained (Video 3). He has been tolerating the lumbar punctures well and is continuing to experience functional improvement.

Clinical Questions

Nusinersen, the antisense oligonucleotide, has been shown to significantly improve motor function outcomes in infants and children with SMA types 1 to 3.

a. True
b. False

Nusinersen is an antisense oligonucleotide that acts on an individuals' *SMN2* to increase exon 7 inclusion and the production of functional SMN protein.

a. True
b. False

Discussion

The CHERISH study of nusinersen in later-onset SMA was designed to assess efficacy in older individuals with SMA type 2 after efficacy was shown in individuals with type 1.[5] Children from 2 to 12 years of age were included if they had symptom onset after 6 months of age, were able to sit independently, and were never able to walk 15 feet or more unaided and had an HFMSE score of 10 to 54. The primary endpoint was the least-squares mean change from baseline in the total HFMSE score at month 15. In the treatment group, there was an approximate 4-point improvement, and in the control group, a 1 point decline in the HFMSE.[9] In the initial dose escalation trial, individuals with SMA type 3 were included, and 17 of these were included in the long-term follow-up study, which showed a small mean improvement in the HFMSE for those individuals with SMA type 3, although the greatest change was seen in those individuals with SMA type 2.[18] At the time of FDA approval for nusinersen, there was no evidence of efficacy or safety in older individuals or individuals with type 3 SMA. After the blanket approval for all types of SMA, numerous individuals with more advanced disease and SMA type 3 have been dosed, and similar results to those of the long-term follow-up study noted above have been seen.[19–22]

CASE: DIAGNOSTIC CONSIDERATIONS IN ADULTS WITH SPINAL MUSCULAR ATROPHY

Case Presentation

A previously healthy 29-year-old man presented for evaluation of weakness. His symptoms started at the age of 17. He noticed he could not keep up with his peers playing sports. He had difficulty climbing stairs and lifting the arms over his head to reach high shelves. His family history was remarkable for 1 brother with similar symptoms. Examination was notable for intact higher mental function and cranial nerve examination. His strength testing using Medical Research Council grading showed normal strength except for bilateral elbow flexion graded at 4+, elbow extension 4−, hip flexion 2, knee extension 3−, and knee flexion 5−. His deep tendon reflexes were symmetrically present in the arms and absent in the legs. He had no scapular winging. His calves were large. His sensory examination was normal. The creatinine kinase (CK) was 1000 U/L. Limb girdle muscular dystrophy genetic panel came back negative. Subsequently, he had an electromyography (EMG) that showed mild neurogenic changes.

Clinical Question

The causes of the calf hypertrophy in this case are likely which of the following:

a. Miyoshi myopathy
b. *ANO5* related limb girdle muscular dystrophy (LGMR 12)
c. Bilateral S1 radiculopathy
d. Spinal muscular atrophy
e. Amyotrophic lateral sclerosis (ALS)

Discussion

This patient has proximal predominant limb muscle weakness, large calf muscles, positive family history, and elevated CK. There is no sensory deficit on his examination. The phenotype apparently looks like a myopathy, which prompted the referring physician to get a limb-girdle panel. In the era of next-generation sequencing, this is an increasingly used first step to establish a diagnosis.

The EMG showed neurogenic changes, which excluded myopathy as a cause. Although S1 radiculopathy is reported as a cause of calf hypertrophy, it will not explain the arm weakness and the CK elevation.[23] Although ALS is another diagnostic consideration, it usually presents with distal predominant asymmetric weakness.

This case underscores the importance of noting that both CK elevation and calf hypertrophy can occur in individuals with a relatively milder form of SMA. The early loss of deep tendon reflexes in the lower extremities may be a clue. In the era of disease-modifying therapies, clinicians need to be vigilant and include SMA in the differential diagnosis for patients presenting with proximal predominant weakness.

Clinical Question

Genetic testing will likely show which of the following:

a. Deletion of the *SMN1* gene with 2 *SMN2* copies
b. Deletion of the *SMN1* gene with 4 *SMN2* copies
c. Androgen receptor gene CAG repeats expansion
d. Dynein, cytoplasmic 1, heavy chain 1(*DYNC1H1*) gene mutation
e. Vesicle-associated membrane protein-associated protein B (*VABP*) gene mutation

Discussion

Disease severity is largely determined by retention of varying copy numbers of the *SMN2* gene, which alters the degree of SMN protein deficiency.[1] The main functional difference between these 2 genes relates to a single nucleotide change at exon 7. The transcript of the *SMN1* is full length and results in stable SMN protein compared with about 10% of transcripts of the *SMN2* gene.[24]

Most individuals with SMA type 1 have 2 copies of *SMN2*; those with SMA type 2 have 3 copies, and those with SMA type 3 have 3 or 4 copies.

Thus, a patient with 2 copies is likely to have a severe disease (SMA type 1) characterized by symptom onset in the first 6 months of life and the inability to sit unassisted. Obviously, this phenotype is changing in this gene-modifying era; children with 2 *SMN2* copies now can sit unsupported and stand, and some walk independently following treatment.

The term adults with SMA is a pragmatic approach to define patients with 5q SMA at age 18 and above. They are best classified based on their functional status at the time of evaluation as ambulatory and nonambulatory. The latter is divided further based on the severity of the weakness to a severe and intermediate phenotype.[25]

The above patient is an adult with symptoms onset in his late teens, and he remained ambulatory. Using the traditional classification, he will be labeled at type 3b (ie, ambulatory with symptoms onset after 3 years of age). Adults with 4 *SMN 2* copies are more likely to remain ambulatory compared with those with 3 *SMN2* copies.[26]

An additional point to highlight is the recognition of other forms of motor neuron disease with proximal predominant muscle weakness (**Table 1**[27]).

CASE: CHALLENGES IN TREATING ADULTS WITH SPINAL MUSCULAR ATROPHY

Case Presentation

This patient is a 27-year-old woman known to have SMA who presented to the clinic to discuss new FDA-approved treatments. She was an outcome of a normal pregnancy and birth. She sat unassisted at the age of 8 months. She never pulled up to a stand or walked. At that point, her pediatrician realized that something was wrong. This realization led to a muscle biopsy, and she was diagnosed around 14 months old. Later genetic testing confirmed she has deletion of the *SMN1* gene and 3 copies of the *SMN2* gene.

Table 1
Proximal predominant non 5q spinal muscular atrophy

Autosomal Dominant	Locus	Main Features
Adult proximal SMA (Finkle)	20q 13.22 *VABP*	Slowly progressive adult onset weakness and atrophy usually start in the legs. Bulbar muscles usually spared
Scapuloperoneal syndrome	12q24 TRPV4	Congenital nonprogressive leg weakness with associated contractures allelic with Charcot-Marie-Tooth type 2C and congenital SMA with contractures
SMA with lower-extremity predominance (SMALED)	14q32 *DYNC1H1*	Nonprogressive, childhood onset, delayed ambulation and leg weakness, and muscle wasting with prominent involvement of the quadriceps muscles
SMA with lower-extremity predominance (SMALED)	9q22.31 *BICD2*	Congenital or early adulthood onset of leg weakness and wasting affecting proximal and distal muscles groups. Ankle contractures, scoliosis, and scapular winging can occur
X Linked		
Bulbospinal muscular atrophy (Kennedy disease)	Xq12 androgen receptor gene	Slowly progressive atrophy and weakness of the bulbar and proximal limb muscles. Distal and asymmetric limb muscles involvement also described. It affects middle-aged men, and characteristic features include facial and perioral fasciculations, gynecomastia, and testicular atrophy
Infantile SMA with arthrogryposis	X p11.3 *UBE1*	Infantile onset of proximal predominant weakness, severe contractures, and arthrogryposis with associated respiratory insufficiency

Abbreviations: BICD2, bicaudal D homolog 2 gene; *DYNC1H1*, dynein, cytoplasmic 1, heavy chain 1; *SMN1*, survival motor neuron; TRPV4, vanilloid transient receptor protein; UBE1, ubiquitin activating enzyme 1; *VABP*, vesicle-associated membrane protein-associated protein B; *VRK1*, vaccinia-related kinase.

Her course over the years was notable for a slow decline in strength and motor function. She has slept on BiPAP since she was 7 years old. She has severe scoliosis and underwent spinal fusion surgery when she was 8 years old. She was able to feed herself until this past year, but now it has become difficult and she has to use plastic utensils because they are lighter.

On examination, she is awake and alert with normal speech. She has facial weakness and difficulty opening her mouth fully. Her tongue was atrophic with fasciculations. She has severe contractures most notable at the elbows and hamstrings. Strength examination reveals diffuse weakness more apparent in the legs with MRC strength in the 2 to 3 range in the arms and 1 to 2 in the legs. She is areflexic with a normal sensory examination.

Clinical Question

The following is true about the FDA-approved treatments for adults with 5q- SMA:

a. The FDA approved nusinersen treatment only for pediatric SMA patients less than the age of 15.

b. The FDA approved nusinersen treatment for all pediatric patients and ambulatory adults only.
c. The FDA approved nusinersen for all pediatric patients and nonambulatory adults only.
d. The FDA approved nusinersen for all ages and types of SMA, including both pediatric and adult individuals.
e. The FDA approved onasemnogene abeparvovec-xioi for treatment of adults with SMA.

Discussion

The FDA approved nusinersen treatment for all ages and types of 5-q SMA in December 2016.[28] The FDA approved onasemnogene abeparvovec-xioi only for children under the age of 2. Following the approval of nusinersen, several challenges faced physicians treating adult patients with SMA. Despite the robust studies in the pediatric population, there was a lack of efficacy data in adults over the age of 15. Moreover, the high cost of the treatment led to rigorous requirements by insurance companies for approval.

It was evident from the previous basic and clinical studies that earlier treatment is associated with better response. Counseling patients is based on extrapolating data from studies of the later-onset SMA in the pediatric population. In addition, some preliminary data from adult with SMA population are encouraging.[29]

Clinical Question

The following approaches are used as options for intrathecal delivery of nusinersen in SMA patients with history of spinal fusion:

a. Fluoroscopy-guided cervical puncture
b. Subcutaneous intrathecal catheter system
c. Computed tomography-guided transformational approach
d. None of the above
e. All of the above

Discussion

Scoliosis is commonly seen in patients with weakness related to chronic neuromuscular diseases, including SMA. The history of spinal fusion surgery to help correct the scoliosis made intrathecal drug delivery another challenge in patients requiring treated with nusinersen. All of the above routes were proposed in case series.[20,30–32]

The long-term safety and effectiveness of these methods are under evaluation. The choice depends on the availability of resources, personnel, and most importantly, patient's preference.

Clinical Question

The following outcome measures can be used to track treatment response in nonambulatory adults with SMA:

a. Revised upper limb module (RULM)
b. Hammersmith Functional Motor Scale Expanded (HFMSE)
c. Pulmonary function test
d. SMA Functional Rating Scale (modified SMAFRS)
e. All of the above

Discussion

Another challenge is the lack of consensus on the best outcome measure to use to help track treatment response. Evaluations are based on the current patient functional status. In this case, all of the above are appropriate for use in a nonambulatory adult with SMA. In general, motor function assessments, strength measurements, lung function testing, and quality-of-life questionnaires are used. The current tools have limitations with flooring effect in patients with very severe weakness and are limited in the assessment of axial muscles, bulbar function, fatigue, and endurance. Applying additional measures and capturing subjective changes may be helpful. It is pertinent to ensure that evaluators are familiar with the use of these scales.[33–36] Given that insurance in the United States will demand documentation of change over time, it is probably best at this stage to apply several measures when evaluating these individuals.

SUMMARY

SMA is now a disease with a rapidly changing natural history. Infants who historically would have died at the age of 2 are now sitting and standing, and some are walking. Children with more advanced disease are either experiencing a stabilization of the disease or a return of abilities that they had recently lost. Preliminary data on safety and efficacy of treatment in adults are promising. Currently, there are 2 treatment options available, and more are anticipated in the near future. More work is needed in the community to help guide decision making in selection of which treatment to use, and continued follow-up in multidisciplinary clinics is needed to monitor the long-term outcomes and safety of these treatments.

SUPPLEMENTARY DATA

Supplementary data related to this article can be found online at https://doi.org/10.1016/j.ncl.2020.03.002.

REFERENCES

1. Kolb SJ, Kissel JT. Spinal muscular atrophy: a timely review. Arch Neurol 2011;68:979–84.
2. Prior TW, Krainer AR, Hua Y, et al. A positive modifier of spinal muscular atrophy in the SMN2 gene. Am J Hum Genet 2009;85:408–13.
3. Finkel RS, McDermott MP, Kaufmann P, et al. Observational study of spinal muscular atrophy type I and implications for clinical trials. Neurology 2014;83:810–7.
4. Kolb SJ, Coffey CS, Yankey JW, et al. Natural history of infantile-onset spinal muscular atrophy. Ann Neurol 2017;82:883–91.
5. Finkel RS, Mercuri E, Darras BT, et al. Nusinersen versus sham control in infantile-onset spinal muscular atrophy. N Engl J Med 2017;377:1723–32.
6. Mendell JR, Al-Zaidy S, Shell R, et al. Single-dose gene-replacement therapy for spinal muscular atrophy. N Engl J Med 2017;377:1713–22.
7. Kolb SJ, Coffey CS, Yankey JW, et al. Baseline results of the NeuroNEXT spinal muscular atrophy infant biomarker study. Ann Clin Transl Neurol 2016;3:132–45.
8. Aragon-Gawinska K, Seferian AM, Daron A, et al. Nusinersen in patients older than 7 months with spinal muscular atrophy type 1: a cohort study. Neurology 2018;91:e1312–8.
9. Mercuri E, Darras BT, Chiriboga CA, et al. Nusinersen versus sham control in later-onset spinal muscular atrophy. N Engl J Med 2018;378:625–35.

10. Al-Zaidy S, Pickard AS, Kotha K, et al. Health outcomes in spinal muscular atrophy type 1 following AVXS-101 gene replacement therapy. Pediatr Pulmonol 2019;54(2):179–85.
11. Hao le T, Duy PQ, Jontes JD, et al. Temporal requirement for SMN in motoneuron development. Hum Mol Genet 2013;22:2612–25.
12. Burghes AH, Beattie CE. Spinal muscular atrophy: why do low levels of survival motor neuron protein make motor neurons sick? Nat Rev Neurosci 2009;10: 597–609.
13. Szunyogova E, Zhou H, Maxwell GK, et al. Survival motor neuron (SMN) protein is required for normal mouse liver development. Sci Rep 2016;6:34635.
14. Finkel RS, Chiriboga CA, Vajsar J, et al. Treatment of infantile-onset spinal muscular atrophy with nusinersen: a phase 2, open-label, dose-escalation study. Lancet 2016;388:3017–26.
15. Bevan AK, Duque S, Foust KD, et al. Systemic gene delivery in large species for targeting spinal cord, brain, and peripheral tissues for pediatric disorders. Mol Ther 2011;19:1971–80.
16. Kantor B, Bailey RM, Wimberly K, et al. Methods for gene transfer to the central nervous system. Adv Genet 2014;87:125–97.
17. Dehay B, Dalkara D, Dovero S, et al. Systemic scAAV9 variant mediates brain transduction in newborn rhesus macaques. Sci Rep 2012;2:253.
18. Darras BT, Chiriboga CA, Iannaccone ST, et al. Nusinersen in later-onset spinal muscular atrophy: long-term results from the phase 1/2 studies. Neurology 2019;92:e2492–506.
19. Montes J, Dunaway Young S, Mazzone ES, et al. Nusinersen improves walking distance and reduces fatigue in later-onset spinal muscular atrophy. Muscle Nerve 2019;60:409–14.
20. Veerapandiyan A, Eichinger K, Guntrum D, et al. Intrathecal nusinersen in older children and adults with spinal muscular atrophy (S5.001). Neurology 2019;92. S5.001.
21. Yeo CJJ, Simeone S, Zhang RZ, et al. Outcome measures for nusinersen efficacy in adults with spinal muscular atrophy (S5.008). Neurology 2019;92. S5.008.
22. Drory V, Fainmesser Y, Abraham A, et al. Nusinersen treatment in adults with SMA–the first year experience at a large center (S5.007). Neurology 2019;92. S5.007.
23. Volpi N, Ginanneschi F, Cerase A, et al. Calf muscle hypertrophy following S1 radiculopathy: a stress disorder caused by hyperactivity with variable response to treatmen. Clin Neuropathol 2018;37:146–50.
24. Arnold WD, Kassar D, Kissel JT. Spinal muscular atrophy: diagnosis and management in a new therapeutic era. Muscle Nerve 2015;51:157–67.
25. Rai W, Elsheikh B. Spinal muscular atrophy. Pract Neurol 2019;18:61–6.
26. Elsheikh B, Prior T, Zhang X, et al. An analysis of disease severity based on SMN2 copy number in adults with spinal muscular atrophy. Muscle Nerve 2009;40: 652–6.
27. Spinal muscular atrophy: disease mechanisms and therapy. In: Sumner CJ, Pushkin S, Ko CP. 1st edition. Academic Press.
28. Waldrop MA, Kolb SJ. Current treatment options in neurology-SMA therapeutics. Curr Treat Options Neurol 2019;21:25.
29. Walter MC, Wenninger S, Thiele S, et al. Safety and treatment effects of nusinersen in longstanding adult 5q-SMA type 3–a prospective observational study. J Neuromuscul Dis 2019;6(4):453–65.

30. Strauss KA, Carson VJ, Brigatti KW, et al. Preliminary safety and tolerability of a novel subcutaneous intrathecal catheter system for repeated outpatient dosing of nusinersen to children and adults with spinal muscular atrophy. J Pediatr Orthop 2018;38:e610–7.
31. Mousa MA, Aria DJ, Schaefer CM, et al. A comprehensive institutional overview of intrathecal nusinersen injections for spinal muscular atrophy. Pediatr Radiol 2018; 48:1797–805.
32. Bortolani S, Stura G, Ventilii G, et al. Intrathecal administration of nusinersen in adult and adolescent patients with spinal muscular atrophy and scoliosis: transforaminal versus conventional approach. Neuromuscul Disord 2019;29:742–6.
33. Mazzone ES, Mayhew A, Montes J, et al. Revised upper limb module for spinal muscular atrophy: development of a new module. Muscle Nerve 2017;55:869–74.
34. Pera MC, Coratti G, Forcina N, et al. Content validity and clinical meaningfulness of the HFMSE in spinal muscular atrophy. BMC Neurol 2017;17:39.
35. Pera MC, Coratti G, Mazzone ES, et al. Revised upper limb module for spinal muscular atrophy: 12 month changes. Muscle Nerve 2019;59:426–30.
36. Kissel JT, Elsheikh B, King WM, et al. SMA valiant trial: a prospective, double-blind, placebo-controlled trial of valproic acid in ambulatory adults with spinal muscular atrophy. Muscle Nerve 2014;49:187–92.

Advances in the Genetic Testing of Neuromuscular Diseases

Perry B. Shieh, MD, PhD

KEYWORDS

- Transcriptome analysis • Exome sequencing • Mitochondrial testing • Mosaicism
- Genome sequencing

KEY POINTS

- Mosaicism of the proband or parent may make certain cases particularly challenging to interpret.
- Testing of the DNA from tissues including muscle may improve diagnostic sensitivity in mosaic patients.
- Whole-exome sequencing of the proband and parents (trio testing) can identify a mosaic parent that may otherwise confound the interpretation of an autosomal-dominant pathogenic variant.
- Testing of the RNA from affected tissue (eg, muscle) can identify intronic mutations that may not be seen on standard genetic testing.
- Genomic rearrangements and intronic mutations are often difficult to diagnose with standard genetic testing, and may require whole-genome sequencing or RNA sequencing.

Video content accompanies this article at http://www.neurologic.theclinics.com.

INTRODUCTION

Traditional clinical genetic testing has been focused, where testing is ordered based on a patient's clinical presentation. Next-generation sequencing (NGS) is a form of high-throughput sequencing that has allowed parallel sequencing of a large number of genes at relatively low cost. Depending on how the testing is configured, testing may be designed to sequence the whole genome of a patient (ie, whole-genome sequencing or WGS), only the protein encoding regions of the genome (ie, whole-exome sequencing or WES), or a set of genes associated with clinically related syndromes (ie, disease-specific panels). Although WES and disease-specific panels are

Department of Neurology, University of California Los Angeles, 300 Medical Plaza, Suite B-200, Los Angeles, CA 90095, USA
E-mail address: pshieh@mednet.ucla.edu

Neurol Clin 38 (2020) 519–528
https://doi.org/10.1016/j.ncl.2020.03.012

now often used for clinical testing, WGS is only performed on a research basis, as the pathogenicity of variants in noncoding genomic sequences can be challenging. With the advent of NGS, however, it is also common to encounter variant DNA sequences that do not match the reference sequence, and as such, the clinical significance is unclear. To minimize overinterpretation, standards for how new variants are to be described and potentially interpreted have been established.[1]

To improve specificity, clinical DNA testing typically focuses on the coding regions of a gene, and clinical testing protocols have generally been optimized to improve the "coverage" of coding regions or other known pathogenic regions of the relevant genes. However, the optimization of these panels varies depending on the laboratory performing the test. Nonetheless, disease-specific panels have become a powerful tool for clinicians and have reduced the diagnostic journey that is challenging even for the most experienced clinicians.

More advanced applications of NGS have also been developed. Although genetic testing has traditionally been performed on DNA isolated from leukocytes, for some conditions it may be more appropriate to perform testing on the DNA or RNA within specific tissues. Tissue-specific gene expression provides a profile of the genetic milieu of that tissue that may be contributing to the pathogenesis of the disease. The relative availability of affected muscle or nerve tissue provides an opportunity for diagnostic testing that may not be as readily available in other conditions. Testing preformed on DNA or RNA isolated from these tissues may provide information that improves the diagnostic yield of genetic testing.

This article presents neuromuscular cases that will illustrate the clinical utility of more advanced applications of NGS, including cases that result from mosaicism, genomic rearrangements, transcriptome sequencing, and discovery of novel genes.

CASE 1: MOSAICISM

Case Presentation

The proband is currently age 16 but originally presented at 8 years of age for an unusual gait. He was born at term via cesarean section secondary to breech presentation. The birth was otherwise uncomplicated, and his hospital course was not prolonged after delivery. The patient appeared to have decreased leg movement during his first few months, however, and started crawling at age 8 months but using only his arms. The patient eventually started walking at 2 years of age, although his parents did not feel that he was steady. His gait improved gradually over the next few years, but he never ran. After 5 years of age, his motor development reached a plateau. He did not have any sensory abnormalities and did not appear to have any cognitive impairment. He was first evaluated in the neurology clinic at age 8. At age 10, he underwent electrodiagnostic testing, which was nondiagnostic.

His family history is notable for identical twin brothers who are 2 years younger than him and appear to have the same condition. He does not have any other siblings. His parents are unaffected, and there is no one else in his extended family with this condition.

On examination, his mental status examination demonstrated normal memory and fund of knowledge for age. Cranial Nerves examination was normal. Motor testing revealed decreased bulk throughout with calf atrophy. Confrontation testing of the upper extremities demonstrated mild weakness of deltoids. Testing of the lower extremities revealed hip flexion MRC grade 4/5, hip extension 5/5, knee extension 3/5, knee flexion 4+/5, dorsiflexion 4+/5, and plantar flexion 1/5. Sensation was normal. He stood with a flexion forward posture (**Fig. 1**A). While ambulating, he walks with his

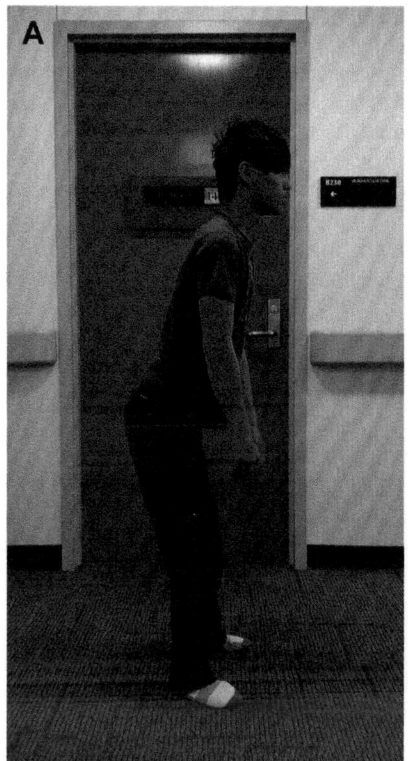

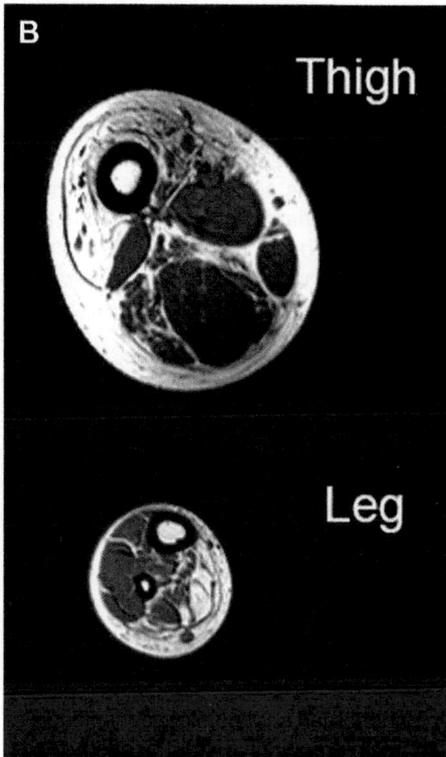

Fig. 1. (*A*) Patient from case 1, 16 years old in this picture, stands with his hip flexed and torso leaning forward. (*B*) MRI of the thigh and lower leg demonstrated fatty replacement of anterior thigh muscles and posterior calf muscles.

hips flexed, rotating his hips and trunk to accommodate this posture (see Video 1 at age 16). His coordination was normal on finger-to-nose testing. Reflexes were absent throughout. CK was 348.

Electrodiagnostic testing performed at age 10 was performed under sedation. This study demonstrated no abnormal spontaneous activity. Motor unit action potentials, however, could not be assessed as the patient was under sedation. However, electrodiagnostic testing on one of his younger brothers at age 15 demonstrated chronic neurogenic changes, including abnormal spontaneous activity and decreased recruitment of giant amplitude motor unit action potentials in distal muscles.

He underwent MRI imaging of the lower extremity, which revealed significant fatty replacement of the muscles in the anterior compartment of the thigh and posterior compartment of the lower leg (**Fig. 1**B).

Given the patient's unusual gait, there was significant suspicion for a hereditary motor neuropathy. The patient underwent extensive genetic testing, including distal hereditary motor neuropathy panel testing and WES – trio testing (testing of proband and both parents). Although variants were identified, they could not be determined to be pathogenic. The patient subsequently underwent WGS, which identified a c.2327 C > T (p.Pro776Leu) variant in the *DYNC1H1* gene, which has been associated with lower extremity dominant spinal muscular atrophy (SMA-LED).[2] The patient and his twin brothers all carried this variant, and their phenotype was similar. This particular variant, however, has not been previously reported. This variant was actually seen on WES – trio testing, because the unaffected father carried the variant. On the WGS analysis, however, the relative representation of the normal allele versus the variant could be quantified in the father's DNA more reliably. The normal allele was represented in approximately 37 out of 47 reads (79%), whereas the c.2327 C > T variant was only represented in the remaining 10 out of 47 reads (21%). This suggests that the father is actually a mosaic, with approximately 42% the cells containing 1 copy of this variant (heterozygous) and the remaining cells sampled having no copies of this variant (homozygous wild type). In retrospect, this imbalance was actually seen in the WES; however, the capture/amplification process in exome sequencing makes quantification less reliable.

Discussion

This case illustrates one of the ways that a patient may present with an autosomal-dominant condition while not having an affected parent. The patient's clinical presentation is similar to patients with variants in *DYNC1H1* that have been described in the literature. What was particularly challenging in this case, however, was that the father had tested positive for the identified autosomal-dominant variant, even though he was phenotypically normal. The imbalanced representation of the normal allele and the variant indicates that he is mosaic, with the lower dose of the mutant allele likely explaining why he was not affected. Thus, the father's apparent incomplete penetrance is actually a result of his mosaicism for this mutation.

CASE 2: INTRONIC MUTATIONS REVEALED THROUGH TRANSCRIPTOME ANALYSIS

Case Presentation

The patient presented as a 7-year-old boy who was experiencing weakness. His parents reported normal development until about 4 years of age when the parents noted a mildly unsteady gait. At 4 years of age, he was noted to rise from the floor with a Gower sign.

His weakness has been slowly progressing, and the parents reported frequent falls. He appears to have normal cognition, does well in school, and has no behavioral issues. His parents are of Greek and Hispanic heritage, and neither parent is affected. There is no family history of anyone with similar symptoms.

On examination, the patient was a thin boy with noticeably low muscle mass. His general examination was normal. Mental Status examination was normal for age. His cranial nerve examination was normal. Motor examination demonstrated proximal upper and lower extremity weakness, graded at 4/5 bilaterally, with relatively normal distal muscle strength. No contractures were noted. Bilateral scapular winging was observed (**Fig. 2**A, B). The sensory examination was normal. Reflexes were mildly diminished at 1+ in the biceps, triceps, patellar, and ankles. Plantar responses were flexor bilaterally. He had normal coordination. His gait demonstrated mild toe walking, and he rose from the floor with a Gower maneuver (Video 2).

His initial serum CK at 4 years of age was elevated at 1207. Testing for Pompe disease, spinal muscular atrophy, and Duchenne was negative. His chromosomal microarray study was also negative.

The patient underwent a muscle biopsy, which demonstrated nonspecific myopathic changes including random fiber size variation and rare degenerating/regenerating fibers. He underwent WES twice, which revealed some variants that were not thought to be significant.

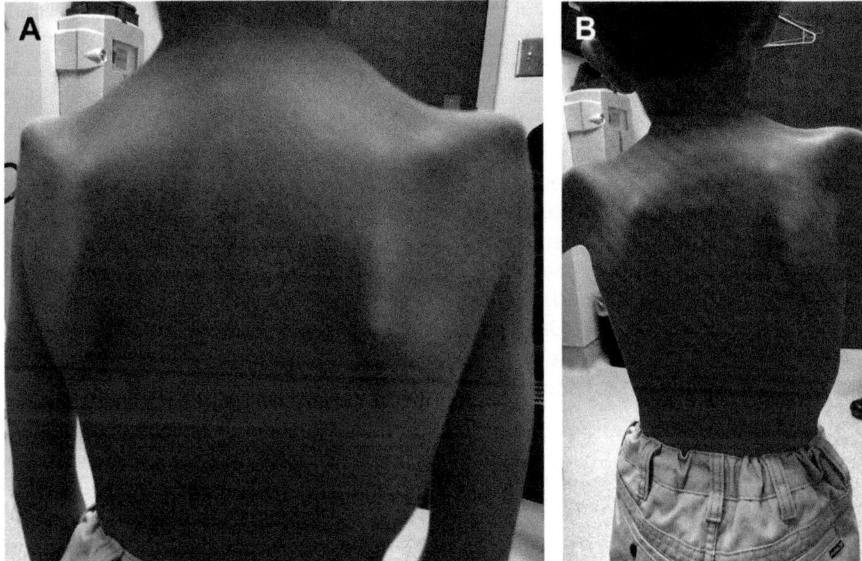

Fig. 2. (*A*) Patient from case 2, with mild prominence of the scapulae. (*B*) With his arms abducted, scapular winging is more prominent.

NGS was performed on RNA that was isolated from muscle tissue (transcriptome analysis or “RNA seq”). This analysis demonstrated a 66 bp insertion between exon 6 and exon 7 of the *LMNA* transcripts. Data from WGS demonstrated that there was de novo 26 bp deletion within intron 6 of *LMNA*, and the 66 bp insertion represented the remaining sequences from intron 6. This resulted in a 22 amino acid insertion within the Lamin A/C protein.

Discussion

The patient presented with early onset proximal weakness and scapular winging, which was clinically consistent with several muscular dystrophies. The absence of any family history suggested that the disease was caused by an autosomal-recessive condition. *LMNA* mutations, however, are typically associated with autosomal-dominant inheritance. In this case, RNA seq was able to prove that the de novo 26 bp deletion within intron 6 of *LMNA* altered the amino acid sequence of the lamin A/C protein, resulting in the patient’s clinical presentation. This case has been reported as part of a case series on transcriptome analysis.[3]

CASE 3: WHOLE GENOME ANALYSIS REVEALS A REARRANGEMENT

Case Presentation

The patient was referred for motor delay when he was 5 years old. He had a normal birth, delivery, and early development. He walked at around 15 months of age. When he was approximately 2 years of age, however, the mother noticed that he was neither running nor jumping and appeared behind in motor capabilities compared with his cousins. He had normal cognition and language development. He was seen by multiple physicians who considered the diagnosis of Duchenne muscular dystrophy (DMD).

On examination, he was shy but otherwise had normal cognition for age. Cranial nerves were normal. The motor examination revealed mildly weak hip flexion but otherwise normal strength on confrontation testing. He rose from the floor with a Gower maneuver. His gait appeared normal. Reflexes were absent throughout, and his plantar responses were flexor. He had mildly limited range of motion at the ankle.

Laboratory testing revealed a serum CK of 21,000. Genetic testing for DMD, including duplication/deletion testing and full sequencing of all 79 exons, was normal. A muscle biopsy demonstrated increased endomysial fibrosis and fiber size variation. Immunohistochemistry demonstrated absence of the dystrophin protein.

He underwent WGS on a research basis, which demonstrated an inversion of a 5 megabase segment that included exons 38 to 79 of the *DMD* gene. This inversion resulted in a truncation of the *DMD* gene after exon 37. Transcriptome analysis performed on RNA isolated from the patient's muscle demonstrated mRNA that was truncated after the exon 37 sequences.

Discussion

This case illustrates a patient with a case of Duchenne Muscular Dystrophy that was clinically apparent and confirmed on immunohistochemistry from the muscle but could not be verified on standard genetic testing. Conventional genetic testing for Duchenne muscular dystrophy typically involves a 2-tiered approach: (1) testing for duplication or deletion most commonly through multiplex ligation-dependent polymerase chain reaction (PCR) amplification (MLPA) followed by (2) direct sequencing of all 79 exons if necessary. Based on the prevalence of mutations,[4] this approach should have a sensitivity of over 95%. Genomic rearrangements and intronic mutations, however, will be missed with this testing. Definitive genetic testing in these types of cases may require WGS and possibly RNA sequencing of the dystrophin transcript to confirm and identify the genetic cause.

CASE 4: GENE DISCOVERY THROUGH WHOLE-EXOME SEQUENCING

Case Presentation

The patient initially presented as a 37-year-old Persian Jewish man with 2 years of progressive weakness. He stated that he had never been athletic, and he had always been thin. Notably, he was never able to throw a ball as far as others but he had just assumed that he was not meant to be athletic. He was prescribed steroids to help increase his muscle bulk, which did not have any significant effect and so were discontinued. Symptoms slowly progressed until 2 years prior to presentation when it became difficult for him to climb stairs, and he noticed he was struggling to get up from a chair. He stated that although he has always been thin, his muscle bulk appeared to be diminishing. He also noted some difficulty with swallowing. The patient otherwise did not have any other medical problems and was not on any medications. His family history was notable for a maternal aunt and maternal uncle who appeared to have similar symptoms. Neither of his parents nor his 2 older sisters were affected. His parents were cousins, however, and there was known consanguinity in his extended family.

At the time of evaluation, his examination revealed diminished muscle bulk in the chest (**Fig. 3**A), pelvis, and thighs (**Fig. 3**B), and he stood with a mildly lordotic posture (**Fig. 3**C).

Cranial nerves were normal. His weakness was generally symmetric and graded as follows: neck flexor 3/5, deltoids 4+/5, biceps 5/5, triceps 4/5, grip 5/5, interossei 4/5, wrist extensors 5/5, hip flexors 4/5, hip extensors 4+/5, hip abduction 5-/5, hip

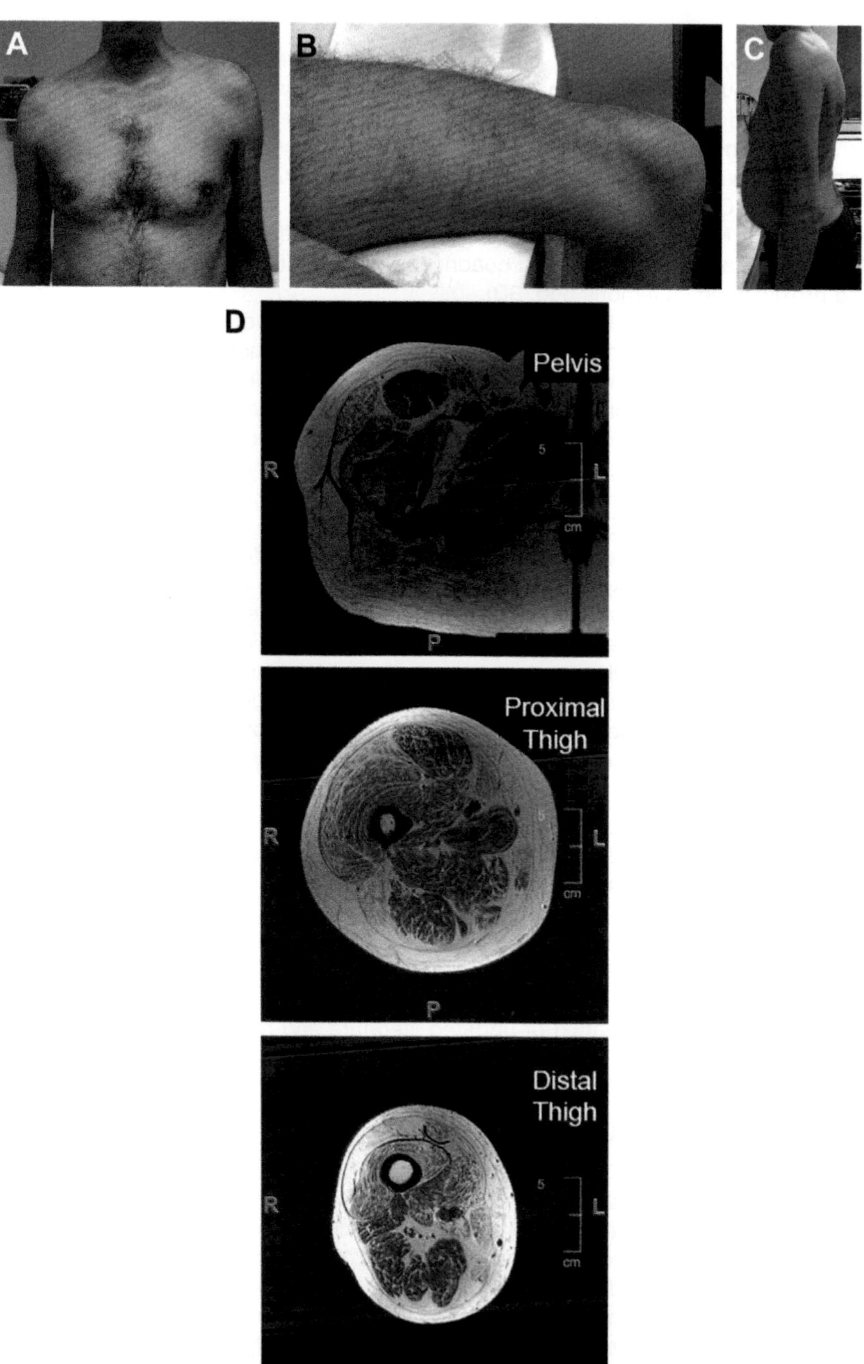

Fig. 3. (*A*) Patient from case 4, with atrophy of pectoral muscles. (*B*) Notable distal quadriceps atrophy. (*C*) Upon standing, the patient has protuberant abdomen from low abdominal muscle tone and a mildly lordotic posture. (*D*) MRI of the pelvis and thigh demonstrate fatty replacement of muscles with relative sparing of the adductor and proximal rectus femoris muscles.

adduction 5/5, hamstrings 5-/5, quadriceps 5-/5, foot eversion 5/5, and foot inversion 5/5. His scapulae were asymmetric, but there was no winging. He struggled to rise from a seated position. Coordination was normal, and sensation was intact. The patient had a slight waddling gait but could jog for a short distance. There was no action or percussion myotonia. He also had an intention tremor.

His serum CK was normal. EMG/NCS demonstrated mild nonirritable myopathic changes. An MRI at 46 years of age demonstrated diffuse muscular atrophy with the gluteus, sartorius, gracilis, and quadriceps, with relative sparing of the adductors and proximal rectus femoris (**Fig. 3**D).

Muscle biopsies of the left quadriceps demonstrated numerous fibers with internalized nuclei, frequent pyknotic nuclear clumps, along with angular atrophic fibers, hypertrophied fibers, and split fibers. Immunohistochemistry for membrane proteins was normal. Clinical testing for facioscapulohumeral muscular dystrophy (FSHD) was nondiagnostic. Clinical WES did not reveal any mutations in genes that were associated with muscular dystrophy. WES of additional affected family members was also not diagnostic.

Reanalysis of the WES data performed later, however, revealed a homozygous c.464 A > G (p.D155S) variant in the *PYROXD1* gene that had not been established to be associated with a specific muscle disease at the time the testing was originally performed. By the time of reanalysis, this gene had been reported to be associated with autosomal-recessive, early onset muscle disease.[5] Review of the WES data from other affected family members demonstrated the same homozygous variant. This patient had similar muscle biopsy findings to those described in the O'Grady and colleagues 2016 report, although he had a milder phenotype than those in the reported cohort. His case has subsequently been reported in a separate case report.[6]

Discussion

Although neuromuscular specific NGS panels are relatively inexpensive and sensitive, there remain novel neuromuscular conditions still being discovered every year. WES continues not only to be a powerful diagnostic tool in identifying genes associated with well-described conditions, but also in identifying new genetic syndromes. Although the clinical WES in this case did not actually lead to the initial discovery of *PYROXD1* association with muscle disease, it highlights the need to periodically reanalyze WES data in the context of updated literature and revised genomic reference databases.

CASE 5: MITOCHONDRIAL MOSAICISM

Case Presentation

This patient came for evaluation at 53 years of age. Her symptoms began in her early 20s, with ptosis, diplopia, and ophthalmoplegia. Symptoms were mild at first, but became progressively worse. In her late thirties, however, she was also told that she may have muscular dystrophy. At the time of presentation, she reported, in addition to her ocular symptoms, she had some neck pain, shoulder pain, and diffuse muscle aches that were worse in proximal muscles. She generally felt more fatigue toward the end of the day, but she denied any dysphagia. Despite these symptoms, she was able to carry out daily activities.

On examination, her mental status was normal. Cranial nerve examination demonstrated moderate ptosis and fixed gaze with no extraocular movements. She had weak eye closure, but facial expressions were otherwise symmetric and intact. Hearing was normal. Manual motor testing revealed mild proximal weakness with grade

4+/5 strength in proximal upper and lower extremities. Distal muscles were essentially normal. Sensation and coordination were normal. Reflexes were present but mildly diminished at 1+ throughout; plantar responses were flexor. She walked with a stooped posture and reduced arm swing bilaterally, but was otherwise steady with normal base and stride length.

Because of the presentation of chronic progressive external ophthalmoplegia, the patient underwent a muscle biopsy, which demonstrated mitochondrial aggregates on NADH and SDH staining, with occasional COX-negative fibers. Muscle tissue was sent for mtDNA sequencing using NGS. This testing demonstrated a single heteroplasmic 4365 bp deletion of the mitochondrial genome (m.9588_13,952 del4365). No nuclear mutations were identified.

Discussion

This is a case of chronic progressive external ophthalmoplegia (CPEO). A single large deletion within the mitochondrial genome was identified, which is typically associated with a more rapid variant of CPEO known commonly as Kearns Sayre Syndrome (KSS). Single deletions presumably arise de novo in the maternal germline or early in embryogenesis, and are typically associated with a more rapid variant of CPEO, with onset of symptoms within the first 20 years of life. Because mutant mtDNA replicates faster than the normal mtDNA, heteroplasmy increases with age, thus accounting for progressive symptoms with age.

This patient appears to have a milder course than what is typically seen in KSS. In contrast with typical CPEO, nuclear gene variants (eg, *POLG1*) are usually not seen in KSS patients. Typically, mtDNA testing is performed on muscle tissue, since testing on blood is often negative. NGS performed with high depth-of-read can improve the test sensitivity in patients with relatively low heteroplasmy of mutant mtDNA.

SUMMARY

Next-generation sequencing has enhanced the diagnostic yield of conventional genetic testing. Certain patients, however, may be particularly challenging and require special testing. This article presented 5 cases that illustrate how more advanced applications of NGS have led to an accurate genetic diagnosis. Although most of these methods are currently only available on a research basis, some may become available for clinical testing in the future as robust standardized algorithms are developed for testing particularly difficult-to-diagnose patients.

DISCLOSURE

The author has served as a consultant for Sarepta, Avexis, Biogen, and Pfizer, and as a speaker for Biogen, Grifols, Avexis, and Alexion.

SUPPLEMENTARY DATA

Supplementary data to this article can be found online at https://doi.org/10.1016/j.ncl.2020.03.012.

REFERENCES

1. Richards S, Aziz N, Bale S, et al. Standards and guidelines for the interpretation of sequence variants: a joint consensus recommendation of the American College of Medical Genetics and Genomics and the Association for Molecular Pathology guideline. Genet Med 2015;17:405–24.

2. Scoto M, Rossor AM, Harms MB, et al. Novel mutations expand the clinical spectrum of DYNC1H1-associated spinal muscular atrophy. Neurology 2015;84:668–79.
3. Lee H, Huang AY, Wang LK, et al. Diagnostic utility of transcriptome sequencing for rare Mendelian diseases. Genet Med 2019. https://doi.org/10.1038/s41436-019-0672-1.
4. Bladen CL, Salgado D, Monges S, et al. The treat-NMD DMD global database: analysis of more than 7,000 Duchenne muscular dystrophy mutations. Hum Mutat 2015;36:395–402.
5. O'Grady GL, Best HA, Sztal TE, et al. Variants in the oxidoreductase PYROXD1 cause early onset myopathy with internalized nuclei and myofibrillar disorganization. Am J Hum Genet 2016;99:1086–105.
6. Woods J, Khanlou N, Lee H, et al. Myopathy associated with homozygous PYROXD1 pathogenic variants detected by genome sequencing. Neuropathology 2020. [Epub ahead of print].

Case Studies on the Genetic and Clinical Diagnosis of Facioscapulohumeral Muscular Dystrophy

Johanna Hamel, MD*, Rabi Tawil, MD

KEYWORDS

- Facioscapulohumeral muscular dystrophy • DUX4 • SMCHD1 • Epigenetic
- Hypomethylation • Muscle pathology

KEY POINTS

- A key requirement for the pathophysiology of facioscapulohumeral muscular dystrophy is hypomethylation of the region containing the DUX4 gene on chromosome 4q35 and a polymorphic polyadenylation signal distal to it.
- Hypomethylation of 4q35 either results from a contraction of the number of repeats in that region or from a mutation in a different gene responsible for methylation on 4q35.
- Patients with large contractions often develop symptoms and signs earlier in life and are at risk of developing extramuscular manifestations.
- Often, a clinical diagnosis of facioscapulohumeral muscular dystrophy can be made and genetic testing is confirmatory. However, in the presence of unusual features, a broad differential diagnosis and workup is important.

INTRODUCTION

Facioscapulohumeral muscular dystrophy (FSHD) is the second most common adult muscular dystrophy and is caused by DUX4 protein, which is toxic to skeletal muscle.[1,2] DUX4 protein is a transcription factor expressed in the germline and silenced in somatic tissue of healthy individuals. *DUX4* (double homeobox 4) is a retrogene, which consists of a sequence of large (3.3 kb) repeats. Healthy individuals have more than 10 repeats with lengths measured in kilobase (>38 kb) and high methylation levels, resulting in a closed chromatin structure preventing gene transcription from within the repeats. In FSHD, a decreased number of repeats and/or hypomethylation result in opening of the chromatin structure and expression of DUX4 (**Fig. 1**). The

Department of Neurology, University of Rochester Medical Center, 601 Elmwood Avenue, Box 673, Rochester, NY 14642, USA
* Corresponding author.
E-mail address: Johanna_Hamel@URMC.Rochester.edu

Neurol Clin 38 (2020) 529–540
https://doi.org/10.1016/j.ncl.2020.03.003

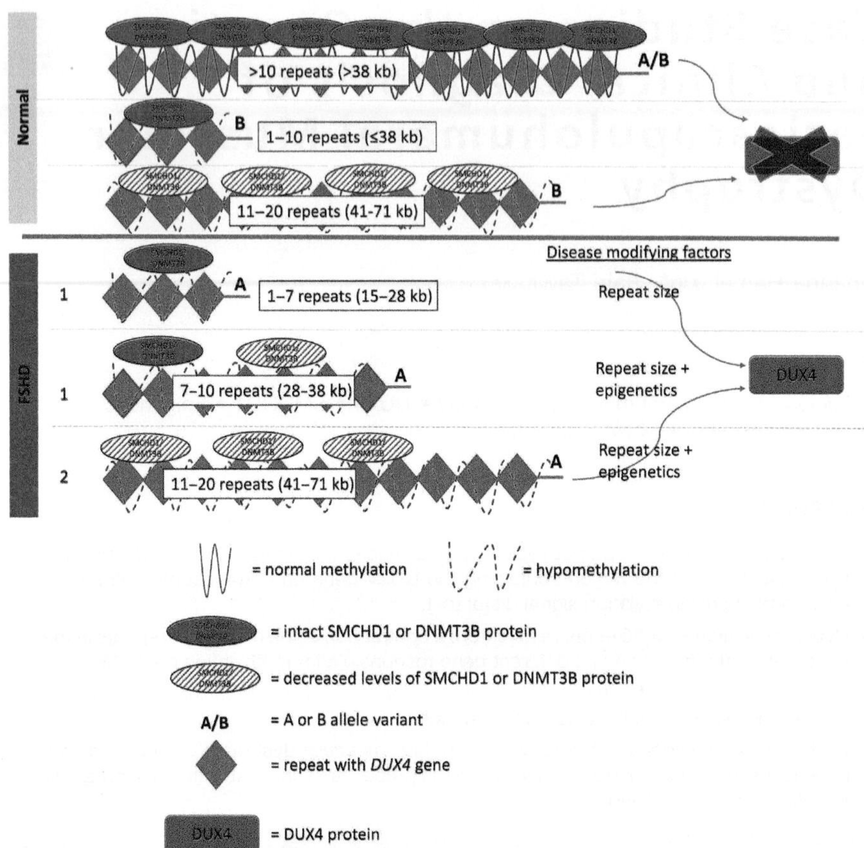

Fig. 1. The spectrum of the genetic mechanisms in FSHD. Normal: in normal individuals both copies of 4q35 contain greater than 10 repeats (>38 kb) with normal methylation or, rarely, a contraction with hypomethylation on a nonpermissive B allele, or rarely a mutation in *SMCHD1* or *DNMT3B* gene is present and repeat arrays are hypomethylated on both 4q35 copies, but with an unstable DUX4 transcript owing to lack of polymorphic polyadenlyation site (PAS) on the B haplotype. FSHD: One copy of 4q35 with a permissive A allele is necessary to cause FSHD1. In FSHD1, one copy of 4q35 is contracted with hypomethylation of the repeat array. In patients with 1 to 6 repeats (<28 kb), the repeat number is associated with disease severity. In patients with 7 to 10 repeats (28–38 kb), nonpenetrance is more common and epigenetic factors (such as mutations in *SMCHD1*) play a larger role. In FSHD2, one copy of 4q35 contains 11 to 20 repeats (41–71 kb) on an A allele with PAS. A mutation in *SMCHD1* or *DNMT3B* gene is present and repeat arrays are hypomethylated on both 4q35 copies.

diagnosis is often made clinically with a typical presentation of facial weakness in combination with scapuloperoneal and abdominal muscle weakness (Beevor sign). Genetic confirmation is typically the first diagnostic step. However, with the discovery of FSHD2 and its underlying epigenetic mechanism, genetic confirmation of FSHD has become more complex. Furthermore, with targeted therapies on the horizon, early diagnosis in minimally symptomatic patients will be important, but more challenging, owing to greater clinical variability in late-onset or mild disease. Here, we present cases to demonstrate the complexity of the genetic mechanism and diagnostic algorithm along with some clinical pitfalls and differential diagnosis. If in doubt, it is helpful to take a step back, redefine carefully the clinical phenotype and possible FSHD mimics, and consider muscle pathology as a diagnostic tool.

CASE 1: DOUBLE TROUBLE

Clinical Presentation

A 39-year-old man first noticed weakness in his upper extremities in his late 20s early 30s. At the time, he was regularly lifting weights and noticed that he was losing milestones. His personal trainer observed a loss of muscle bulk in his biceps, triceps, and pectoralis region. At the time of evaluation, the weakness had progressed to the point that he had difficulty lifting any weight above his head. His lower extremities were less affected, with mild difficulty climbing stairs. He had no facial weakness, dysphagia, ptosis, cardiac manifestations, shortness of breath, or other symptoms. Interestingly, at about age 25, although he had no symptoms yet, he was coincidentally found to have an elevated creatine kinase (CK) in the 7000s, which had remained at a similar high level since. He knew of no other family member with muscle weakness. On examination, he had no facial weakness, no truncal weakness, and no kyphotic or lordotic features. He had symmetric weakness and atrophy of shoulder muscles with mild scapular winging and proximal muscle weakness in the upper and lower extremities, including hip flexion and knee flexion and extension with normal strength of the tibialis anterior muscle. Because of the pattern of shoulder and proximal arm weakness, FSHD genetic testing was obtained and revealed a contraction with 9 repeats (35 Kb) on chromosome 4q35 and a diagnosis of FSHD1 was confirmed.

Clinical Questions

What is most unusual about this diagnosis of FSHD?

1. Symmetric muscle weakness
2. Proximal weakness in the lower extremities with intact distal strength
3. Lack of facial weakness
4. No family history
5. A baseline CK of more than 7000 while asymptomatic

What additional diagnostic studies would you obtain next?

1. Determination of A or B allele associated with repeat contraction on chromosome 4q35
2. Genetic testing for limb girdle muscular atrophy
3. Both 1 and 2

DISCUSSION

FSHD typically presents with weakness of the facial and periscapular muscles, and distal weakness in the lower extremity, often referred to as the scapuloperoneal pattern. Typical features include asymmetry early on, involvement of abdominal muscles with a protuberant abdomen, and a positive Beevor sign. Later in the disease, it affects individuals more symmetrically and the proximal muscles of the lower extremities become weak, with 20% of patients requiring a wheelchair.[3] However atypical presentations or milder forms of the disease can occur, specifically with borderline repeat sizes, making the diagnosis more challenging. Taken together, scapular winging in combination with weakness of facial muscles such as the orbicularis oculi and oris, with absent ptosis and spared extraocular muscles, along with a positive Beevor sign is highly suggestive of and nearly pathognomonic for FSHD. The presented case has many features in line with a diagnosis of FSHD, such as periscapular weakness and atrophy, with the absence of other features such as bulbar symptoms or systemic manifestations. A lack of facial weakness and asymmetry, and the presence of early proximal weakness of the lower extremities are unusual, but not exclusive of FSHD. FSHD can occur sporadically or may not manifest or be diagnosed in family members with larger repeats and mild disease. Therefore, a lack of a family history does not exclude the diagnosis. The most striking feature in this case is the persistently elevated CK of greater than 7000. In FSHD, the CK levels typically do not exceed 1000 on repeated measurements. The elevated CK along with predominant weakness of shoulder and hip girdle muscles prompted additional diagnostic workup in this case.

Determination of the Facioscapulohumeral Muscular Dystrophy Haplotype

Each repeat on chromosome 4q35 contains a copy of *DUX4*, which is not transcribed in healthy somatic tissues (see **Fig. 1**, **Fig. 2**). The normal number of repeats ranges from 11 to 100 (>38 kb). Patients with FSHD1 carry a smaller number of 1 to 10 repeats

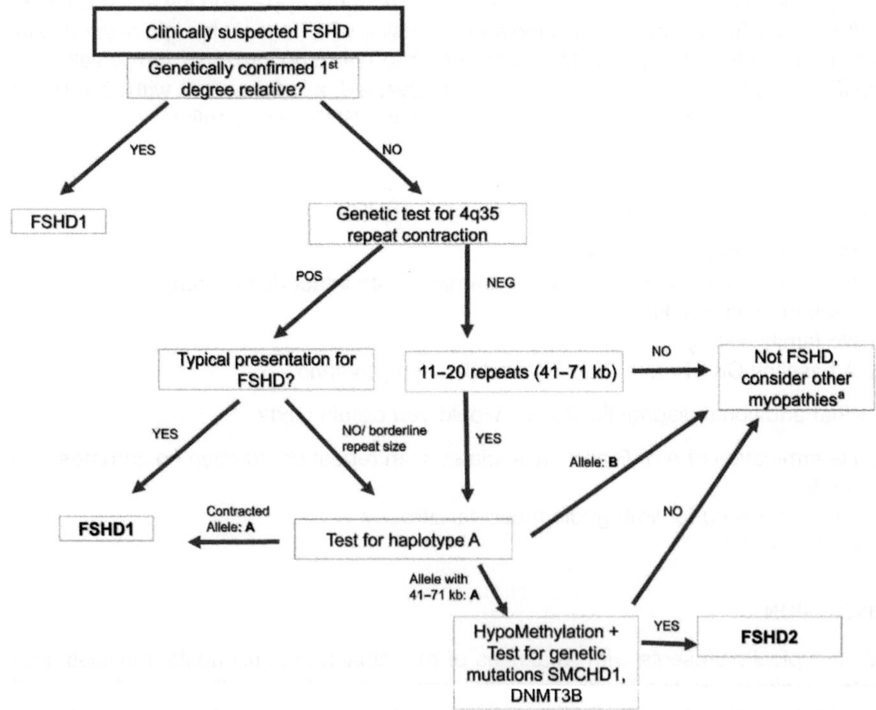

Fig. 2. Diagnostic algorithm for genetic confirmation of FSHD. [a] Other myopathies, such as limb girdle muscular dystrophy (LGMD), acid maltase deficiency, mitochondrial myopathy, congenital myopathies, and inclusion body myositis. (*Adapted from* Tawil R, Kissel JT, Heatwole C, et al. Evidence-based guideline summary: Evaluation, diagnosis, and management of facioscapulohumeral muscular dystrophy: Report of the Guideline Development, Dissemination, and Implementation Subcommittee of the American Academy of Neurology and the Practice Issues Review Panel of the American Association of Neuromuscular & Electrodiagnostic Medicine. Neurology 2015; 85:357; with permission.)

(≤38 kb), referred to as a contraction. The contraction results in hypomethylation and opening of the chromatin structure, resulting in transcription of *DUX4* RNA, which is the root cause of the disease. However, the transcribed *DUX4* full-length messenger RNA is only stable when it comes with a polymorphic polyadenylation signal (PAS). Distal to the last repeat, the chromosome comes in 2 haplotypes: A or B. The A haplotype contains a PAS, whereas the B haplotype does not.[4] Hence, a repeat contraction must occur on the specific permissive A haplotype to cause the disease, whereas contraction on a B variant does not cause the disease.[5] Commercial testing typically does not report out the haplotype. However, in unusual cases, where the phenotype could be explained by another disease, a false-positive genetic test result needs to be excluded. The patient in this vignette was tested and revealed an A haplotype, consistent with a genetic diagnosis of FSHD.

Determination of Comorbid Disease

The unusually high CK level and proximal lower extremity weakness prompted additional testing for limb girdle muscular dystrophies. Genetic testing revealed heterozygous pathogenic mutations in Anoctamin 5, and along with his clinical pattern of weakness and elevated CK, this finding was consistent with a diagnosis of limb girdle muscular dystrophy type 2L. Over the following 12 years, his muscle weakness progressed more rapidly than typically expected with FSHD and he required a wheelchair. On examination 12 years later, he showed no facial weakness, had marked symmetric periscapular and proximal weakness of both upper and lower extremities, but remained without ankle dorsiflexion weakness. Moreover, he now had a protuberant abdomen with a positive Beevor sign and hyperlordosis. Overall, it seems to be difficult to parse out distinct phenotypes because there is overlap between the 2 diseases. However, most disabling was the proximal weakness of the lower extremities that, in light of preserved ankle dorsiflexion, seems most consistent with his anoctaminopathy. Moreover, FSHD1 with 9 repeats (35 kb) are typically associated with later disease onset or milder disease.

Conclusion

Although the FSHD clinical pattern can seem to be pathognomonic, in the presence of unusual features or laboratory results, other diagnoses need to be considered, even in the presence of the appropriate genetic diagnosis of FSHD. This investigation becomes more important when therapies become available targeting genetic mechanisms of FSHD or other diseases mimicking FSHD.

CASE 2: THE COMPLEXITY OF GENETIC TESTING

Clinical Presentation

A 64-year-old man presented with about 3 years of difficulty walking, climbing stairs, and exercise intolerance. He had difficulty rising from a chair, lifting objects above his head such as a 10-pound suitcase, and his muscles felt strained with walking or climbing stairs. In addition to these symptoms, he always had difficulty with balance and was unable to walk a straight line. He had no difficulty swallowing or breathing and no visual symptoms. The patient had a history of cataracts and lipomas. His brother also had lipomas. On examination, he revealed mild facial weakness. He had scapular winging, but with normal orientation of the clavicles. He had symmetric muscle atrophy and weakness in the bilateral upper and lower extremities involving shoulder abduction, external rotation, elbow flexion and extension, hip flexion, and full strength distally, including ankle dorsiflexion. He was unable to sit up from supine without the use of his arms owing to abdominal muscle weakness. In addition, he had bilateral appendicular and truncal ataxia with slightly scanned speech and an ataxic gait. Laboratory testing revealed a slightly elevated CK, glycosylated hemoglobin of 5.4, and a lactate of 2.7. Electrodiagnostic studies showed a nonirritable myopathy, and an axonal polyneuropathy. Commercial genetic testing for FSHD had already been performed and revealed one 38 kb allele and one more than 48 kb allele, consistent with FSHD1. As part of an FSHD research study, the patient underwent extended genotypic characterization. Repeat genetic testing in a research laboratory revealed the following results:

Chromosome 4q alleles: 70 Kb A (19 repeats)/112 Kb A (32 repeats)
Chromosome 10 alleles: 33 Kb B (8 repeats)/65 Kb A (18 repeats)

Clinical Questions

Does this patient have FSHD?

1. Yes, he has FSHD1
2. No, he does not have FSHD1, but he could have FSHD2
3. No, he does not have either FSHD1 or 2

What other diagnostic testing would you recommend (more than one can apply)?

1. Genetic testing for limb girdle muscular dystrophy
2. Muscle biopsy
3. Muscle MRI
4. Methylation levels of chromosome 4q35
5. Genetic test for a mutation in SMCHD1 gene

Discussion

Chromosomes 4 and 10 carry similar repeats, but the repeat section on chromosome 10 is not involved in the pathomechanism of FSHD. However, it can interfere with genetic testing in FSHD. In this case, for example, the short repeat (33 Kb) on chromosome 10 was a compound repeat composed of repeats from both chromosomes 4 and 10, owing to chromosome translocation. This was likely the source of the result from the commercial genetic test for FSHD previously performed on this patient, which measured a 4q short fragment of 38 Kb.

Because the repeat size on both 4q35 alleles are greater than 10 (>38 kb), the patient does not have FSHD1. However, patients with repeats in the normal range on an a Allele background, but typically lower than general average (≤20),[6] can have a mutation on a different gene regulating methylation, the most common is a mutation in the SMCHD1 gene[6,7] (see **Fig. 1**). As a result, DNA methylation and chromatin relaxation is not only seen on the contracted allele, as in FSHD1, but both alleles of chromosome 4q35 and chromosome 10 are hypomethylated. Patients with this genotype and clinical symptoms and signs are termed as FSHD2, and they are not readily clinically distinguishable from patients with FSHD1. Therefore, the patient in this case could still have FSHD2. To further determine this diagnosis, a possibility is to test for the SMCHD1 gene mutation. However, other variants have been reported to result in hypomethylation (DNMT3B).[8] Moreover, if both 4q35 alleles have a B haplotype, this would not result in DUX4 expression, because the polymorphic PAS is absent on B haplotypes to stabilize the DUX4 transcript. Therefore, in this circumstance, evaluating methylation levels can determine if DUX4 transcription is possible. The methylation levels in this patient were normal and excluded the possibility of FSHD2 (see **Fig. 2**).

At that point, the differential diagnosis had to be revisited: In the interim, the patient's brother was evaluated for similar symptoms and a muscle biopsy revealed a mitochondrial myopathy. Subsequently, the patient's muscle biopsy showed similarly abundant ragged red fibers. Considering the patient's additional features of cerebellar ataxia, mild neuropathy and lipomas, the diagnosis of a mitochondrial myopathy was plausible. Lipomas have been described in mitochondrial myopathies.[9] Further genetic testing was not available to further identify the mitochondrial genotype. He was advised to continue aerobic exercise and started on nutritional supplements including coenzyme Q10, carnitine, and vitamin E and to avoid therapies with toxic effects on mitochondria such as valproic acid and statins.

Conclusion

Genetic testing for FSHD has become more complicated (see **Fig. 2**), specifically when assessing for FSHD2. The 2 key ingredients that result in FSHD are the presence of a permissive A haplotype and hypomethylation on 4q35 resulting from either contraction of the number or repeated (FSHD1) or from a mutation in gene responsible for methylation on 4q35 (FSHD2):

FSHD1:
 A allele + 4q35 repeat contraction (1–10 repeats [10–38 kb])
FSHD2:
 A allele + 11 to 20 repeats (41–71 kb) on 4q35 + mutation affecting methylation levels (SMCHD1 or DNMT3B)

THE GENETIC AND CLINICAL SPECTRUM OF FACIOSCAPULOHUMERAL MUSCULAR DYSTROPHY

Case 3a: Infantile Facioscapulohumeral Muscular Dystrophy

Case presentation

A boy was born at full term with a complicated delivery with meconium aspiration. Subsequently, he was noted to have motor developmental delay (walked at 15 months), sensorineural hearing loss (at age 2), and exudative vascular retinopathy (age 5), consistent with Coats syndrome. He was noted to sleep with his eyes open, but otherwise revealed no signs of weakness, participating in swimming, running, and jumping. His parents noted cognitive symptoms, including irritability, low frustration tolerance, delayed language acquisition, obsessive–compulsive disease–type counting and ordering rituals, and stereotypies; later, he was diagnosed with Tourette syndrome. He had mild bifacial weakness predominantly affecting eye closure, but otherwise a normal motor examination. There was no other affected family member. His parents googled "Coats syndrome" and "hearing loss" and requested genetic testing for FSHD. His test result revealed 10 kb (1 repeat) on one 4q35 allele.

Clinical questions

FSHD1, contraction size and disease severity. Select the correct answers.

1. FSHD1 can manifest at any age throughout a lifetime.
2. Patients with very large contractions typically have earlier onset of disease and more extramuscular complications, such as Coats disease and hearing loss
3. Coats disease and hearing loss can manifest at variable age and may be missed on newborn screening
4. Screening for extramuscular manifestations should be guided by repeat size and not necessarily a patient's age

Discussion

Twenty-five percent of patients with FSHD have abnormal retinal blood vessels on examinations. However, symptomatic retinal disease, or Coats disease, manifests as retinal telangiectasias and leakage, which can result in exudative retinal detachment with partial visual loss and blindness. Coats disease is a rare manifestation that occurs in about 0.8% of patients with FSHD1 with larger contractions of 18 kb or less (4 repeats).[10] Similarly, high-frequency sensorineural hearing loss has been described in 32% of subjects with a repeat size of 20 kb or less with a negative association of repeat size and hearing loss.[11] Early-onset FSHD is typically associated with larger contractions, significant facial weakness, and a muscular phenotype similar to adult onset, although they are typically more severe and more likely to lose ambulation at an earlier age.[12] Rare cases of FSHD1 with seizures and cognitive deficits have been reported. Interestingly, the patient presented here did not develop respiratory, limb, or truncal weakness over the course of 15 years. This finding is in contrast with a study that reported scapular weakness in all patients with early-onset FSHD (n = 48).[12] The phenotypic variability seen in early onset FSHD may be due to epigenetic effects. A high percentage of de novo mutations have been reported (73%) with 12% with mosaic inheritance.[13] Treatment approaches for Coats disease include photocoagulation and cryotherapy in mild disease to vitreoretinal surgery or enucleation in advanced stages. Early detection of hearing loss in children is important to avoid impaired language and social development with appropriate interventions, such as hearing aids or sign language. The patient reported here received cryotherapy and Avastin injection twice and has remained stable since. He was provided with hearing aids at age 2 years. Care guidelines recommend referring patients with larger deletions to a retina specialist. Children with FSHD should be screened for hearing loss at diagnosis and yearly thereafter.[14]

Case 3b: Late-Onset Camptocormia

Case presentation

A 76-year-old woman presented with progressive axial muscle weakness. At age 50, she started to have a stooped posture when carrying trays and developed scoliosis after menopause. In her 70s, she had difficulty climbing stairs and most recently noticed difficulty whistling. On examination, she had weak neck flexion (grade 3 on the Medical Research Council [MRC] scale), notable atrophy of the pectoralis and neck muscles, and her clavicles were horizontal. She had scapular winging bilaterally. There was weakness of shoulder forward flexion (grade 4 on the MRC scale), external rotation and hip flexion, hip extension, and ankle dorsiflexion. She had marked camptocormia. She had a minimally elevated CK (157 U/L; reference range, 34–145 U/L). Her electromyogram was normal without muscle fiber irritability. There was no family history of FSHD. Testing for FSHD1 was positive with one allele with 35 kb and one with greater than 48 kb.

Differential diagnosis for late onset camptocormia "bent spine syndrome" includes:

1. Inflammatory myopathy
2. Late-onset nemaline myopathy
3. FSHD
4. Amyotrophic lateral sclerosis
5. All of the above

Discussion

A retrospective study analyzing patients manifesting with camptocormia as the first symptom by Ghosh and Milone[15] showed that FSHD was the most common genetically determined myopathy in these patients (specifically when facial weakness was present), whereas inclusion body myositis (IBM) was the most common acquired myopathy. Other inflammatory myopathies were seen as well. A high proportion of patients with camptocormia had abnormal respiratory studies. Muscle biopsy had a high yield in demonstrating myopathic changes. Late-onset sporadic nemaline myopathy can present with camptocormia and was found in 2 of 52 patients by Ghosh and Milone. To further evaluate for this diagnosis, a muscle biopsy would be indicated to demonstrate rods. Amyotrophic lateral sclerosis as a cause of camptocormia in this case was unlikely given normal electromyography without evidence of widespread denervation and reinnervation. The case presented here, in contrast with case 3a, demonstrates the other end of the spectrum, namely, late onset and mild disease, or disease with more atypical features, such as camptocormia as the leading sign.

Conclusion

- FSHD can occur at any age
- Larger contraction is associated with earlier disease onset and multisystemic features

CASE 4: FACIOSCAPULOHUMERAL MUSCULAR DYSTROPHY MIMICS

Case Presentation

A 54-year-old man who presented with facial, shoulder, and leg weakness, as well as difficulty breathing and swallowing. He first noted facial weakness at age 45. Over the following years, he developed progressive weakness in his arms and legs with scapular winging, was unable to lift his arms above his head, and mostly relied on a wheelchair for ambulation. In addition, he developed respiratory weakness requiring nightly biphasic positive airway pressure. There was no other affected family member. He had no cardiac disease. On examination, he had paraspinal weakness with kyphosis and lumbar lordosis. Physical examination showed facial weakness, scapular winging, proximal and distal weakness in all 4 limbs with the weakest muscles being finger flexion (grade 3 on the MRC scale), hip flexion (grade 2 on the MRC scale), and asymmetric weakness of knee extension. His initial biopsy of the biceps muscle showed inflammation with invasion of non-necrotic fibers. He was treated with immunosuppression without benefit. Because of his lack of response to treatment and his pattern of weakness, he underwent genetic testing for FSHD 1.

Clinical questions

What is the most likely differential diagnosis?

1. Dermatomyositis sine dermatitis
2. Polymyositis
3. IBM
4. FSHD2

Discussion

The initial symptom of progressive facial weakness was concerning for FSHD. However, the presence of dysphagia, dyspnea, and fairly rapid progression was unusual. Nevertheless, because of facial weakness and overall pattern of limb weakness FSHD2 testing was done, which was also negative. Repeat muscle biopsy of the tibialis anterior muscle as part of a research protocol revealed inflammation, invasion of non-necrotic fibers, rimmed vacuoles, and mitochondrial changes. Electron microscopy (EM) showed subsarcolemmal and perinuclear collection of myeloid bodies, membranous whorls, mitochondria and lipofuscin. His muscle biopsy with invasion of non-necrotic fibers was most consistent with an inflammatory myopathy, either polymyositis or IBM. The rimmed vacuoles with mitochondrial changes were most consistent with IBM. EM findings supported the diagnosis of IBM, even in the absence of filamentous inclusions. His dysphagia was also consistent with IBM.

Although the overall pattern of involvement was consistent with FSHD, there were 2 red flags. The first is the presence of wrist and finger flexor weakness, which is classic for IBM. In FSHD, distal weakness in the upper extremities almost invariably involves the wrist and finger extensors. The second is the presence of inflammation with invasion of non-necrotic fiber on muscle biopsy. Inflammation is common in FSHD as well, but is often perivascular and does not show invasion of non-necrotic fibers. Restrictive lung disease does occur in patients with FSHD, especially in patients with significant truncal and hip girdle weakness, larger repeat contractions, and more severe disease.[16]

Conclusion

A careful examination of the pattern of weakness can help to differentiate myopathies with overlapping phenotypes. It is important to remember that a single biopsy may not reveal the full pathologic picture. When in doubt, NT5C1A antibody testing has replaced the need for repeat muscle biopsy in many cases but, if negative, one may consider repeating the muscle biopsy.

CASE 5: CHALLENGES OF GENETIC VARIANTS OF UNKNOWN SIGNIFICANCE

Case Presentation

A 57-year-old man presented with a few years of shoulder weakness, with difficulty combing his hair and lifting objects above shoulder level. In addition, he had difficulty climbing stairs and squatting. Although the weakness was noted just within recent years, he recalled that his wedding suit 25 years ago had to be tailored specifically owing to abnormal sloping of his shoulders. He had no bulbar or respiratory weakness and no double vision or ptosis. He had a history of elevated liver function tests of unknown etiology and paroxysmal atrial fibrillation. There was no family history of neuromuscular diseases. On examination, he had no facial weakness, but asymmetric scapular winging. He had atrophic muscles of the shoulder girdle and pectorales muscles. His clavicles were horizontal with forward sloping shoulders. He had normal strength in the deltoids and other proximal muscles of the upper extremities. His abdomen was protuberant with a positive Beevor sign. He had truncal weakness with hyperlordotic gait and mild scoliosis. He had mild weakness of hip flexion. On needle examination, he revealed myopathic units and increased insertional activity in the cervical paraspinal muscles. His CK was mildly elevated at 262. Biopsy of his left deltoid muscle showed increased variability of fiber size, occasional scattered pyknotic nuclear clumps, and slight type 1 predominance. The nicotinamide adenine dinucleotide reaction showed a slight amount of targetoid and moth-eaten fibers. Overall these changes were not diagnostic. His genetic testing was negative for FSHD1 and FSHD2.

Clinical Questions

What other additional tests would you order?

1. Echocardiogram
2. Serum lactate
3. Serum aldolase
4. Forced vital capacity

5. Dried blood spot for acid α-glucosidase testing

Discussion

The patient underwent genetic testing (next-generation sequencing that covered >170 genes implicated in muscle diseases any specific panel) and a single variant, not previously reported, was found in the SYNE1 (Nesprin1) gene that was predicted to be pathogenic. Mutations in this nuclear membrane protein gene was reported in a few small families to cause Emery-Dreifuss muscular dystrophy (EDMD) type 4.[17] The classic EDMD1 is an X-linked condition that causes muscular dystrophy with severe contractures, as well as significant cardiac involvement. The other forms of EDMD are typically milder variants, but there is limited information about the spectrum of manifestations in EDMD4. Despite the remaining uncertainties about the pathogenicity of the variant, the distribution of weakness in EDMD and FSHD are similar, and it was felt that there was a link between this genetic variant and the patient's phenotype. Moreover, the patient had recurrent atrial fibrillation in the absence of underlying coronary artery disease, again potentially connecting the SYNE1 variant with his cardiac disease. However, he developed shortness of breath and a forced vital capacity measurement revealed respiratory weakness (sitting, 2.62 L; 57% of predicted, and 49% of predicted when supine). This result prompted testing for α-glucosidase activity in blood (dry blood spot test), which was low at 2.00 (reference value, >3.88 pmol/punch/h). He started enzyme replacement therapy every other week. He has noted improved function with using higher weights at the gym, with walking, and improved endurance when swimming. His strength has not further declined with continued proximal upper extremity strength in the 4+ range in shoulder testing with scapular winging.

SUMMARY

Pompe's disease is an important and treatable differential diagnosis in FSHD, specifically in patients with respiratory symptoms early in the disease. In FSHD respiratory weakness can be asymptomatic and recently has been demonstrated to be more common than initially thought.[16,18] It is recommended to obtain a forced vital capacity measurement at baseline in FSHD, or in this case, when it may help to define the phenotype. This case also illustrates the challenges when encountering variants of unknown significance and emphasizes the importance of not discontinuing the diagnostic workup prematurely when encountering these variants of unknown significance.

REFERENCES

1. Flanigan KM, Coffeen CM, Sexton L, et al. Genetic characterization of a large, historically significant Utah kindred with facioscapulohumeral dystrophy. Neuromuscul Disord 2001;11(6–7):525–9.
2. Deenen JC, Arnts H, van der Maarel SM, et al. Population-based incidence and prevalence of facioscapulohumeral dystrophy. Neurology 2014;83(12):1056–9.
3. Statland JM, Tawil R. Risk of functional impairment in Facioscapulohumeral muscular dystrophy. Muscle Nerve 2014;49(4):520–7.
4. Lemmers RJ, de Kievit P, Sandkuijl L, et al. Facioscapulohumeral muscular dystrophy is uniquely associated with one of the two variants of the 4q subtelomere. Nat Genet 2002;32(2):235–6.
5. Lemmers RJ, van der Vliet PJ, Klooster R, et al. A unifying genetic model for facioscapulohumeral muscular dystrophy. Science 2010;329(5999):1650–3.

6. Lemmers RJ, Goeman JJ, van der Vliet PJ, et al. Inter-individual differences in CpG methylation at D4Z4 correlate with clinical variability in FSHD1 and FSHD2. Hum Mol Genet 2015;24(3):659–69.
7. Lemmers RJ, Tawil R, Petek LM, et al. Digenic inheritance of an SMCHD1 mutation and an FSHD-permissive D4Z4 allele causes facioscapulohumeral muscular dystrophy type 2. Nat Genet 2012;44(12):1370–4.
8. van den Boogaard ML, Lemmers R, Balog J, et al. Mutations in DNMT3B modify epigenetic repression of the D4Z4 repeat and the penetrance of facioscapulohumeral dystrophy. Am J Hum Genet 2016;98(5):1020–9.
9. Musumeci O, Barca E, Lamperti C, et al. Lipomatosis incidence and characteristics in an Italian cohort of mitochondrial patients. Front Neurol 2019;10:160.
10. Statland JM, Sacconi S, Farmakidis C, et al. Coats syndrome in facioscapulohumeral dystrophy type 1: frequency and D4Z4 contraction size. Neurology 2013;80(13):1247–50.
11. Lutz KL, Holte L, Kliethermes SA, et al. Clinical and genetic features of hearing loss in facioscapulohumeral muscular dystrophy. Neurology 2013;81(16):1374–7.
12. Mah JK, Feng J, Jacobs MB, et al. A multinational study on motor function in early-onset FSHD. Neurology 2018;90(15):e1333–8.
13. Goselink RJ, Schreuder TH, Mul K, et al. Facioscapulohumeral dystrophy in children: design of a prospective, observational study on natural history, predictors and clinical impact (iFocus FSHD). BMC Neurol 2016;16:138.
14. Tawil R, Kissel JT, Heatwole C, et al. Evidence-based guideline summary: evaluation, diagnosis, and management of facioscapulohumeral muscular dystrophy: report of the guideline development, dissemination, and implementation subcommittee of the American Academy of Neurology and the Practice Issues Review Panel of the American Association of Neuromuscular & Electrodiagnostic Medicine. Neurology 2015;85(4):357–64.
15. Ghosh PS, Milone M. Camptocormia as presenting manifestation of a spectrum of myopathic disorders. Muscle Nerve 2015;52(6):1008–12.
16. Moreira S, Wood L, Smith D, et al. Respiratory involvement in ambulant and non-ambulant patients with facioscapulohumeral muscular dystrophy. J Neurol 2017;264(6):1271–80.
17. Zhang Q, Bethmann C, Worth NF, et al. Nesprin-1 and -2 are involved in the pathogenesis of Emery Dreifuss muscular dystrophy and are critical for nuclear envelope integrity. Hum Mol Genet 2007;16(23):2816–33.
18. Henke C, Spiesshoefer J, Kabitz HJ, et al. Respiratory muscle weakness in facioscapulohumeral muscular dystrophy. Muscle Nerve 2019;60(6):679–86.

Congenital Myasthenic Syndromes

Stanley Jones P. Iyadurai, MSc, PhD, MD, FAAN*

KEYWORDS

- Congenital myasthenic syndrome • Neuromuscular transmission
- Inherited neuromuscular junction disorder • Repetitive nerve stimulation

KEY POINTS

- Congenital myasthenic syndromes are rare, inherited neuromuscular disorders that result from mutations in components of the neuromuscular junction.
- Congenital myasthenic syndromes can present at any age: birth, infancy, adolescence, or adulthood.
- Congenital myasthenic syndromes, especially in adults, may be misdiagnosed or undiagnosed owing to the nonspecific nature of symptoms at presentation; therefore, a high degree of clinical suspicion is necessary.
- Specific electrodiagnostic studies aimed at evaluating the neuromuscular junction may be helpful in diagnosing congenital myasthenic syndromes.
- Mutations in more than 30 different genes can cause congenital myasthenic syndromes; identifying the specific genetic type may have implication in choice of treatment options available.

Video content accompanies this article at http://www.neurologic.theclinics.com.

INTRODUCTION

Congenital myasthenic syndromes (CMS) comprise a rare heterogeneous group of diseases that impair neuromuscular transmission (NMT) and are characterized by fatigability and transient or permanent weakness of ocular, facial, bulbar, or limb muscles. Symptoms are often present from birth or early childhood, although, more rarely, may develop in adolescence or adulthood. The CMS have a wide range of phenotypes and severity—from mild weakness to permanent disabling muscle weakness to respiratory failure.

Department of Neurology, Johns Hopkins All Children's Hospital, St Petersburg, FL, USA
* Institute for Brain Protection Services, 601 5th Street South, Suite 510, St Petersburg, FL 33701.
E-mail address: stanley.iyadurai@gmail.com

Neurol Clin 38 (2020) 541–552
https://doi.org/10.1016/j.ncl.2020.03.004
neurologic.theclinics.com

Caused by genetic mutations in any of the numerous genes encoding for components of the neuromuscular junction (NMJ), CMS are classified by where in the NMJ the mutated component is located: presynaptic, synaptic, or postsynaptic. An additional category of CMS includes mutations in glycosylation-related genes that encode proteins that help to stabilize the NMJ through glycosylation. Taken together, mutations in more than 30 genes have been implicated in CMS phenotypes. Because of the large number of gene mutations that can cause CMS, clinical features, age of onset, symptoms, and response to treatment vary widely and can make diagnosis difficult. Of people diagnosed with CMS, only 50% to 70% have a confirmed genetic diagnosis.[1] Advances in genetic testing have made genetic diagnosis faster and more cost effective, which is imperative; the location of the defect in the NMJ based on the underlying causative mutation has implications for differences in response to treatment.

The prevalence of CMS is estimated at 9.2 per 1,000,000 children less than 18 years of age[2]; however, the prevalence is likely underestimated because many cases of CMS remain misdiagnosed or go undetected in people with mild symptoms. In addition, although less common, owing to extensive use of gene sequencing panel-based testing, more and more adults are being diagnosed with CMS (specifically, the group of patients with seronegative myasthenia gravis). Despite the rarity and diagnostic challenges of CMS, mor than 1000 independent kinships have been identified carrying pathogenic variants worldwide.[3] As more individuals with CMS are reported, appropriate treatment strategies may be identified and refined to maximize benefit. Although this goal seems to be noble, there are no treatments approved by the US Food and Drug Administration for patients with CMS. Historically, several medications have been used to treat patients with CMS (and they have shown clinical improvement). Although there is no specific treatment option available or favored, some neuromuscular clinicians favor an algorithmic approach to currently used therapeutic options.

Despite the low cost and the ready availability of gene panel testing, CMS remains undiagnosed and underdiagnosed in many cases. Some of the reasons are that (1) CMS remains a rare neuromuscular disorder and many neuromuscular providers have not seen a single case of CMS (or they have missed the diagnosis). (2) Many adult providers are of the opinion that CMS must be a childhood phenomenon and therefore do not expect see such a diagnosis in the adult patient, although CMS can present as an adult. (3) The wide variability of symptoms and age of presentation, makes no 2 cases similar, making it more difficult for the provider to make an educated guess for a diagnosis. (4) The fluctuation of symptoms is quite abundant in such a way that, when the patient comes to the provider, no obvious signs are present. (5) The symptoms are mild, so much so that they are seen as soft signs by the provider and are often discarded in the overall evaluation. (6) Even when suspected, the right choice of electrodiagnostic study is not performed, precluding the diagnosis. (7) Although fatigue is one of the most common symptoms in the neurology/neuromuscular clinic, it remains the least favorite (and nonspecific) symptom of neuromuscular doctors (in general), which overwhelmingly seems to be the most common symptom in CMS, and thus overlooked. (8) Certain types of CMS (especially limb-girdle type) are misdiagnosed as limb-girdle muscular dystrophy or congenital myopathy. (9) There is often an absence of a family history in many of these patients (CMS is predominantly a recessive disorder, with rare exceptions). (10) Unawareness of significant electrodiagnostic findings such as repetitive compound muscle action potential (R-CMAP), or repetitive nerve stimulation (RNS) after fatigue of the muscle using continuous repetitive stimulation paradigms by the evaluating neurologist/neuromuscular physician. (11) Clinical suspicion for a diagnosis of seronegative myasthenia gravis (and a steroid trial to follow) is more favored than a diagnosis of CMS by the neuromuscular physician, because the opinion that something can be done about the disease self-serves the treating physician, and there is a feeling that nothing can be done about a genetic disorder. The cases presented herein highlight some of the clinical and teaching points and provide a broader awareness of CMS, a rare neuromuscular disorder. It should be borne in mind that proper diagnosis can lead to proper treatment, at least, as noted in these cases to near recovery of normal function, highlighting the point that CMS, although a genetic disorder, may be treatable. Several anecdotal treatment options and approaches to treat patients with CMS are present among treating neuromuscular clinicians. However, one of the major drawbacks in the field is that there are no randomized, double-blind, placebo-controlled clinical trials in patients with genetically confirmed CMS, to date, to demonstrate the efficacy of these anecdotal treatment options.

CASES

Case 1: Right Cervical Radiculopathy in a 55-Year-Old Man

Case presentation

A 55-year-old man with no significant past medical history presented to the neuromuscular clinic with a 6-month history of progressive distal right arm weakness, without any loss of sensation. He denied any family history of muscle weakness or fatigability. The neurologic examination was significant for static left eye ptosis, equal pupils with no delayed light reflex, intact extraocular movements, weakness of the right wrist, finger extensors, and intrinsic hand muscles; normal reflexes; and a normal sensory examination.

The patient's workup included noncontrast MRI of the brain that showed nonspecific T2 changes. Visual evoked potential was within normal limits. MRI of cervical spine showed mild multilevel cervical stenosis. MRI of bilateral brachial plexii was normal. Creatine kinase and aldolase were mildly elevated at 401 IU/L (normal, <200 IU/L) and 8.1 IU/L (normal, <7.8 IU/L), respectively. The rest of the laboratory workup, including the acetylcholine receptor antibodies panel, muscle-specific kinase (MuSK) antibodies, rapid plasma reagin, folate, vitamin B_6, vitamin B_{12}, methylmalonic acid, homocysteine, amino acids, long chains fatty acids, lactic acid, and pyruvic acid levels were all within normal ranges. Urine protein electrophoresis, serum protein electrophoresis, and immunofixation electrophoresis did not identify any abnormal protein peaks.

Patients with CMS usually have:

A. Antibodies against acetylcholine receptor (binding type)
B. Antibodies against acetylcholine receptor (blocking type)
C. Antibodies against MuSK antigen
D. Antibodies against LRP4 antigen
E. No antibodies against either acetylcholine receptor or MuSK or LRP4 antigen
   Correct Answer: E

Nerve conduction velocities were normal. However, the presence of a single satellite, CMAP (also known as R-CMAP) amplitude peaks after the main CMAP amplitude peaks was noted on all the motor nerve tested. The R-CMAP morphology was similar to that of the main CMAP, consisting of a negative then a positive peak, but of smaller amplitude (**Fig. 1**). Electromyography of distal upper extremity muscles revealed myopathic units and early recruitment patterns. RNS of the median nerve at 2 Hz did not show a decremental response for the main

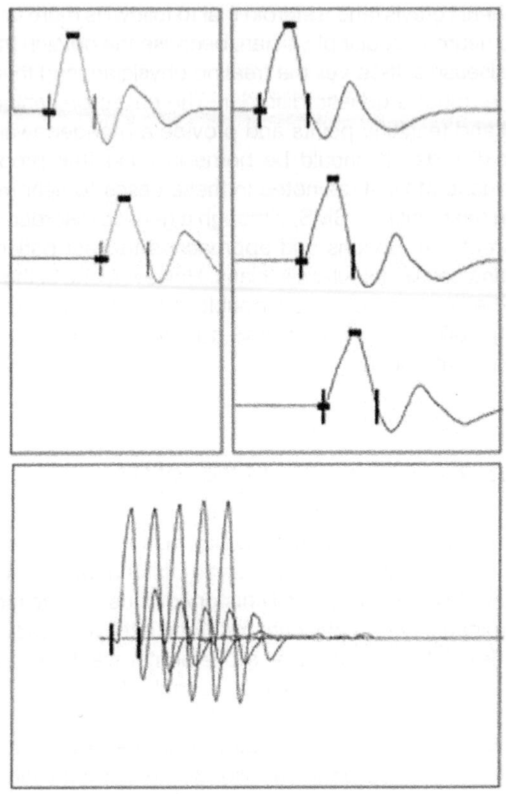

Fig. 1. Demonstration of R-CMAP amplitude peak (*top*) in a patient with slow channel syndrome. Decrement of the R-CMAP peak, without significant change in the primary CMAP peak.

CMAP amplitude. However, the R-CMAP amplitude showed a decremental response (see **Fig. 1**).

Genetic evaluation revealed a mutation in the beta subunit of the acetylcholine receptor subunit corresponding to a previously described slow channel syndrome mutation (exon 7, Val252Phe).

The patient was started on fluoxetine at 10 mg/d and titrated up to 80 mg/d. Within 6 months of initiation of treatment, he regained normal strength.

Clinical questions

Why was the clinical presentation so late, in this inherited disorder?
What is the significance of the R-CMAP?
What is the reason for the elevated creatine kinase?
What is the treatment option for slow channel syndrome?

Discussion

Although it seems to be a late diagnosis, it is not uncommon in slow channel syndrome for patients to manifest weakness much later in life. In early part of their life, they usually learn adaptive measures to deal with their issues and never comes up as an issue. The careful observation of the R-CMAP peak is critical in this diagnosis. Only another

CMS, acetylcholinesterase deficiency causes, R-CMAP, thus narrowing the differential diagnosis in this clinical setting. This discrimination is important because pyridostigmine can make acetylcholinesterase deficiency worse, whereas in slow channel syndrome, it makes a modest difference in the early stages, but fails to work later. The elevated creatine kinase is due to a phenomenon called endplate myopathy. In slow channel syndrome, upon treatment with fluoxetine, this myopathy can be normalized. Although it is not fully understood how fluoxetine works in the slow channel syndrome (some theories that it shortens the channel open time have been offered), it seems to be the best treatment option at this time. With treatment, most often, one can observe reversal of their deficits to normalcy.

Case 2: A 37-Year-Old Woman with "Conversion Disorder"

Case presentation

A 37-year-old woman was seen in the neuromuscular clinic with complaints of episodic extremity weakness and exertional fatigue, described as difficulty walking, running, and lifting objects starting at age 15. She also complained of occasional double vision and difficulty swallowing. She mentioned that she could not efficiently comb her hair and could not lift her children. She did not report any family history of similar problems. Her initial examination at age 29 was reported to be normal. Further workup at that time showed a normal creatine kinase level, negative acetylcholine receptor binding and MuSK antibodies. Although her EMG was reported to be myopathic in nature, slow (3 Hz) RNS showed no significant decrement on stimulation of the ulnar, spinal accessory, or facial nerves. A muscle biopsy showed nonspecific findings.

She was seen 8 years later at age 37 with similar complaints. At this time, examination showed bilateral fatigable and fluctuating ptosis (**Fig. 2**), dysconjugate gaze (Video 1), and mild facial asymmetry. The remainder of the motor examination was normal. Cerebellar and sensory examination was normal as well.

The most compelling aspect(s) of this case that increases the clinical suspicion for CMS is/are:

A. Fatigue
B. Weakness

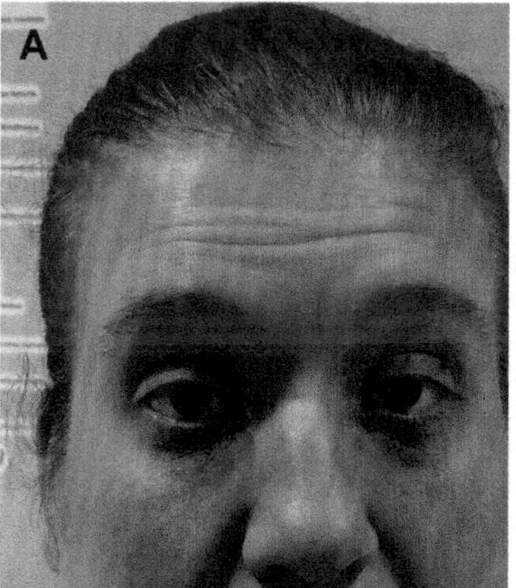

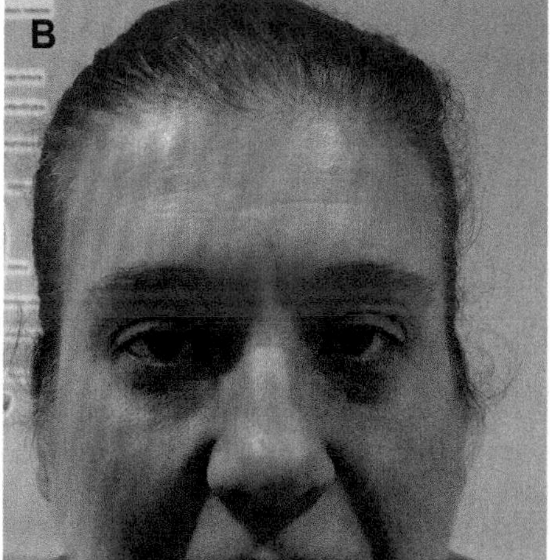

Fig. 2. (*A, B*) Fluctuating ptosis during casual observation in a patient with Rapsyn mutation.

C. Fatigable weakness
D. Family history
E. History and examination suggestive of fatigable weakness and negative antibodies to acetylcholine receptor and MuSK antigen
   Correct Answer: E

RNS of the median nerve at 3 Hz showed a nonsignificant decrement of 6.5% at baseline, which improved to 0.7% immediately after a brief 30-second exercise and reached significant decrement of 12.3% at 240 seconds after exercise. The details of underlying electrodiagnostic testing is published elsewhere.[4] In this case, the median nerve was chosen for RNS, given that it is better tolerated and devoid of artifacts, although facial and spinal accessory nerves could have been tested as well. Although prominent, fatigable extraocular muscle weakness was noted on examination, the ptosis was subtle in comparison on examination. Prominent weakness or fatigability was not noted upon shrugging of shoulders. Therefore, testing of facial or spinal accessory was deemed more invasive or ineffective and was not favored.

A diagnosis of CMS was entertained, and genetic testing was performed. Genetic testing revealed homozygous mutation in the Rapsyn gene, corresponding with a change in Asn88Lys. The patient was started on pyridostigmine 60 mg 3 times a day, with significant improvement in her strength and activities of daily living.

Clinical questions

Is fluctuation of examination findings common in CMS?
Do you expect normal RNS findings in CMS?
What are the roles of exercise and fatigue in electrodiagnostic evaluation in CMS?

Discussion

Fluctuating findings are very common in CMS, sometimes may seem very normal. However, because fatigue is the cornerstone of findings in CMS, attention should be paid to neuromuscular examination with the goal of fatiguing the muscle in mind. Because rest helps these patients, examining after a period of rest may sometimes seem to provide normal findings. Normal RNS findings may be seen in CMS. However, if the muscle is fatigued enough, one may be able to pick up deficits. Postexercise RNS is a nice way to establish decrement in CMS. In other situations, repetitive testing of the affected muscles is also useful. In certain cases of CMS (such as mutations in choline acetyltransferase gene), fatiguing the muscle by electrophysiologic means (at 10 Hz for 5 minutes) has been helpful in identifying the decrement indicative of NMJ disorder.[5]

Case 3: "Multifocal Motor Neuropathy" in a 63-Year-Old Woman

Case presentation

A 63-year-old woman was referred to a neuromuscular clinic for bilateral weakness of the hands and wrists, with significant weakness on the right. Based on the initial evaluation, multifocal motor neuropathy was suspected, and the patient was placed on monthly treatment with intravenous immunoglobulin. However, no significant improvement was noted with treatment with intravenous immunoglobulin over a 1-year period.

An examination of the head, eyes, ears, nose, and throat was significant for narrow facies, without any ptosis, diplopia, or extraocular movement deficits. Strength examination revealed significant wrist and finger extension weakness bilaterally, right worse than the left. Repeat electromyographic evaluation was significant for the observation of short duration motor unit action potential, in multiple distal muscles of the right hand, suggestive of a distal myopathy. Further evaluation of family history at this point revealed multiple other family members with similar problems with weak wrists and fingers (including a 24-year-old niece and a 58-year-old nephew).

Slow channel syndrome refers to:

A. The acetylcholine receptor complex (composed of 5 subunits) is slow to open upon binding by the 2 acetylcholine molecules, and behaves as a bad channel, resulting in improper NMT.
B. The acetylcholine receptor complex (composed of 5 subunits) is slow to close upon binding by the 2 acetylcholine molecules, and behaves as a bad channel, resulting in improper NMT.
C. The sodium channel is slow to open and causes improper NMT.
D. The potassium channel is slow to open and causes improper NMT.
E. The sodium channel is slow to close and causes improper NMT

Correct Answer: B

GM1 antibodies were negative. Genetic evaluation of DNA from affected and unaffected family members revealed a previously described slow channel syndrome mutation (in the alpha subunit of the acetylcholine receptor gene; dominant; CHRNA1, exon 5, c.517G > A [p.Gly173Ser] with complete concordance). Intravenous immunoglobulin was discontinued. The patient and the other affected family members were treated with fluoxetine, at a starting dose of 20 mg/d, to a final amount of 60 mg/d.

Significant improvement of strength was noted in all the affected family members treated with fluoxetine, in about 6 months. Strikingly, the 58-year-old nephew who was restricted to a wheel chair, upon treatment with fluoxetine, is now able to walk and even run short distances. The 24-year-old niece who could not extend her fingers or pick up a gallon of milk with her fingers and hand or hang on to an overhead beam for even a single second, upon treatment with fluoxetine, is now able to extend her fingers forcefully (**Fig. 3**), lift a glass of water with her fingers and hand (**Fig. 4**), and can cling on to an overhead beam for more than 50 seconds. These 3 cases clearly demonstrate reversibility of the weakness owing to slow channel syndrome, upon treatment with fluoxetine.

Clinical questions

Is distal weakness a common finding in CMS?
Are most CMS recessive in nature?
Does treatment in CMS result in reversal of deficits?

Discussion

Proximal weakness and fatigable ptosis are most commonly seen in CMS. However, slow channel syndrome is notorious for displaying distal extensor weakness at the level of wrist and fingers with sparing of lower extremities. In this scenario, slow channel syndrome remains an exception to the classical proximal weakness seen in CMS. Most CMS are recessive in nature; however, there are few dominant ones, which include slow channel syndromes (mutations in the alpha, beta, and delta subunits in the acetylcholine receptor gene), SYT2 (synaptotagmin), and SNAP25B mutation CMS. It seems that treatment of slow channel CMS with fluoxetine indeed does lead to reversal of prior deficits, which is not always seen in other CMS.

Case 4: A "Collapsing" 10-Year-Old Girl

Case presentation

A 10-year-old girl was referred to the pediatric neuromuscular clinic for evaluation of muscle weakness. As described by the mother, the child had an uneventful birth

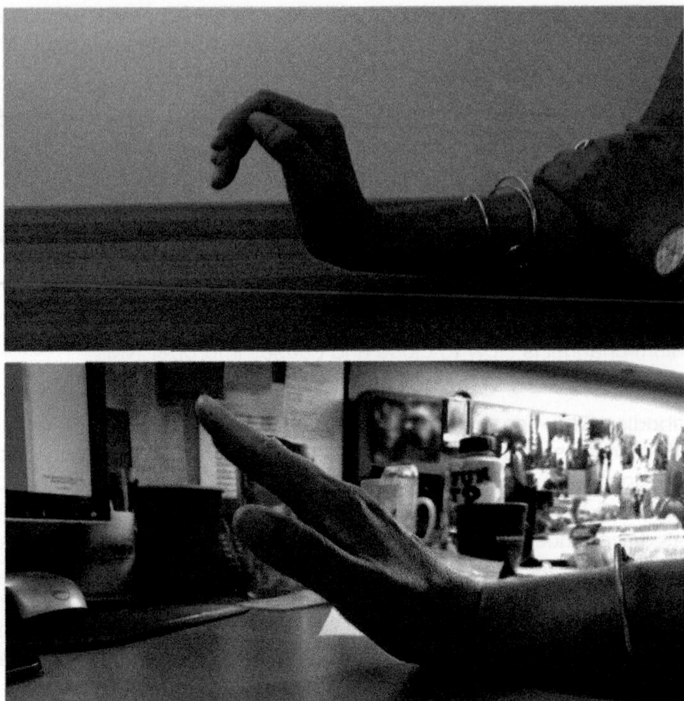

Fig. 3. Finger extension before (*top*) and after (*bottom*) treatment with fluoxetine in a patient with slow channel syndrome.

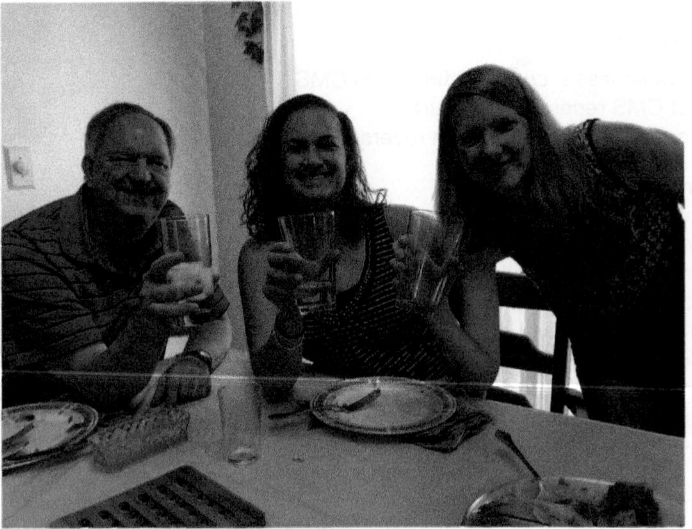

Fig. 4. Lifting a glass of water after treatment with fluoxetine in 3 patients in the same family, all with slow channel syndrome (which was an impossible task before treatment with fluoxetine).

and normal early development, and had maintained good health until recently. However, the child was noted to be on the heavier side and did not particularly like running, either as a task or as an exercise. The physical education teacher called the mother one day to report that her daughter had collapsed while attempting to run a required 1-mile run at school. Later, the mother, who witnessed one of these episodes, described this episode that would happen in school when the child was asked to run—her daughter would collapse after running about a 30-foot distance and would take a 30- to 40-minute recovery period to be able to walk again. No pain was reported. No weakness of arms or facial muscles was reported. Neurologic examination revealed a mildly obese girl with a normal cranial nerve examination (with no extraocular movement deficits, no diplopia, no fatigable ptosis, no facial weakness, and no hoarseness of voice), normal strength, normal reflexes, normal cerebellar examination, and downgoing toes. However, when asked to run along the corridor of the examination room, the child collapsed after running (slowly) for about 20 to 25 feet.

Initially, periodic paralysis was suspected and electrodiagnostic studies (short and long exercise testing) were set up to evaluate for channel dysfunction. However, the initial nerve conduction study on the median nerve showed a normal primary CMAP amplitude followed by a R-CMAP amplitude peak. Additional electrodiagnostic studies showed a significant decrement of the abductor pollicis brevis primary CMAP amplitude upon stimulation of the median nerve in slow RNS paradigm (while the amplitudes of the R-CMAP amplitude peak remained constant). Short and long exercise testing was within normal limits.

Classically, muscle channelopathies are characterized by:

A. Constant pain sensation
B. Constant numbness (loss of sensation)
C. Episodic, paroxysmal, or periodic manifestations of muscle weakness
D. Symptoms of dysautonomia
E. MRI lesions seen on the lumbar spine

Correct Answer: C

Genetic analysis revealed a novel mutation in the alpha subunit of the acetylcholine receptor gene, in a similar location for a slow channel syndrome mutation previously reported in the beta subunit of the acetylcholine receptor gene. In addition, analysis of acetylcholine receptor antibodies was positive (>100 units; upper limit of normal, 0.02 units), and a diagnosis of coincident slow channel syndrome and acetylcholine receptor antibody positive myasthenia gravis was made. Pyridostigmine treatment did not show any significant response. The patient underwent thymectomy and was started on steroids and fluoxetine, sequentially. Fluoxetine was later discontinued because the patient could not tolerate the medication. The patient is currently doing well on immunomodulatory therapy without any episodes of collapse.

Clinical questions

Can slow channel syndrome CMS and acetylcholine receptor antibody positive myasthenia gravis coexist?

If in such a case, what should be the priority for treatment?

Is there something as acquired slow channel syndrome?

Discussion

There have been prior observations of a CMS patient, later developing acetylcholine receptor antibody-positive myasthenia gravis (Miriam Freimer, MD, personal communication, 2018). However, this occurrence would be deemed unusual. Having said that, there has been no systematic analysis of whether patients with CMS develop antibodies with time, in later stages. One hypothesis is that the altered configuration of the mutant acetylcholine receptor protein (a dominant negative form) may trigger development of antibodies; such a theory has not been either proven or discarded. If in such a case of coincident mutant slow channel syndrome CMS and acetylcholine receptor antibody-positive myasthenia gravis, this author's opinion is that priority should be given to treatment of antibody-mediated process, because since untreated antibody-mediated processes lead to destruction of NMJs and endplates, owing to compliment-mediated damage. It is unclear if an acquired slow channel syndrome (purely mediated by antibodies) exist; however, it has been discussed in literature before, during the time when genetic testing was not broadly available.[6] So, it remains a question. However, this author believes that such a state might exist.

Case 5: Two Siblings with Congenital Myasthenic Syndromes

A 22-year-old woman was referred to the neuromuscular clinic for excessive fatigue and eyes getting tired out. She reported a history when she was 2 years old, she was seen by an ophthalmologist for a lazy eye, which then became normal. At 8 years of age, she was seen by a neuromuscular specialist for possible myasthenic gravis, owing to eyelid weakness. At this time, RNS studies showed a significant decrement at slow (2 Hz) RNS paradigm, which was readily corrected by injection of edrophonium. Acetylcholine receptor and MuSK antibodies were negative, and apparently, the patient was started on pyridostigmine, which the patient had discontinued herself, at age 10.

At the time of presentation at 22 years of age, the patient had bilateral fatigable ptosis (Video 2) (completely recoverable after a single blink), bilateral ophthalmoparesis to lateral gazes (without diplopia), decreased muscle bulk overall, fatigable proximal weakness in both upper and lower extremities. An ice pack test readily reversed the ptosis deficit (Video 3), so did a brief rest.

When 2 siblings from the same family (born of the same mother and father) manifest a neuromuscular condition such as CMS, the most appropriate conclusion about the mode of inheritance is:

A. A recessive condition
B. A dominant condition
C. A mitochondrial disorder
D. Either a dominant, recessive, or a mitochondrial disorder
E. An X-linked disorder

Correct Answer: D

Genetic evaluation revealed compound heterozygous mutations in the epsilon subunit of the acetylcholine receptor gene (1 deletion and 1 point mutation), suggestive of recessive acetylcholine receptor deficiency CMS. The patient was placed on pyridostigmine, 60 mg 3 times a day, in addition to long-acting pyridostigmine at bed time. She was able to perform many of the daily activities without any trouble at this regimen and has and gone on to become a pediatric occupational therapist.

Six years later, at age 28, she noted that her benefits had plateaued and in fact may have lost some strength she had gained. She noticed that she had fatigue when she had to move patients in wheel chairs, and that she could not perform squats anymore. At this time, she was seen by a different neuromuscular physician, who enrolled her in an extended access protocol for treatment of patients with CMS with 3,4-diaminopyridine phosphate (amifampridine phosphate), in addition to her pyridostigmine

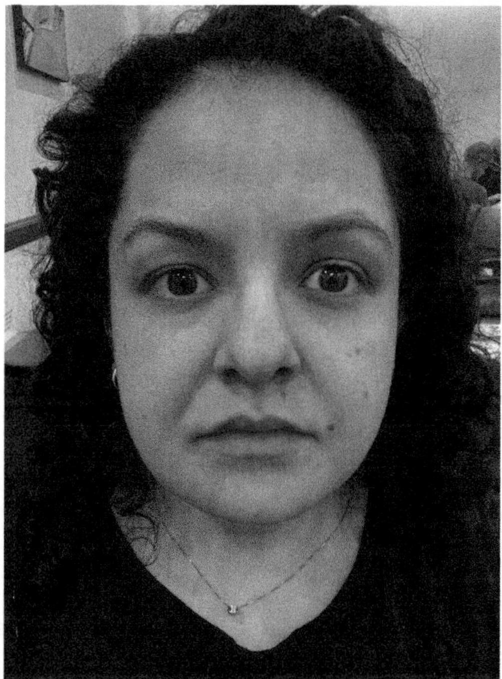

Fig. 5. "Wide open eyes" after treatment with pyridostigmine and amifampridine phosphate in a patient with mutation in the epsilon subunit of the acetylcholine receptor.

treatment. Since the initiation of treatment with amifampridine phosphate, she has noted an improvement in strength, a decrease in fatigue, and the ability to do things that she could not do before (like squatting) and states that her eyes are now wide open (**Fig. 5**).

Clinical questions

Is the ice pack test specific to myasthenia gravis (antibody mediated)?
What is the relevance of rectification of ptosis deficits with a quick, single blink?
Can pyridostigmine and amifampridine phosphate be used together?

Discussion

An ice pack test (cold conditions ameliorating symptoms of myasthenia gravis) is not specific to antibody-mediated myasthenia gravis. It can show a similar result in CMS (certain types, such as epsilon mutation) as well. The relevance of quick rectification of ptosis in CMS after a quick blink is unclear. However, the rectification seems to be much faster and fuller in extent than the rectification that happens in antibody-mediated myasthenia gravis. There are limited data that suggest that both pyridostigmine and amifampridine can be used together in certain myasthenic conditions. It should be borne in mind that, although both treatments result in increased amount of acetylcholine in the synaptic space, the mechanism by which these drugs achieve this effect is different—one by inhibition of acetylcholinesterase enzyme and the other by blocking potassium channels (allowing the neuron to remain depolarized longer).

SUMMARY

CMS are a heterogeneous group of inherited disorders that affect NMT. Genetic mutations in more than 30 genes that encode for components in the NMJ result in CMS. The clinical phenotype and presentation vary quite widely. Electrodiagnostic studies are helpful in diagnosis of CMS. Genetic studies are helpful in identifying what specific mutation underlies the CMS presentation. Understanding the specific subtype is helpful in providing optimal treatment, and to prevent harm (as in avoidance of acetylcholinesterase inhibitors in acetylcholine esterase deficiency). Careful evaluation of the patient and focused electrodiagnostic testing are of paramount importance in evaluation of a suspected CMS patient. Specific treatment options in specific CMS subtypes seems to be helpful in restoring muscle function, although no randomized, double-blinded, placebo-controlled clinical trials exist in genetically confirmed patients with CMS.

REFERENCES

1. Kinali M, Beeson D, Pitt MC, et al. Congenital myasthenic syndromes in childhood: diagnostic and management challenges. J Neuroimmunol 2008;201-202:6–12.
2. Parr JR, Andrew MJ, Finnis M, et al. How common is childhood myasthenia? The UK incidence and prevalence of autoimmune and congenital myasthenia. Arch Dis Child 2014;99(6):539–42.
3. Chaouch A, Beeson D, Hantai D, et al. 186th ENMC international workshop: congenital myasthenic syndromes 24-26 June 2011, Naarden, The Netherlands. Neuromuscul Disord 2012;22:566–76.
4. LoRusso SJ, Iyadurai SJ. Decrement with high frequency repetitive nerve stimulation in a RAPSN congenital myasthenic syndrome. Muscle Nerve 2018;57(3): e106–8.
5. Ohno K, Tsujino A, Brengman JM, et al. Choline acetyltransferase mutations cause myasthenic syndrome associated with episodic apnea in humans. Proc Natl Acad Sci U S A 2001;98(4):2017–22.
6. Wintzen AR, Plomp JJ, Molenaar PC, et al. Acquired slow-channel syndrome: a form of myasthenia gravis with prolonged open time of the acetylcholine receptor channel. Ann Neurol 1998;44(4):657–64.

Diabetic Lumbosacral Radiculoplexus Neuropathy (Diabetic Amyotrophy)

Melanie D. Glenn, MD[a,*], Duaa Jabari, MD[b]

KEYWORDS

- Diabetic amyotrophy • Lumbosacral radiculoplexus neuropathy
- Proximal diabetic neuropathy • Bruns-Garland syndrome

KEY POINTS

- Diabetic lumbosacral radiculoplexus neuropathy might easily be recognized in the neuromuscular clinic by its typical clinical history and examination findings; however, patients may present with a variety of unexpected clinical features that can make the diagnostic process challenging.
- The syndrome is self-limiting, but recovery can be slow and is often incomplete.
- There is no clear evidence that immunotherapy is beneficial in improving neurologic outcome.
- The investigative process requires differentiating this syndrome from other treatable conditions to avoid unnecessary or potentially harmful treatments or procedures.
- This article provides a series of interesting cases to highlight the challenges of diagnosing diabetic lumbosacral radiculoplexus neuropathy.

Video content accompanies this article at http://www.neurologic.theclinics.com.

INTRODUCTION

Diabetic lumbosacral radiculoplexus neuropathy (DLSRPN; also known as diabetic amyotrophy, proximal diabetic neuropathy, or Bruns-Garland syndrome) is characterized by acute onset of severe, proximal, unilateral pain of the hip, buttocks, or thigh, progressing to sensory disturbance of the affected limb and followed by weakness and atrophy of the proximal lower extremity muscles. The process often spreads to the contralateral limb within weeks to months.[1] It is frequently accompanied by weight loss and, as the name implies, is frequently associated with diabetes. The initial pain can be debilitating and last for weeks to months while weakness usually continues to

[a] Neuromuscular Medicine, Auckland 0624, New Zealand; [b] Neuromuscular Medicine, University of Kansas Medical Center, 3901 Rainbow Boulevard MS 2012, Kansas City, KS 66160, USA
* Corresponding author.
E-mail address: mel.doerflinger@gmail.com

Neurol Clin 38 (2020) 553–564
https://doi.org/10.1016/j.ncl.2020.03.010

progress for several months more after the pain has subsided. Cases of weakness progressing up to 18 months have been described. The distribution of weakness and sensory loss depends on the lumbosacral roots involved, but most patients have both proximal and distal weakness and require assistance with ambulation.[1] Involvement of the upper extremities or the thoracic region is also encountered in some cases (Video 1). Almost all patients will improve spontaneously after reaching a nadir, but recovery is slow and often incomplete, with around 10% of patients requiring the use of a wheelchair 2 years after onset.[2]

This article aims to explore common and uncommon features of radiculoplexus neuropathy and discusses the diagnostic workup and management decisions with the following case examples.

CASE 1: UNILATERAL LOWER EXTREMITY PAIN AND WEAKNESS IN A DIABETIC PATIENT

An 84-year-old man with diabetes mellitus and bladder cancer presented with a 6-month history of left lower extremity weakness affecting the proximal muscles. Six months before the onset of weakness, he had developed left thigh pain that did not resolve with pain medications or epidural injections. Bladder cancer was diagnosed 4 years prior, with ureteral recurrence within 2 years and recent recurrence in the left kidney.

On physical examination, he had atrophy of the left thigh muscles and weakness in left hip flexion (4/5), hip adduction (4/5), and knee extension (2/5). The left patellar reflex was absent. Sensory perception was decreased in the lateral aspect of the left thigh and the upper part of the medial aspect of the left leg.

MRI of the lumbar spine showed only mild degenerative changes. Left thigh MRI showed diffuse edema in the rectus femoris, vastus lateralis, and vastus intermedius.

Question

What should be the next step in this patient's management?

A. Inform the patient that this is diabetic amyotrophy, during which most patients improve over time.
B. Obtain an electrodiagnostic study.
C. Refer to physical therapy.
D. Obtain a contrast-enhanced pelvis MRI.

Answer: D

Considering the malignancy, which is on the same side as the weakness, the most important step is to obtain a pelvic MRI to evaluate for malignant infiltration of the left lumbosacral plexus. Pelvic MRI was done for this patient and did not show such infiltration. With negative MRI, the likely diagnosis was DLSRPN (diabetic amyotrophy), and the other choices were all appropriate at that point.

Discussion

Lumbosacral radiculoplexus neuropathy typically starts with sudden onset of unilateral pain in the thigh and hip, which may spread to the other side in weeks to months.[1] As the pain subsides, weakness becomes more apparent.[1] Sensory loss is usually length dependent on examination (possibly because of concomitant peripheral polyneuropathy), but it could simply follow the roots involved as in this case. This case illustrates a typical clinical presentation of DLSRPN, but the associated history of malignancy should not be dismissed. Brejt and colleagues[3] illustrated a number of cases of malignant infiltration of the lumbosacral plexus in patients with pelvic malignancies. The symptomatic presentations described are indistinguishable from diabetic radiculoplexus neuropathy.

MRI findings in lumbosacral radiculoplexus neuropathy include T2 hyperintensity and enhancement of the lumbosacral roots, plexus, and nerves in addition to T2 hyperintensity of the affected muscles.[4] Cross-sectional area of the roots and nerves is significantly enlarged in diabetic amyotrophy compared with controls.[5] These changes can be seen in other disorders (eg, radiculitis, demyelinating polyneuropathies), and MRI should not be used to confirm the diagnosis of lumbosacral radiculoplexus neuropathy but rather to exclude certain other possibilities such as compression or malignant infiltration, as in this case.

Treatment should focus on pain control and rehabilitation in addition to diabetic control (typically the condition affects patients with well-controlled diabetes mellitus and no history of end-organ damage).[6] Immunomodulatory treatment has not proved to be effective in hastening improvement of strength.[7] However, steroids in the early phase may reduce pain and enhance cooperation with physical therapy. Considering that some patients may continue to worsen for 18 months before they improve, rehabilitation remains essential even if the patient is seen 2 years after the onset. In cases such as this one, where there is a history of pelvic malignancy, continued monitoring in collaboration with the patient's oncologist is essential, particularly if the progression of symptoms persists longer than expected.

CASE 2: BILATERAL LOWER EXTREMITY WEAKNESS IN ASSOCIATION WITH LIVER DISEASE

A 33-year-old woman with alcoholic liver disease was referred to the neuromuscular clinic for evaluation of lower extremity weakness. She had "muscle aches" in the thighs 3 months before her visit, followed within 1 to 2 weeks with weakness and muscle atrophy in the thighs. She also reported sharp pain in the feet along with numbness in the feet and legs and, to a lesser degree, the thighs. She had no symptoms in the upper extremities.

Prior workup included normal brain and entire spine MRI. Cerebrospinal fluid (CSF) protein was 220 mg/dL with normal cell count. Creatine kinase (CK) was normal while aspartate aminotransferase (112 IU/L) and alanine aminotransferase (61 IU/L) levels were elevated. Muscle biopsy of the vastus lateralis muscle was inconclusive.

The patient was treated with intravenous immunoglobulin (IVIG) and prednisone before her visit, without benefit.

Examination showed mild bilateral lower extremity muscle atrophy, more pronounced in the thigh muscles. There was weakness in bilateral hip flexion (4/5), hip abduction (4+/5), knee extension (4−/5), knee flexion (4/5), and ankle dorsiflexion (4/5). Strength was normal in the upper extremities. Reflexes were absent in the lower extremities and normal in the upper extremities. She had sensory loss to small fiber modalities up to the knee, but no definite sensory loss on vibration or proprioception examination.

An electrodiagnostic study showed normal nerve conduction results. Needle electromyography (EMG) showed active denervation and reinnervation in the tibialis anterior, gastrocnemius, and vastus lateralis; and reinnervation only in the semitendinosis and tensor fasciae latae. The upper extremity study was normal.

Question

What is the next step in this patient's management?

A. Continue IVIG and prednisone considering the CSF protein elevation.
B. Hold treatment, refer to physical therapy, and continue to monitor closely.
C. Repeat muscle biopsy and send a myositis antibody panel.
D. Refer for combined nerve and muscle biopsy for evaluation of vasculitic neuropathy.

Answer: B

- The patient presentation is consistent with nondiabetic radiculoplexus neuropathy. The best next step will be to stop immunomodulatory treatment and refer her to physical therapy.
- Elevated CSF protein is frequently seen with radiculoplexus neuropathy and should not be used to differentiate it from chronic inflammatory demyelinating polyneuropathy (CIDP).
- Because proximal weakness can be prominent in lumbosacral radiculoplexus neuropathy, myopathy is also a consideration. However, the normal strength of the upper extremities, presence of significant sensory symptoms and neuropathic pain, normal CK, and lack of myopathic changes on needle EMG all make myopathy less likely (**Table 1**).
- There was no weakness in the upper extremities or electrodiagnostic evidence for demyelinating neuropathy or vasculitic neuropathy.

Discussion

Presentation of nondiabetic lumbosacral radiculopathy is very similar to the diabetic variant, which indicates that diabetes is likely a risk factor and not a cause.[8,9] There is no sufficient literature to determine other risk factors, but other metabolic disorders (hepatic and renal impairment) are frequently encountered in the neuromuscular clinic in association with lumbosacral radiculoplexus neuropathy. More studies are needed to form a conclusion. In the authors' experience, diabetic patients with other metabolic factors (such as renal impairment and liver failure) may have more severe weakness, including significant weakness of the upper extremities, which may sometimes be confused with demyelinating neuropathy. These patients still have spontaneous recovery, which may be misinterpreted as a response to immunomodulatory therapy if such therapy is initiated.

Our patient improved over the following months and her strength was normal 5 months after the initial visit.

Table 1
Comparison of lumbosacral radiculoplexus neuropathy and acquired myopathy

	LSRPN	Acquired Myopathy
Weakness	Proximal and distal in most cases	Mostly proximal
Symmetry	Mostly asymmetric (but not all)	Mostly symmetric
Arms involvement	Relatively spared (but not always)	Arms are usually weak
Sensory symptoms	Present	Not expected
Reflexes	Affected	Normal (unless advanced)
Electrodiagnostic study	Neurogenic changes	Myopathic changes
CK level	Normal or mildly elevated	Variable

CASE 3: PAINLESS PROGRESSIVE WEAKNESS

A 67-year-old man with no significant medical history presented to the neuromuscular clinic with progressive weakness of his right leg starting 6 months prior. He reported inability to stand on toes on the right side. There was no weakness in the other extremities, and there was no sensory loss or neuropathic pain. Intermittent soreness in the lower back was reported.

Physical examination showed weakness in right knee flexion, planter flexion, toe extension and flexion (all 4/5), and hip flexion and abduction (4+/5). Reflexes were absent in the right lower extremity and left patella and normal in the upper extremities. There was no sensory loss. He was unable to stand on toes on the right but able to stand on heels. He was also noted to have fasciculations, limited to both calves and with percussion only.

Laboratory testing revealed CK of 315 IU/L and hemoglobin A_{1c} of 6.7% (no history of diabetes). Nerve conduction study did not show evidence of peripheral neuropathy. Needle EMG revealed multilevel active denervation with reinnervation in both lumbosacral and cervical regions but not the thoracic paraspinals. Cervical spine MRI showed marked spinal canal and neuroforaminal stenoses (**Fig. 1**). Lumbar spine MRI showed moderate to severe canal and neuroforaminal stenoses at L3-L4 level (**Fig. 2**).

Question

What is the next step in management?

A. Refer the patient to a spine surgeon for evaluation.
B. Refer the patient to the amyotrophic lateral sclerosis (ALS) clinic.
C. Monitor the patient for 3 to 6 months.
D. Start a trial of IVIG for possible motor neuropathy.

Answer: C

- Lumbosacral radiculopathy secondary to degenerative spinal disease is expected to be associated with pain in most cases. Furthermore, the denervation found on needle EMG in this case was diffuse and not limited to 1 or 2 nerve root distributions (**Table 2**).

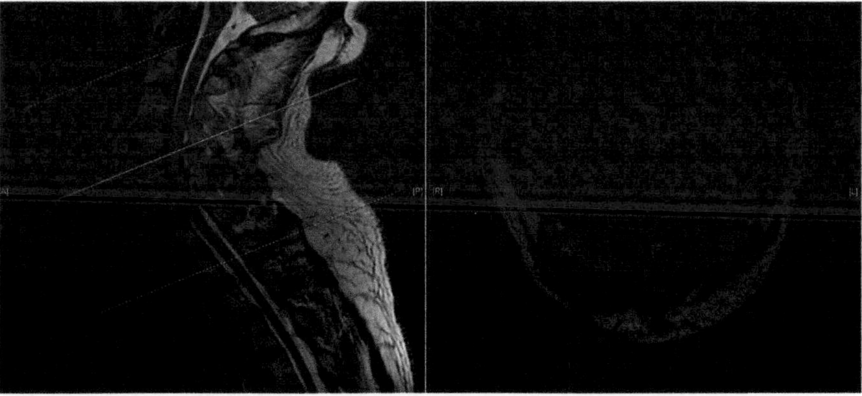

Fig. 1. Noncontrast T2-weighted cervical spine MR image showing multilevel central canal stenoses on sagittal view.

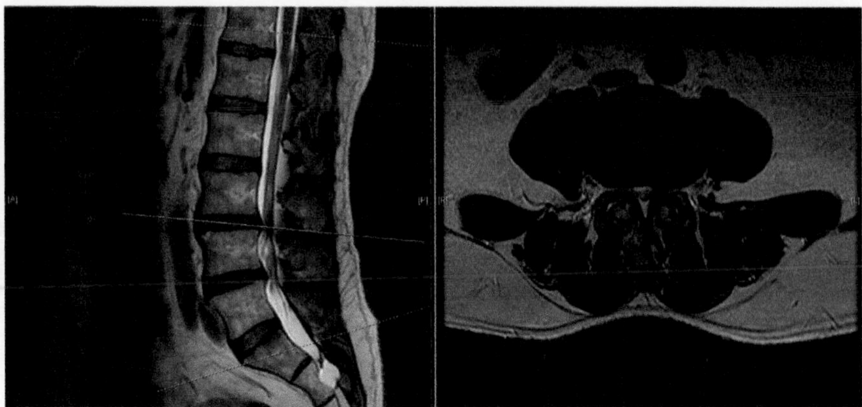

Fig. 2. Noncontrast T2-weighted lumbar spine MR image showing marked central canal stenosis and left more than right neuroforaminal stenoses at the L3/L4 level.

- Although progressive painless distal weakness is concerning for ALS, the findings on examination of this patient were not yet sufficient to establish the diagnosis. The patient did not have upper motor neuron signs or weakness in the other extremities. Mildly elevated CK is often seen in ALS but can also be seen with other causes of active denervation and can also be idiopathic. One additional clue to consider is that the weakness affected the posterior compartment of the leg, whereas in ALS it is more typical for the anterior compartment to be affected first (ie, foot drop) (**Table 3**).
- Autoimmune multifocal motor neuropathy typically starts in the upper extremities in middle-aged patients (more common in men), and it is likely to be more rapidly progressive and not confined to one limb 6 months after onset.

Discussion

DLSRPN can be the presenting manifestation that leads to an initial diagnosis of diabetes, as in this case. In lumbosacral radiculoplexus neuropathy, proximal

Table 2
Comparison of lumbosacral radiculoplexus neuropathy and radiculopathy secondary to spine disorder

	LSRPN	Radiculopathy Secondary to Spinal DJD
Onset	Acute/subacute	Chronic (unless there is acute event)
Pain	Constant	Starts radicular and intermittent
Roots involvement	Upper lumbar root involvement is common	Most commonly L5-S1
SNAPs	Usually abnormal	Normal
MRI	Can be helpful if negative	Correlation with clinical and electrodiagnostic data is important

Abbreviations: DJD, degenerative joint disease; SNAP, sensory nerve action potential.

Table 3
Comparison of lumbosacral radiculoplexus neuropathy and motor neuron disease

	LSRPN	Motor Neuron Disease
Onset	Acute/subacute	Insidious
Weakness pattern	Variable	Variable (but mostly distal)
Course	Spontaneous improvement	No improvement
Pain	Mostly painful (but not all)	Mostly painless
Upper motor neuron signs	No upper motor neuron signs	Mostly present (but not in progressive muscular atrophy and some other variants)
Fasciculations	Uncommon	Common and diffuse
Electrodiagnostic study	Abnormal SNAPs may help	Normal SNAPs

weakness is the predominant complaint in most patients; however, it has been widely reported that proximal and distal weakness can occur abruptly together, arguing that the previously often used term "proximal diabetic neuropathy" is imprecise.[1] This patient had both proximal and distal weakness on examination, even though distal weakness was his main complaint. Also, as illustrated in this case, lumbosacral radiculoplexus neuropathy can be painless.[10] It is estimated that for every 10 to 20 cases of painful diabetic amyotrophy there is 1 painless case.[11]

Our patient was referred to physical therapy and for management of his newly diagnosed diabetes. He showed improvement in his strength 3 months after the initial visit and normal strength 6 months after. The final diagnosis was DLSRPN.

CASE 4: PROGRESSIVE WEAKNESS OF ALL EXTREMITIES

A 55-year-old man with uncontrolled diabetes mellitus and obesity presented to establish care in the neuromuscular clinic. He had scrotal gangrene 2 years prior followed by progressive weakness, neuropathic pain, and sensory loss in all extremities. His initial examination from that time showed asymmetric weakness in all extremities with distal sensory loss and areflexia. The weakness was more distal than proximal in the upper extremities, but the hip flexion was weaker than the ankle dorsiflexion in the lower extremities. He was not able to ambulate even with a walker. An electrodiagnostic study showed predominately axonal polyneuropathy with mild slowing, which did not meet most criteria for CIDP. He was admitted to the hospital and underwent lumbar puncture, which showed normal cell count in the CSF but protein of 179 mg/dL. He was treated with plasma exchange followed by maintenance of IVIG. While in the hospital he developed a cranial nerve III palsy.

Improvement in strength was slow, and there was no clear improvement in neuropathic pain or sensory deficit. In fact, his sensory examination showed worse findings than what was reported on his initial evaluation 2 years before. His recent strength examination was mostly normal, except for mild distal weakness in finger abduction and ankle dorsiflexion (4+/5). He had been on IVIG 1 g/kg every 3 weeks. His renal function had worsened within the last year, most recently with a creatinine of 1.5 mg/dL and glomerular filtration rate of 51 mL/min.

Question

What should be the next step in the management of this patient?

A. Change the IVIG dose to 0.5 g/kg every 10 days to decrease the risk of further deterioration in renal function.
B. Start rituximab to stop IVIG.
C. Start azathioprine with low-dose steroids and stop IVIG.
D. Hold IVIG without starting any additional treatment but with close monitoring.

Answer: D

This case represents a challenge in differentiating radiculoplexus neuropathy from CIDP. The patient presented with progressive weakness in all extremities with sensory loss and areflexia, clinical features that can be seen with both diseases. What favors radiculoplexus neuropathy in this patient is the presence of proximal more than distal weakness in the lower extremities and no definite response to immunomodulatory treatment. Rather, he had slow improvement in strength over more than a year. In addition, the persistent neuropathic pain and worsening of sensory deficit along with cranial nerve III palsy all suggest a diabetic association. Elevated CSF protein, which is widely considered a sign of demyelinating polyneuropathy, is not specific and has been reported in radiculoplexus neuropathy at numbers even higher than seen in this patient.[12] Axonal and demyelinating polyneuropathy is seen in diabetes, and nerve conduction study can easily meet the less strict criteria for primary demyelination.

Considering these factors, along with renal function deterioration, IVIG was held and the patient was monitored for 6 months with no change in his neurologic examination at the time of this writing. The longer this stability lasts, the more likely he has dealt with radiculoplexus neuropathy. Nonetheless, caution and monitoring are still needed.

Discussion

While upper extremity sparing may favor lumbosacral radiculoplexus neuropathy over CIDP, such involvement in radiculoplexus neuropathy is well reported and may be seen in one-third of cases.[11] When all extremities are involved in radiculoplexus neuropathy, diffuse areflexia would be expected. Initial onset in the upper extremity has been reported, although this is a less common presentation of radiculoplexus neuropathy.[13,14]

Table 4
Comparison of lumbosacral radiculoplexus neuropathy and acquired demyelinating neuropathy

	LSRPN	Demyelinating Neuropathy
Limb involvement	Arm sparing can be a clue (arm involvement is present in up to one-third of cases)	Arms are usually involved
Pain	Severe pain that can be proximal	Less painful and usually distal
Symmetry	Usually asymmetric	More symmetric
Reflexes	Preserved reflexes in the arms in most cases	Diffuse areflexia
Electrodiagnostic	Axonal or axonal and demyelinating	Primary demyelinating with secondary axonal changes
CSF	Not helpful to differentiate these entities because both can show significant CSF protein elevation	

Nerve and Muscle Center of Texas

Differentiating radiculoplexus neuropathy from CIDP is especially important in diabetic patients considering the risks associated with IVIG and corticosteroid treatment in this population. Such differentiation (**Table 4**) can be very difficult at times. When this is the case, frequent re-evaluation of the diagnosis is highly recommended.

CASE 5: POSSIBLE VASCULITIC NEUROPATHY

A 75-year-old man with hypertension was referred to the neuromuscular clinic for management of possible vasculitic neuropathy. Eleven months before his visit, he developed back pain radiating to the left leg. He had a lumbar spine MRI that showed degenerative changes and was referred to surgery. He developed weakness and atrophy in the left thigh and leg while waiting for the surgery, which was performed 2 months after symptom onset and resulted in no clear benefit. He then developed recurrent pain in the lower back accompanied by paresthesia and numbness in the right lower extremity followed by weakness of the limb. The right leg weakness was progressive, and he began using a wheelchair 5 months after the onset. He was seen by neurology and rheumatology, and began treatment with corticosteroids for possible vasculitic neuropathy 6 months after the onset. CSF analysis was unremarkable. CK, C-reactive protein, and erythrocyte sedimentation rate were normal. He had a sural nerve biopsy, which showed mild loss in the myelinated fibers without evidence for inflammation or vasculitic changes. He was referred to rehabilitation and was walking with a walker by the time of his initial presentation to the neuromuscular clinic. At that time, he was still on 20 mg of prednisone daily.

His examination showed asymmetric weakness in the lower extremities, which involved both proximal and distal muscles. Hip flexion was 4–/5 on the right and 4/5 on the left. Knee extension was 2/5 on the right and 3/5 on the left. Dorsiflexion was 0/5 on the right and 1/5 on the left. Ankle plantar flexion was 5/5 on the right and 4+/5 on the left. He had normal strength in the upper extremities except for slight weakness in finger abduction. Reflexes were absent in the lower extremities except for the left ankle, which was normal. Reflexes were normal in the upper extremities. Sensory loss was present in the right foot and leg to both small and large fiber modalities. Left foot sensory examination was normal.

Electrodiagnostic study showed absent sensory responses in the legs with low motor responses and active denervation in proximal and distal muscles of the lower extremities.

Question

What is the recommended treatment approach at this point?

A. Add rituximab.
B. Add cyclophosphamide.
C. Stop prednisone and initiate no further therapy.
D. Stop prednisone and start IVIG.

Answer: C

Although pain, sensory changes, and weakness can be seen with both vasculitic neuropathy and lumbosacral radiculoplexus neuropathy, there are a few features in this case indicating that the patient was dealing with the latter. The severe proximal lower extremity weakness and relative sparing of the upper extremities is not usual for vasculitic neuropathy, which tends to be more distal in nature. Vasculitic neuropathy is likely to affect the upper extremities to a significant degree if left untreated for 6 months. The isolated mild weakness in finger abduction was suspected to be due to a different cause (eg, ulnar neuropathy, which is not

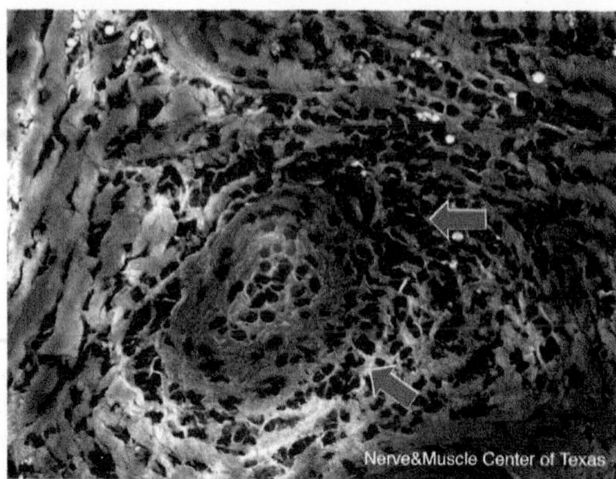

Fig. 3. Perivascular inflammatory infiltrate (yellow arrows).

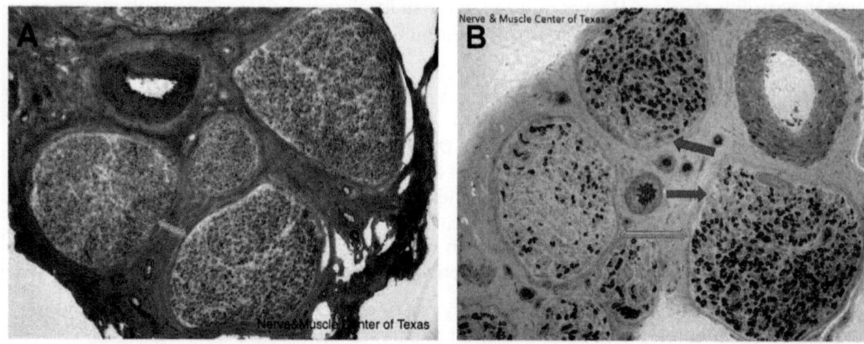

Fig. 4. Gomori-Trichrome stain (*A*) and toluidine blue stain (*B*) of peripheral nerve biopsy showing variable degree of fiber loss among fascicles (*yellow left-right arrows*) and asymmetric loss within some fascicles (*blue arrows*).

Table 5
Comparison of lumbosacral radiculoplexus neuropathy and vasculitic neuropathy

	LSRPN	Vasculitic Neuropathy[a]
Weakness	Proximal muscles are usually involved early on	Distal weakness
Pain	Severe pain proximally (lower back, hip, and thigh)	Severe pain distally
Upper extremities	Might be spared	Not spared for long without treatment
Electrodiagnostic study	Active denervation proximally and distally	Active denervation distally

[a] Purpuric skin rash and multisystemic involvement are typical for vasculitis except when it is confined to the peripheral nervous system.

uncommon with wheelchair use). There was also no pathologic evidence of vasculitis, and inflammatory markers were normal. The correct approach would be to stop prednisone because of lack of evidence for vasculitis and refer the patient to physical therapy.

Discussion

Vasculitic changes are reported in nerve biopsies in lumbosacral radiculoplexus neuropathy. Raff and colleagues[15] documented multiple areas of nerve ischemia and perivascular inflammation within the lumbosacral plexus in a postmortem study. Early in the disease course, epineural and perivascular inflammation around the small vessels has also been reported (microvasculitis)[16,16] (**Fig. 3**), but these changes can also be seen in diabetic polyneuropathy along with asymmetric axonal loss (**Fig. 4**). Relying only on these changes to make the case of vasculitic neuropathy may result in unnecessary treatments. Vasculitic neuropathy is likely to have clinical features different from those of radiculoplexus neuropathy (**Table 5**). In addition, radiculoplexus neuropathy does not respond to the usual treatment of vasculitis. Corticosteroids were shown to be helpful only with pain control in radiculoplexus neuropathy but not with neurologic improvement.[7]

SUMMARY

Diabetic LSRPN is a neuromuscular disorder with characteristic clinical features that have been well described in the literature. However, as illustrated in the cases described herein, patients with less typical presentations, including distal weakness, upper extremity involvement, painless course, and lack of diabetes, can present a diagnostic challenge. Thoughtful and thorough investigation and a sound knowledge of the variable presentations of LSRPN will assist the neurologist in making the correct diagnosis, thereby avoiding unnecessary or potentially harmful treatment or procedures.

SUPPLEMENTARY DATA

Supplementary data to this article can be found online at https://doi.org/10.1016/j.ncl.2020.03.010.

REFERENCES

1. Barohn RJ, Sahenk Z, Warmolts JR, et al. The Bruns-Garland syndrome (diabetic amyotrophy) revisited 100 years later. Arch Neurol 1991;48:1130–5.
2. Dyck PJ, Windebank AJ. Radiculoplexus neuropathy: new insights into pathophysiology and treatment. Muscle Nerve 2002;25(4):477–91.
3. Brejt N, Berry J, Nisbet A, et al. Pelvic radiculopathies, lumbosacral plexopathies, and neuropathies in oncologic disease: a multidisciplinary approach to a diagnostic challenge. Cancer Imaging 2013;13(4):591–601.
4. Filosto M, Pari E, Cotelli M, et al. MR neurography in diagnosing nondiabetic lumbosacral radiculopathy. J Neuroimaging 2013;23(4):543–4.
5. His R, Poh F, Bryarly M, et al. Quantitative assessment of diabetic amyotrophy using magnetic resonance neurography—a case-control analysis. Eur Radiol 2019;29(11):5910–9.
6. Shaibani A, Jabari D, Weimer LH. Diabetic amyotrophy. San Diego (CA): Medlink Neurology; 2019. Available at: https://www.medlink.com/article/diabetic_amyotrophy.

7. Dyck PJ, O'Brien PC, Bosch EP, et al. Results of a controlled trial of IV methylprednisolone in diabetic lumbosacral radiculoplexus neuropathy (DLRPN): a preliminary indication of efficacy. J Peripher Nerv Syst 2005;10(s1):21.
8. Dyck PJ, Engelstad JN, Norell J, et al. Microvasculitis in nondiabetic lumbosacral radiculoplexus neuropathy (LSRPN): similarity to the diabetic variety (DLSRPN). J Neuropathol Exp Neurol 2000;59:525–38.
9. Dyck PJ, Norell JE, Dyck PJ. Non-diabetic lumbosacral radiculoplexus neuropathy. Natural history, outcome and comparison with the diabetic variety. Brain 2001;124:1197–207.
10. Graces-Sanchez M, Laughlin RS, Dyck PJ, et al. Painless diabetic motor neuropathy: a variant of diabetic lumbosacral radiculoplexus neuropathy. Ann Neurol 2011;69(6):1043–54.
11. Pasnoor M, Dimachkie MM, Barohn RJ. Diabetic neuropathy Part 2: proximal and asymmetric phenotypes. Neurol Clin 2013;31(2):447–62.
12. Imtiaz KE, Lekwuwa G, Kaimal N, et al. Elevated cerebrospinal fluid protein in diabetic lumbosacral radiculoplexus neuropathy. QJM 2011;105(11):1119–23.
13. Katz JS, Saperstein DS, Wolfe G, et al. Cervicobrachial involvement in diabetic radiculoplexopathy. Muscle Nerve 2001;24:794–8.
14. Massie R, Mauermann ML, Staff NP, et al. Diabetic cervical radiculoplexus neuropathy: a distinct syndrome expanding the spectrum of diabetic radiculoplexus neuropathies. Brain 2012;135(10):3074–88.
15. Raff MC, Sangalang V, Asbury AK. Ischemic mononeuropathy multiplex associated with diabetes mellitus. Arch Neurol 1968;18:487–99.
16. Dyck PJ, Norell JE, Dyck PJ. Microvasculitis and ischemia in diabetic lumbosacral radiculoplexus neuropathy. Neurology 1999;53:2113–21.

ALS: Management Problems

Jonathan R. Brent, MD, PhD[a], Colin K. Franz, MD, PhD[b,c], John M. Coleman III, MD[d], Senda Ajroud-Driss, MD[e,*]

KEYWORDS

- ALS • Dysphagia • Dysarthria • Spasticity • Noninvasive ventilation
- Respiratory failure • Secretion management • Sialorrhea

KEY POINTS

- Multidisciplinary care of patients with amyotrophic lateral sclerosis (ALS) in specialized clinics improves survival.
- Early initiation of noninvasive ventilation improves quality of life and prolongs survival.
- Early implementation of airway clearance techniques in patients with bulbar ALS may improve noninvasive ventilation compliance and prevent respiratory infections.
- Addressing dysarthria and pseudobulbar affect may improve social isolation of ALS patients.
- Spasticity may be difficult to treat in ALS patients and may require the trial of different agents.

Video content accompanies this article at http://www.neurologic.theclinics.com.

INTRODUCTION

Amyotrophic lateral sclerosis (ALS) causes significant morbidity but despite the fact that it is an incurable disease, symptomatic management has evolved in the past decade, and aggressive symptom management can improve survival and patient quality of life.

CASE 1: PROGRESSIVE NEUROMUSCULAR RESPIRATORY FAILURE

A 48-year-old man diagnosed with limb-onset ALS with right lower extremity weakness and foot drop presents to clinic for 3-month follow-up. During the visit he

[a] Department of Neurology, Feinberg School of Medicine, Northwestern University, 303 East Chicago Avenue, Chicago, IL 60611, USA; [b] Department of Physical Medicine and Rehabilitation, Northwestern University Feinberg School of Medicine, Chicago, IL, USA; [c] Department of Neurology, Shirley Ryan AbilityLab, Northwestern University Feinberg School of Medicine, Chicago, IL, USA; [d] Division of Pulmonary and Critical Care Medicine, Northwestern University Feinberg School of Medicine, Chicago, IL, USA; [e] Department of Neurology, Feinberg School of Medicine, Northwestern University, Chicago, IL, USA
* Corresponding author.
E-mail address: s-ajroud@northwestern.edu

Neurol Clin 38 (2020) 565–575
https://doi.org/10.1016/j.ncl.2020.03.013

mentions he is waking up more tired in the morning and getting more fatigued during the day. At his last clinic visit his forced vital capacity (FVC) was 79% upright and his maximal inspiratory pressure (MIP) was −89 mm Hg. Today in clinic his FVC is 61% upright and his MIP is −62 mm Hg.

Clinical question: What are the criteria required to initiate a patient with ALS on a respiratory assist device (RAD) for noninvasive ventilation support?

1. FVC less than 50%
2. MIP less than −60
3. Overnight oximetry, with oxygen saturation less than 88% for 5 minutes (not continuous)
4. Arterial blood gas, with P_{CO_2} more than 45 mm Hg
5. All of the above

Answer: 5.

Discussion

In the United States, under Centers for Medicare & Medicaid Services guidelines, for people living with neuromuscular disease (ALS, muscular dystrophy, or spinal cord injury), noninvasive ventilation can be initiated with only 1 of the above criteria. People with neuromuscular respiratory do not require a polysomnogram or sleep study to qualify for noninvasive ventilation (**Fig. 1**).

Summary

Chronic neuromuscular respiratory failure is the most common cause of morbidity and mortality in ALS patients, due to progressive diaphragm weakness. Diaphragm weakness has an impact on the following respiratory functions:

- Inspiratory muscle strength, which contributes most to ventilation
- Expiratory muscle strength, required for airway clearance and secretion management
- Bulbar muscle function, which protects the airway from recurrent aspiration[1]

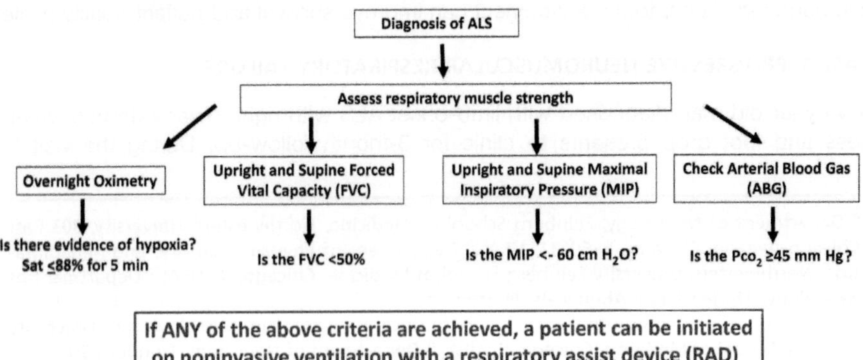

Fig. 1. Decision tree, management of respiratory failure in ALS.

Noninvasive ventilation is proved to extend life in people living with ALS on average 205 days.[2]

All patients with ALS qualifying and requiring noninvasive ventilation must be initiated on therapy with the proper machine. All patients require a device, either a RAD or home mechanical ventilator, that can provide full (ventilatory) support, meaning the machine provides a back-up respiratory rate. There are various different modes of ventilation available, but every one must include a respiratory rate.

CASE 2: INEFFECTIVE COUGH AND SECRETION MANAGEMENT

A 57-year-old woman with bulbar-onset ALS, with persistent secretions and weak cough, presents to clinic. She currently is on noninvasive ventilation with excellent adherence and compliance. She denies any shortness of breath. She has had progressive difficulty with swallowing and having increased episodes of choking and aspiration. When aspiration occurs, she has difficulty clearing her secretions. Her most recent FVC was 23% with mask, but this value likely reflects difficulty with upper airway weakness.

With the upcoming cold and flu season, in addition to an annual flu shot, what are other airway clearance options?

1. Lung volume recruitment
2. Manual assisted cough
3. Nebulizer machine
4. Suction machine
5. High-frequency chest wall oscillation (therapy vest)
6. Mechanical insufflation/exsufflation (cough assist)
7. All of the above

Answer: 7.

Discussion

Progressive neuromuscular respiratory weakness in ALS leads to impairment with clearing secretions and coughing and can lead to respiratory infections, increasing morbidity and mortality.[3] Techniques to assist with secretion clearance are widely recommended and include mucus-mobilizing techniques and assisted cough techniques (**Fig. 2**).[4]

Summary

Assessing effective airway clearance starts with an assessment of peak cough flow. An effective cough is essential to clear airway secretions from the proximal airways. When cough is ineffective secondary to diaphragm muscle weakness, there are a variety of therapies available to help mobilize secretions.[5]

In addition to respiratory therapies to help mobilize secretions, management of excessive secretions is important. Many people living with ALS struggle with excessive oral secretions, or sialorrhea, and this can come in 2 different types, thick and copious or thin and watery. Management approaches are different in each case.

A classic example of excessive thin watery secretions is a patient with tongue weakness and immobilization, unable to redistribute secretions throughout the mouth. Treatment options include[6]

1. Anticholinergic medications (glycopyrrolate, scopolamine, sublingual atropine, and amitriptyline): doses should be escalated as tolerated, and multiple therapies can be used at the same time. With anticholinergic medications, need to monitor for constipation and urinary retention.

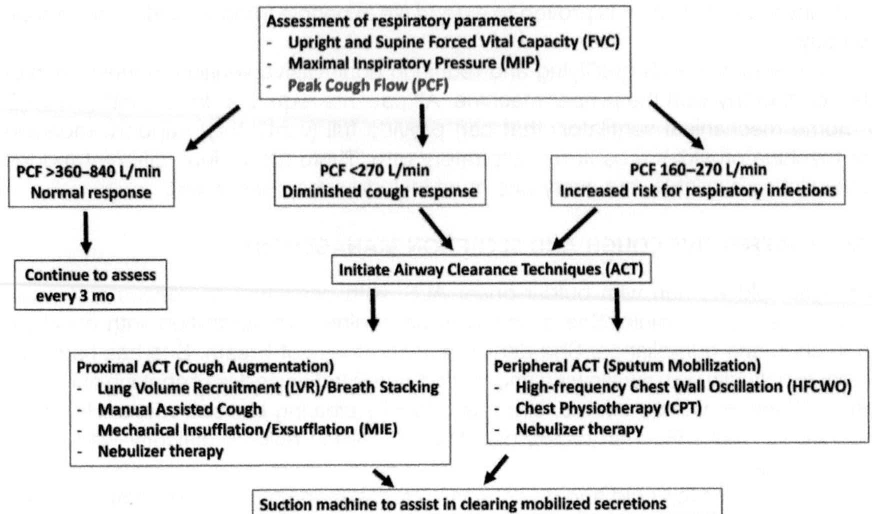

Fig. 2. Airway clearance techniques in ALS.

2. Botox injections: performed by otolaryngology surgeons and can be to either or both the submandibular glands and/or parotid glands. This is an effective therapy and typically lasts 2 months to 3 months.[7]
3. Ligation: surgical removal of salivary glands
4. Radiation: evolving therapy, typically requires 5 days of treatment and patient must be able to lay flat[8]

Excessive thick secretions commonly occur in patients with bulbar disease, who have excessive thick secretions. These can be secondary to medications (anticholinergic), dehydration, or mouth breathing. Treatment options include

1. Increasing overall hydration status: people living with ALS tend to always not take enough hydration, whether due to difficulty swallowing or difficulty with mobility to get to the washroom.
2. Increasing oral hydration with nebulizer therapy or humidifiers: with nebulizer therapy, it is recommended to use saline solution to help moisturize thick oral secretions. Increasing humidification in the home if a patient is on noninvasive ventilation is helpful.

Respiratory failure is the most common cause of death in people living with ALS. Respiratory infections can severely diminish respiratory reserve in patients with already reduced function. Comprehensive airway clearance, from management of excessive secretions to mobilization and removal of excessive secretions, is key to maintain optimal respiratory function.

CASE 3: DYSARTHRIA

A 58-year-old man presents with 1 year of progressive dysarthria and dysphagia. The patient initially was having difficulty pronouncing words. The patient denies word-finding difficulties but instead speech was noted by family to be slurred and much slower than his baseline. The patient also notes that eating is taking longer and occasionally he coughs on dry solids. He denies any weakness of arms and legs but does have generalized fatigue. Additional complaints include bouts of laughter and crying that seem difficult to control. Examination demonstrates weakness of the palate, tongue atrophy, and tongue fasciculation. The speech is very slow and nasal (Video 1).

Clinical Questions

1. What currently are the most important interventions to help treat dysarthria in ALS?
   A. Text-to-speech apps to allow patients to select words and phrases from customized menus
   B. Exercises to strengthen the muscles of the palate, tongue, and mouth
   C. Surgical palatal lift and/or prostheses
   D. Brain-machine interface that can translate thoughts into speech
2. When should interventions to treat ALS dysarthria be discussed?
   A. Before a patient has any symptoms of ALS
   B. As early as possible within the disease course
   C. Only once a patient has lost all ability to speak
   D. When dysarthria progresses despite conservative treatments, such as speech therapy
3. Which of the following is correct?
   A. Speech-to-text apps work the best for patients with severe dysarthria.
   B. It is important for patients to learn about options, such as voice banking, as soon as possible.
   C. It is important to avoid talking about interventions for dysarthria until it is absolutely necessary.
   D. Exercises to strengthen speech muscles can reverse dysarthria in most patients

Answers: 1, A; 2, B; 3, B.

Discussion

- Dysarthria may be a presenting symptom in ALS with bulbar onset, which includes approximately 20% of patients.[9] Nonetheless, eventually at some point in their disease, 80% to 95% of ALS patients cannot meet their daily communication needs with natural speech. This makes it challenging for patients to communicate their needs to caregivers, which is a major factor in quality of life.[10] The dysarthria most often is of mixed etiology, with spasticity from corticobulbar dysfunction and flaccidity with atrophy from bulbar dysfunction contributing, although either presentation can predominate early in the disease.[11]

Summary

The major interventions for dysarthria in ALS focus on training the patient and family to use assistive and augmentative communication.[11–13]

- Low-technology options, such as a writing board, may be used early in the disease in patients with functional limbs.
- The most commonly used tools include text-to-speech apps, where patients can type or choose words/phrases on a tablet screen.
- If motor function precludes manipulating a tablet screen with the limbs, patients can use eye gaze software that tracks eye movements to control a cursor on the screen.

Proactive, early introduction of these tools is essential for several important reasons.

- Some of the apps include customizable menus and often have a significant learning curve. This requires patients and their families to practice and tailor the functionality of the program to their needs over time.

Some text-to-speech devices allow patients to bank their own voice, and, for this to be most beneficial, the voice must be recorded when speech is most intelligible. Although patients and families often ask for specific strengthening exercises to improve speech, the role of exercise in the management of bulbar dysfunction in ALS is not well understood.[14] Because of the detrimental effect of fatigue, patients usually are taught to save their voice for specific times that are highest priority and to minimize fatigue by using speech amplification devices, such as portable microphones. Additionally, patients and families can reduce fatigue by pursuing nonverbal communication wherever possible. Several centers have reported improved dysarthria with surgical palatal lift or prostheses but the evidence supporting their use is limited.

CASE 4: DYSPHAGIA

A 62-year-old woman, who presented with left foot drop 18 months ago and 6 months ago, developed left hand weakness, dysphagia, and dysarthria. In the last year, the patient's weight declined from 160 to 125. Initially the patient had decreased appetite but in the last 6 months she has had dysphagia first for solids and then for all oral intake. When she tries to eat, the food gets stuck in her throat and she coughs. She tried to eat more slowly and cut her food up but eventually meals took over an hour. She also complains of excessive drooling and trouble catching her breath during meals.

Clinical Questions

1. When should enteral nutrition be discussed with an ALS patient?
   A. When a patient has reached 50% of the baseline/premorbid weight
   B. The timing is individualized but should be introduced as early as possible. This is best approached over multiple visits with a goal of having a firm plan well before it is needed urgently.
   C. Once the FVC has reached less than 30%
   D. Only once a patient has lost 10% of baseline/premorbid weight despite speech therapist evaluation and nutrition supplementation
2. What are the key deciding factors regarding which procedure a patient will have to place a gastrostomy tube?
   A. FVC
   B. Patient preference
   C. Center expertise
   D. All of the above
3. Which of the following is correct?
   A. To be able to receive gastrostomy via percutaneous endoscopic gastrostomy (PEG), a patient must be able to lay flat.
   B. Swallowing therapy is able to reverse dysphagia in a majority of patients.
   C. Once a patient receives gastrostomy, it is essential to no longer eat or drink by mouth to prevent aspiration.
   D. Consensus guidelines recommend dysphagia screening at least annually in all ALS patients.

Answers: 1, B; 2, D; 3, A.

Discussion

Management of weight loss and nutrition in ALS

- ALS patients who are malnourished have 30% increase in risk of death for each 5% of weight lost and more than 7-fold increased risk of death overall.[15,16] For this

reason, ensuring that all ALS patients are treated proactively for dysphagia and weight loss is among the most impactful treatment goals in their overall care plan.
- Consensus guidelines support quarterly assessments of dysphagia initially with screening questions.[1] Any dysphagia complaints should prompt evaluation by speech therapist, who can perform bedside and videofluoroscopic assessments.

Summary

It is important to stress to patients that the presence of dysphagia does not have to preclude all oral intake.

- Especially early in the course of disease, behavioral adaptations, such as modification of food and/or liquid consistency, upright eating, and chin-tuck maneuvers, can minimize the chance of aspiration.[17] These techniques also are useful later in the disease because they can enable some patients to experience select foods for pleasure.
- Nutritionists can help monitor caloric intake and often recommend nutritional supplements to help maintain body weight
- If patients have lost more than 10% of their premorbid bodyweight, enteral nutrition is the appropriate intervention.

Enteral nutrition actually may slow disease progression and improve survival.[1] The discussion about enteric nutrition should be started as early in the disease course as is reasonably possible. Patients and their families benefit from time to process all of the options.

The options include

- PEG
- Radiologically inserted gastrostomy (RIG)[18]

Importantly, respiratory function is used to help guide the timing of initiation and the specific procedure the patient will receive.[19]

- PEG tube placement requires a patient to receive sedation and is performed in a supine position. This becomes more dangerous in patients with poor respiratory function. For this reason, most centers attempt PEG tube insertion before the FVC declines to less than 50%.[1,20]
- RIG can be performed in an upright position and can be done without sedation.
- If FVC is less than 50%, PEG still can be performed with additional support and monitoring by anesthesia. Many centers, however, first stabilize the patient on noninvasive ventilation and then pursue RIG.
- Nonetheless, center and patient preference ultimately guide this decision, with the goal of a successful procedure as early as is appropriate.

CASE 5: PSEUDOBULBAR AFFECT

A 58-year-old man presented with bulbar-onset ALS; his symptoms started about 1 year prior to diagnosis with slurred speech that was worse when he was tired. He also noticed episodes of incontrollable laughing with a minimal trigger. His wife said that that certain commercials on TV make him cry easily. He would not describe himself as an emotional person but these episodes were embarrassing to the patient to the point that he limited his social interactions out of fear of having these sudden and inexplicable outbursts in public (Video 2).

What is the correct answer?

A. These episodes of incontrollable laughing or crying, or pseudobulbar affect (PBA), depend on the patient mood.
B. PBA affects only ALS patients.
C. The only Food and Drug Administration (FDA)-approved treatments for PBA are selective serotonin reuptake inhibitors (SSRIs) and tricyclic antidepressants (TCAs).
D. A combination dextromethorphan and quinidine (Nuedexta) has been shown to reduce the frequency of PBA episodes and improve the quality of life of patients in a large, phase 3, multicenter randomized trial.

Answer: D.

Discussion and Summary

Management of pseudobulbar affect

PBA, also known as emotional lability and pathologic laughing and crying, falls under the umbrella term of involuntary emotional expression disorder.[21] It is characterized by sudden outbursts of involuntary and exaggerated laughter and/or crying.[22] These episodes are disproportionate or separate from a patient's undelaying mood or social context.[23] PBA affects up to 50% of patients with ALS[22] and is more prevalent in patient with the bulbar form of the disease. It has significant impact on quality of life and often leads to social isolation. PBA is not specific to ALS and can be seen in multiple sclerosis, dementia, traumatic brain injury, stroke, and Parkinson disease.[23] The anatomic substrate of this syndrome is not well understood but applying advanced neuroimaging and neurophysiologic techniques suggests that, irrespective of the pathology, disturbed circuitry involved in the initiation and modulation of emotional output with cortico-ponto-cerebellar network dysfunction seems central to its pathophysiology.[24]

- SSRIs and TCAs used to be the most frequently used off-label treatment of PBA.
- In 2010, dextromethorphan (20 mg) and quinidine sulfate (10 mg) become the first FDA-approved treatment of PBA. Dextromethorphan is metabolized rapidly by the hepatic first-pass metabolism through cytochrome P450 (CYP)-2D6, and adding a low-dose quinidine as a CYP-2D6 inhibitor increases its bioavailability. A large, phase 3, randomized placebo-controlled trial showed that this combination reduced the frequency and the severity of PBA episodes and improved patient quality of life[25]; side effects include dizziness, nausea, diarrhea, and somnolence,[25] and they can be minimized by starting the treatment at 1 tablet at bedtime for 1 week followed by 1 tablet twice a day. There also is a mild non-arrhythmogenic QT prolongation,[25] and caution should be used with this drug in patients with cardiac disease; an electrocardiogram prior and 2 weeks after treatment initiation may be needed to establish safety. A small randomized, blinded, crossover study also showed that dextromethorphan/quinidine improved speech and swallowing in ALS patients, suggesting that it may have a neuroprotective effect[26]; further study is needed to verify this finding.[27]

CASE 6: SPASTICITY

A 37-year-old man recently diagnosed with lower limb–onset ALS complains of increasing right leg stiffness, decreased walking endurance, and painful muscle spasms that occur mainly at night. In retrospect, his symptoms began approximately 9 months previously, when he noticed frequent muscle twitching in his legs and felt his right legs stiffen up when he tried to run to catch his train to work in the morning. His symptoms have progressed gradually since then to include difficulty holding a pen or typing with this right hand. On general examination, his blood pressure was 106/68 mm Hg, heart rate was 58 beats per minute, and respiratory rate was 16 breaths per minute. The neurologic examination was notable for diffuse but asymmetric lower extremity weakness without marked muscle atrophy. He also has weakness in the right hand intrinsic muscles, including the first dorsal interosseous and abductor pollicies brevis but sparing the abductor digiti minimi. He still can overcome mild resistance on manual muscle testing in his right knee extensors, but he walks right knee–flexed during the midstance phase of gait cycle. He abnormally has increased deep tendon reflexes in all limbs and an exaggerated jaw jerk reflex. His sensory examination is normal.

Regarding the case, what are the clinical features that are most supportive of an ALS diagnosis?

1. Progressive motor deficits
2. Asymmetric weakness pattern
3. Split hand pattern of weakness in right hand (ie, greater involvement of the thenar/lateral hand then of the hypothenar/medial hand intrinsic muscles)[1]
4. Combination of upper and lower motor neuron clinical features
5. All of the above

Answer: 5.

Discussion

At different stages in their disease, ALS patients have different functional limitations to be addressed. At this early stage, the patient remains independent for ambulation, but his right leg stiffness and muscle spasms are causing him pain and decreasing his walking endurance. In addition to following American Academy of Neurology guidelines regarding management and care of the patient with ALS, personalized consideration is needed for his upper motor neuron features that include right leg muscle spasticity. Spasticity refers to a velocity-dependent increase in muscle tone. This is demonstrated in Video 3 as there is normal tone with slow passive range of motion of the knee but a clear spastic catch and release near the end range on a more rapid passive motion (see Video 3). This can be graded and monitored most commonly with the Modified Ashworth Scale.[28] Symptomatic treatment of spasticity should be goal directed. In this case, the goals are to decrease painful muscle spasms and improve his stiff-legged gait pattern. Conservative treatment with skilled physical therapy that includes stretching and education on proper limb positioning and relaxation techniques should be offered as first-line therapy. Currently there are 4 FDA-approved prescription oral agents for the management of spasticity:

1. Baclofen (γ-aminobutyric acid $[GABA]_B$ receptor agonist)
2. Tizanidine (α_2-adrenergic agonist)
3. Dantrolene (blocks the release of Ca^{++} from the sarcoplasmic reticulum in muscle)
4. Diazepam (facilitates activation of $GABA_A$ receptor subtype)

Which antispasticity oral medication should be offered to this patient?
Answer: 1.

Summary

There is no high-quality evidence to choose 1 class of antispasticity agent over another in ALS. In ALS multidisciplinary clinics, however, the most common antispasticity medication is baclofen[29,30] The initial dose is 5 mg to 10 mg, 2 to 3 times a day, and can be titrated up to 20 mg, 4 times a day, but the highest doses rarely are needed for ALS. In addition, for this case, the relatively low normal blood pressure value is an argument against selecting tizanidine. Tizanidine is in the same drug class as common antihypertensive medications, such as clonidine, and therefore could increase risk for orthostatic hypotension. In theory, dantrolene has the lowest risk of central nervous system side effects because its mechanism of action is peripheral, but in practice it is rarely used in ALS patients over concerns that it exacerbates weakness and its association with hepatic toxicity.[31] Diazepam tends to be avoided due to concerns for respiratory depression.[30]

SUPPLEMENTARY DATA

Supplementary data to this article can be found online at https://doi.org/10.1016/j.ncl.2020.03.013.

REFERENCES

1. Miller RG, Jackson CE, Kasarskis EJ, et al. Practice parameter update: the care of the patient with amyotrophic lateral sclerosis: drug, nutritional, and respiratory therapies (an evidence-based review): report of the Quality Standards Subcommittee of the American Academy of Neurology. Neurology 2009;73(15):1218–26.
2. Bourke SC, Tomlinson M, Williams TL, et al. Effects of non-invasive ventilation on survival and quality of life in patients with amyotrophic lateral sclerosis: a randomised controlled trial. Lancet Neurol 2006;5(2):140–7.
3. Hanayama K, Ishikawa Y, Bach JR. Amyotrophic lateral sclerosis. Successful treatment of mucous plugging by mechanical insufflation-exsufflation. Am J Phys Med Rehabil 1997;76(4):338–9.
4. Lechtzin N, Wolfe LF, Frick KD. The impact of high-frequency chest wall oscillation on healthcare use in patients with neuromuscular diseases. Ann Am Thorac Soc 2016;13(6):904–9.
5. Boitano LJ. Management of airway clearance in neuromuscular disease. Respir Care 2006;51(8):913–22 [discussion: 22–4].
6. Jackson CE, McVey AL, Rudnicki S, et al. Symptom management and end-of-life care in amyotrophic lateral sclerosis. Neurol Clin 2015;33(4):889–908.
7. Squires N, Humberstone M, Wills A, et al. The use of botulinum toxin injections to manage drooling in amyotrophic lateral sclerosis/motor neurone disease: a systematic review. Dysphagia 2014;29(4):500–8.
8. Assouline A, Levy A, Abdelnour-Mallet M, et al. Radiation therapy for hypersalivation: a prospective study in 50 amyotrophic lateral sclerosis patients. Int J Radiat Oncol Biol Phys 2014;88(3):589–95.
9. Swinnen B, Robberecht W. The phenotypic variability of amyotrophic lateral sclerosis. Nat Rev Neurol 2014;10(11):661–70.
10. Korner S, Sieniawski M, Kollewe K, et al. Speech therapy and communication device: impact on quality of life and mood in patients with amyotrophic lateral sclerosis. Amyotroph Lateral Scler Frontotemporal Degener 2013;14(1):20–5.
11. Beukelman D, Fager S, Nordness A. Communication support for people with ALS. Neurol Res Int 2011;2011:714693.
12. Hanson EK, Beukelman DR, Yorkston KM. Communication support through multimodal supplementation: a scoping review. Augment Altern Commun 2013;29(4):310–21.
13. Brownlee A, Palovcak M. The role of augmentative communication devices in the medical management of ALS. NeuroRehabilitation 2007;22(6):445–50.

14. Plowman EK. Is there a role for exercise in the management of bulbar dysfunction in amyotrophic lateral sclerosis? J Speech Lang Hear Res 2015;58(4):1151–66.
15. Desport JC, Preux PM, Truong TC, et al. Nutritional status is a prognostic factor for survival in ALS patients. Neurology 1999;53(5):1059–63.
16. Marin B, Desport JC, Kajeu P, et al. Alteration of nutritional status at diagnosis is a prognostic factor for survival of amyotrophic lateral sclerosis patients. J Neurol Neurosurg Psychiatry 2011;82(6):628–34.
17. Dorst J, Ludolph AC, Huebers A. Disease-modifying and symptomatic treatment of amyotrophic lateral sclerosis. Ther Adv Neurol Disord 2018;11. 1756285617734734.
18. ProGas Study Group. Gastrostomy in patients with amyotrophic lateral sclerosis (ProGas): a prospective cohort study. Lancet Neurol 2015;14(7):702–9.
19. Yang B, Shi X. Percutaneous endoscopic gastrostomy versus fluoroscopic gastrostomy in amyotrophic lateral sclerosis (ALS) sufferers with nutritional impairment: a meta-analysis of current studies. Oncotarget 2017;8(60):102244–53.
20. EFNS Task Force on Diagnosis and Management of Amyotrophic Lateral Sclerosis, Andersen PM, Abrahams S, Borasio GD, et al. EFNS guidelines on the clinical management of amyotrophic lateral sclerosis (MALS)–revised report of an EFNS task force. Eur J Neurol 2012;19(3):360–75.
21. Cummings JL, Arciniegas DB, Brooks BR, et al. Defining and diagnosing involuntary emotional expression disorder. CNS Spectr 2006;11(S6):1–7.
22. Gallagher JP. Pathologic laughter and crying in ALS: a search for their origin. Acta Neurol Scand 1989;80(2):114–7.
23. Schiffer R, Pope LE. Review of pseudobulbar affect including a novel and potential therapy. J Neuropsychiatry Clin Neurosci 2005;17(4):447–54.
24. Finegan E, Chipika RH, Li Hi Shing S, et al. Pathological crying and laughing in motor neuron disease: pathobiology, screening, intervention. Front Neurol 2019; 10:260.
25. Pioro EP, Brooks BR, Cummings J, et al. Dextromethorphan plus ultra low-dose quinidine reduces pseudobulbar affect. Ann Neurol 2010;68(5):693–702.
26. Smith R, Pioro E, Myers K, et al. Enhanced bulbar function in amyotrophic lateral sclerosis: the nuedexta treatment trial. Neurotherapeutics 2017;14(3):762–72.
27. Green JR, Allison KM, Cordella C, et al. Additional evidence for a therapeutic effect of dextromethorphan/quinidine on bulbar motor function in patients with amyotrophic lateral sclerosis: A quantitative speech analysis. Br J Clin Pharmacol 2018;84(12):2849–56.
28. Bohannon RW, Smith MB. Interrater reliability of a modified Ashworth scale of muscle spasticity. Phys Ther 1987;67(2):206–7.
29. Mayadev AS, Weiss MD, Distad BJ, et al. The amyotrophic lateral sclerosis center: a model of multidisciplinary management. Phys Med Rehabil Clin N Am 2008; 19(3):619–31, xi.
30. Rocha JA, Reis C, Simoes F, et al. Diagnostic investigation and multidisciplinary management in motor neuron disease. J Neurol 2005;252(12):1435–47.
31. Utili R, Boitnott JK, Zimmerman HJ. Dantrolene-associated hepatic injury. Incidence and character. Gastroenterology 1977;72(4 Pt 1):610–6.

Therapeutic and Diagnostic Challenges in Myasthenia Gravis

Thy Nguyen, MD[a,*], Cecile L. Phan, MD[b], Emilio Supsupin Jr, MD[c], Kazim Sheikh, MD[d]

KEYWORDS

• Neuromuscular junction disorder • Myasthenia gravis • Ptosis • Weakness

KEY POINTS

- A proportion of patients with double-seronegative myasthenia gravis (MG) will carry antibodies to low-density lipoprotein receptor-related protein 4 (LRP4). Patients with LRP4-MG typically have a benign course and respond to treatments similar to patients with acetylcholine receptor (AChR).
- The course of pregnant patients with MG is highly variable. Optimal care of patients with MG of childbearing age includes prepregnancy planning, regular obstetric follow-up, multidisciplinary care for labor, and close post-partum observation/management.
- Patients with refractory MG are defined by lack of response to traditional therapy and/or continued manifestations of the disease despite adequate treatment. Eculizumab is an appropriate therapeutic modality to consider in patients with refractory AChR.
- Thymic abnormalities are common in patients with MG. Thymomas can be detected in 10% to 15% of patients with MG. Thymectomy is the treatment of choice for thymomatous MG. For nonthymomatous, early onset, AChR MG, thymectomy has recently been proved to be beneficial within 5 years of disease onset. Benefit of thymectomy in seronegative patients and patients with muscle-specific tyrosine kinase (MuSK) MG and LRP4-MG is uncertain.
- Patients with MuSK MG display a distinct clinical phenotype, involving a predilection for weakness in bulbar, neck, and proximal arm muscles. The pathophysiology is believed to be immunoglobulin G4–mediated disease, hence treatment responses differ. Patients with MuSK MG respond to plasma exchange, corticosteroids, and rituximab. Their course may be more refractory. They have less clinical response to acetylcholinesterase inhibitors and intravenous immunoglobulin than their AChR MG counterparts.

[a] Department of Neurology, McGovern Medical School, University of Texas Houston Health Science Center, 6431 Fannin Street, MSE R 462, Houston, TX 77030, USA; [b] 7-125 Clinical Sciences Building, 2J2.00 WC Mackenzie Health Sciences Centre, 8440 112 St. NW, Edmonton, Alberta, T6G 2R7 Canada; [c] Department of Diagnostic and Interventional Imaging, 6431 Fannin St. 2.103 MSMB, Houston, Texas 77030, USA; [d] Department of Neurology, McGovern Medical School, University of Texas Houston Health Science Center, 6431 Fannin street, MSE R454 Houston, TX 77030, USA

* Corresponding author.

E-mail address: thy.p.nguyen@uth.tmc.edu

Neurol Clin 38 (2020) 577–590
https://doi.org/10.1016/j.ncl.2020.03.005
0733-8619/20/Published by Elsevier Inc.

INTRODUCTION

Myasthenia gravis (MG) is the most common autoimmune neuromuscular disorder. This article highlights several cases that the practicing neurologist may encounter in the treatment of MG. Diagnostic uncertainty continues to be an issue in patients who are seronegative to the 2 most common antibodies, acetylcholine receptor (AChR) and muscle-specific tyrosine kinase (MuSK). Specific populations of patients with MG, including, MuSK MG, thymomatous MG, refractory MG, and pregnant women, also require special consideration. This article reviews unique cases and an update on current management.

CASE 1: RECURRENT PTOSIS AFTER OCULOPLASTIC SURGERY

Clinical Presentation

A 62-year-old man presented with asymmetric, right eyelid ptosis for 5 years. He underwent corrective cosmetic ptosis surgery 5 months before his evaluation. After a few weeks, he noticed the ptosis had recurred. He also reported occasional diplopia that seems skewed, fluctuating, and improved with closing either eye. He denied dysarthria, dysphagia, dyspnea, or limb weakness.

Neurologic Examination

On neurologic examination, right eye ptosis is noted and worsens within 1 minute of sustained upgaze. After 5-minute ice pack test, ptosis improved significantly (**Fig. 1**). There is also diplopia on sustained upgaze that seems skewed after 15 seconds. Otherwise, he has full strength in his facial and limb muscles without fatigability.

Diagnostic Studies

Laboratory studies were negative for AChR antibodies. Single-fiber electromyography (SFEMG) was performed, which showed abnormal jitter (**Fig. 2**).

Question 1: what is considered the most sensitive diagnostic test for MG?

1. AChR antibodies
2. MuSK antibodies
3. Repetitive nerve stimulation
4. SFEMG

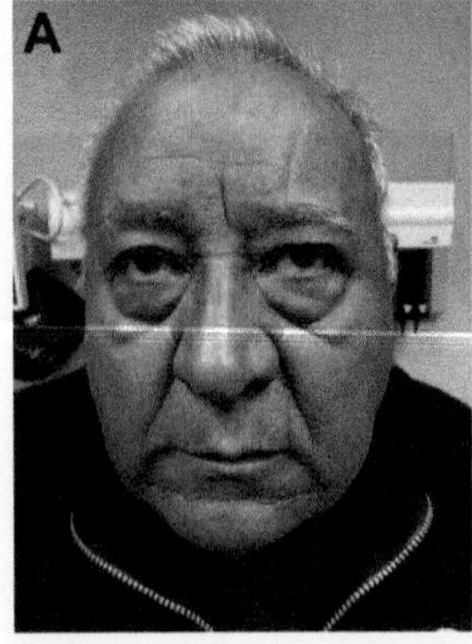

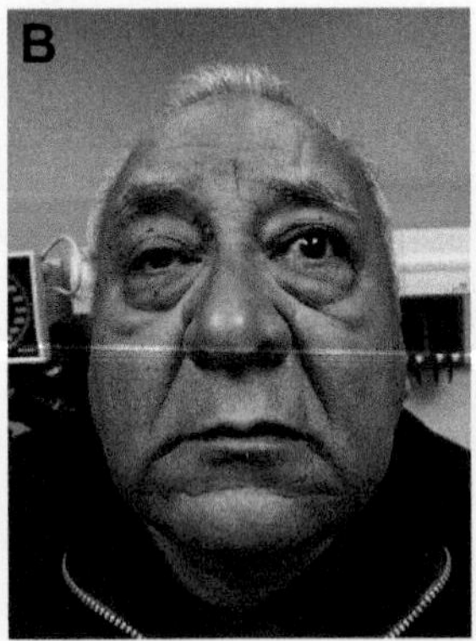

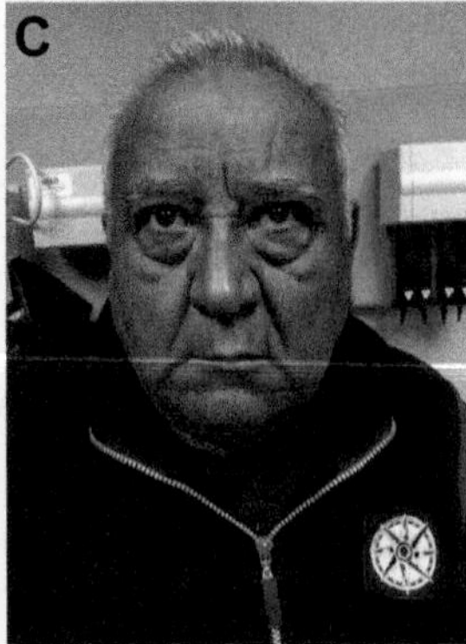

Fig. 1. (*A*) Patient's appearance at baseline. (*B*) Enhanced ptosis of the right eyelid after sustained upgaze for 60 seconds. (*C*) Resolution of enhanced ptosis after 5-minute ice-pack test.

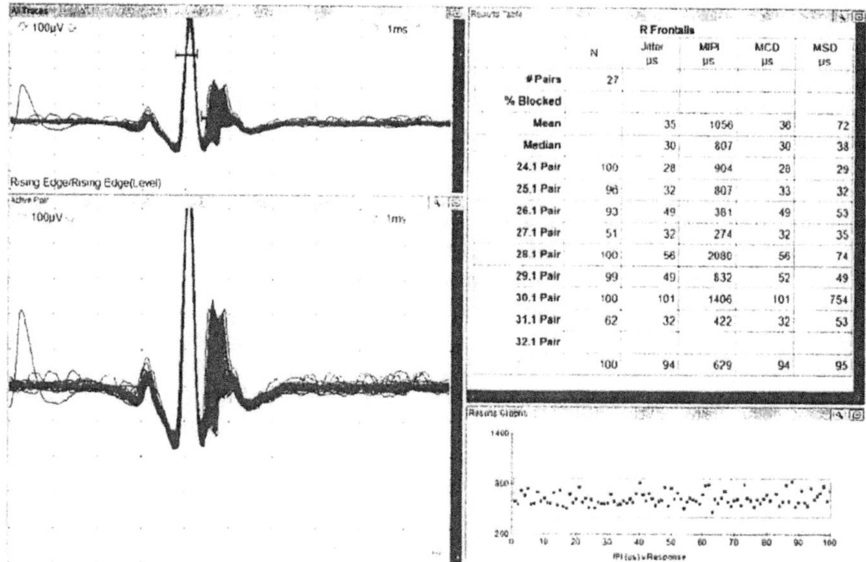

100µV
1ms
Rising Edge/Rising Edge(Level)
100µV
1ms
R Frontalis
N
Jitter µs
MIPI µs
MCD µs
MSD µs
#Pairs 27
% Blocked
Mean 35 1056 36 72
Median 30 807 30 38
24.1 Pair 100 28 904 28 29
25.1 Pair 98 32 807 33 32
26.1 Pair 93 49 381 49 53
27.1 Pair 51 32 274 32 35
28.1 Pair 100 56 2080 56 74
29.1 Pair 99 49 832 52 49
30.1 Pair 100 101 1406 101 754
31.1 Pair 62 32 422 32 53
32.1 Pair
100 94 679 94 95
1400
800
200
0 10 20 30 40 50 60 70 80 90 100

Fig. 2. Variability of occurrence of the second potential compared with triggering potential, significantly higher than the upper limit of normal in concentric jitter individual pairs collected from the frontalis muscle.

Discussion/Answer

Besides the clinical examination, there are several ancillary diagnostic tests available to confirm MG. AChR antibodies are present in up to 85% of patients with generalized MG but in only 50% of patients with pure ocular symptoms. MuSK antibodies are present in up to 40% to 60% of patients with AChR-negative MG and in approximately 6% to 7% of all patients with MG. They very rarely exist in purely ocular MG. Repetitive nerve stimulation sensitivity varies, with ranges of 50% to 85% depending on the number of muscle/nerve pairs studied, as well as the physiologic\state of muscle during testing (baseline or postexercise exhaustion).[1,2] SFEMG is considered the most sensitive, diagnostic confirmatory test for MG, with up to 99% sensitivity in a clinically weak muscle.[3] Sensitivity of SFEMG depends on the type of needle used, concentric or single fiber. In addition, sensitivity will vary based on the muscle selected and experience of the operator.[4]

Clinical Course

SFEMG confirmed the clinical diagnosis of ocular MG. The patient was initially tried on pyridostigmine. He did not respond to treatment. Because ptosis was significantly affecting his quality of life and limiting his driving, prednisone was discussed as an additional option for treatment. Given the significant side-effect profile of prednisone, the patient wanted to do further testing if possible to confirm his diagnosis.

Diagnostic Studies

The patient's serum was sent for low-density lipoprotein receptor-related protein 4 (LRP4) antibodies, which were positive.

Discussion

Two-thirds of patients with MG present with ocular symptoms. Most will develop generalized MG within the first 2 years. After 2 to 3 years of pure ocular symptoms, it is less likely to develop generalized disease. The initial therapy is usually acetylcholinesterase inhibitors such as pyridostigmine. However, pyridostigmine may alleviate symptoms of ptosis more than diplopia. For diplopia, prednisone is considered effective in greater than 80% of patients with ocular MG.[5] In addition, some centers believe that initiation of prednisone may reduce the rate of secondary generalization. A retrospective case series revealed that 50% of untreated (prednisone-naïve) patients with ocular MG developed generalized symptoms, whereas only 13% of prednisone-treated patients ocular MG generalized.[6]

Anti-LRP4 antibodies have recently been detected in a portion of patients with double-seronegative MG (DSNMG) who do not carry AChR or MuSK antibodies.[7–9] Together with agrin, LPR4 plays an important role in neuromuscular junction formation, maintenance, and MuSK activation. The sensitivity of LRP4 antibodies in patients with DSNMG varies from 0% to 50% in several series.[7,10,11] However, in patients with DSNMG with only ocular symptoms, the sensitivity of LRP4 antibodies is estimated up to 34%. The wide variation in sensitivity is likely due to ethnicity or antibody detection techniques. Patients with LRP4-MG generally have milder disease, with most presenting with Myasthenia Gravis Foundation of America class 1 or 2 status.[10,11] Response rate to acetylcholinesterase inhibitors and/or prednisone is greater than 90%.[11]

The abovementioned patient was counseled on the confirmation of ocular MG diagnosis with SFEMG and positive LRP-4 antibodies. The good prognosis and response to treatment were also discussed. The patient opted to undergo treatment with prednisone, and his ocular symptoms improved with a dose of 10 mg daily.

CASE 2: RAPID PRESENTATION OF MYASTHENIA GRAVIS SYMPTOMS

Clinical Presentation

A 42-year-old, previously healthy, woman presented to clinic with 2 weeks of visual symptoms. She reported onset of blurry vision, followed by binocular diplopia, which worsened with fatigue or stress. Her symptoms were significantly better on awakening. She also reported drooping of the left eyelid. She subsequently developed limb weakness and difficulty lifting her head over the next 2 weeks. The patient did not endorse dysarthria, dysphagia, or dyspnea.

Neurologic Examination

Cranial nerve examination revealed left eye ptosis after sustained upgaze of 10 seconds. This significantly improved with rest and ice pack test. She was also noted to have right exophoria on cover-uncover testing. Otherwise, the remaining cranial nerve examination was unremarkable. She had mild weakness of neck extension that was fatigable but had full strength in all other limb muscles without fatigability.

Diagnostic Testing

AChR-binding antibodies were positive, 7.7 nmol per liter. Normal values are less than 0.3 nmol per liter. Computed tomography (CT) of the chest was ordered (**Fig. 3**).

Clinical Course

She was referred to an oncology center with extensive experience in treating thymoma. After multidisciplinary planning, the decision was made to initiate chemotherapy before resection due to the concern for invasive nature of the thymic mass

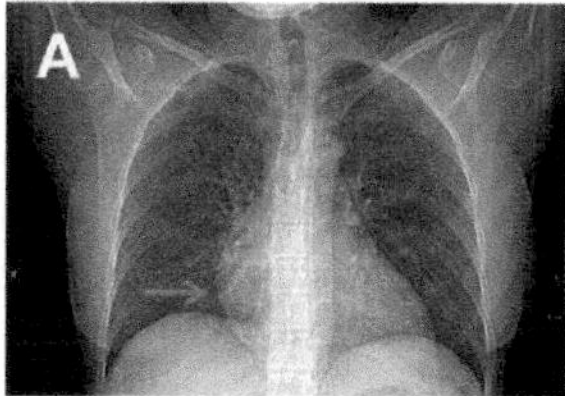

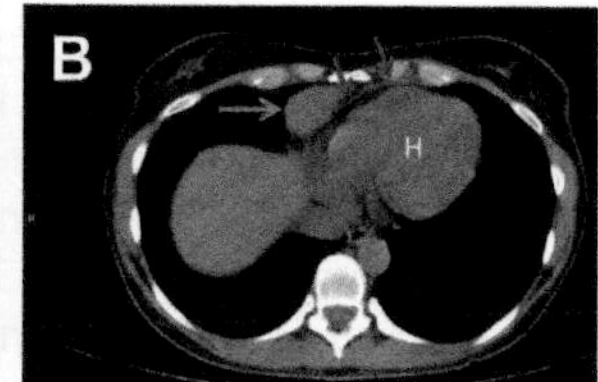

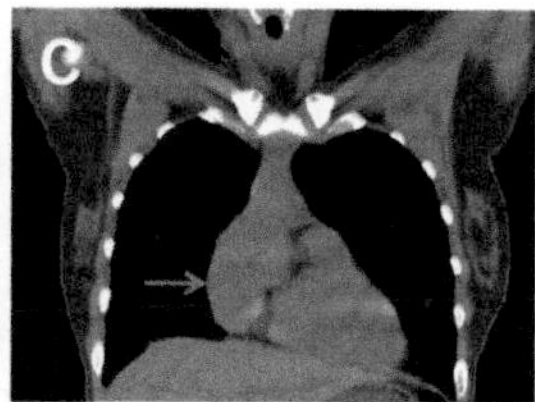

Fig. 3. (*A, C*) Chest radiograph and coronal view of CT chest demonstrates fullness of the cardiac silhouette. (*B*) CT chest without contrast revealed a large 6.7 × 4.5 × 11.2 cm mass inseparable from the thymus. On axial view, red arrows depict pericardium and blue arrows depict anterior mediastinal mass. H indicates the heart.

in the pericardium. She underwent 4 cycles of chemotherapy with cyclophosphamide, doxorubicin, cisplatin, and prednisone. Following chemotherapy, the tumor size was reduced to 5 × 3 cm on imaging. She subsequently underwent thymectomy (**Fig. 4**). Pathology revealed World Health Organization stage 1 (noninvasive) thymoma with B3 histology type (predominantly epithelial cells having a round or polygonal shape and exhibiting no or mild atypia, admixed with a minor component of lymphocytes).

Question 1: what is the most common thymic finding in patients with MG?

1. Normal thymus
2. Thymic atrophy
3. Thymic hyperplasia
4. Thymoma

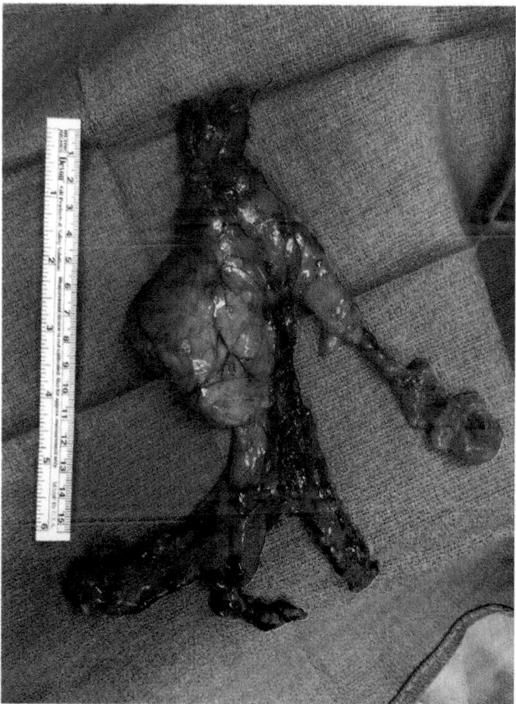

Fig. 4. Gross pathology of the thymus (image taken during surgery).

Discussion

As early as the 1930s, thymectomy was considered as a treatment modality for MG.[12] The thymus gland was considered as a major pathologic cause of MG for several reasons. First, most patients with AChR MG have thymic abnormalities. Thymic hyperplasia is the most common thymic abnormality found in MG, in up to 70%. Thymoma is found in 10% to 15% of patients with MG. Involuted thymus may be found in older patients. Second, pathologic evaluation of thymus reveals follicular hyperplasia or ectopic B-cell germinal centers particularly in early onset MG. Third, removal of the thymus in thymomatous and nonthymomatous AChR-positive MG has been shown to improve outcomes.[13–15] For certain nonthymomatous MG subgroups, such as seronegative, LRP4, MUSK, late-onset, and pure ocular disease, benefit of thymectomy is uncertain.[16–19]

For thymomatous MG, thymectomy is the standard of care. A large retrospective case series of 197 patients with thymomatous MG revealed no clinical or pathologic features that predicted outcome of complete stable remission (CSR). Overall, about 10% of patients with thymomatous MG achieved CSR. The rate of recurrence following thymectomy in thymomatous MG was 10%. Recurrence occurred from 3 to 29 years following the initial surgery. The type of procedure (video assisted or transcervical thymectomy) was not a predictor of recurrence. Patients with stage 1 or noninvasive disease had a lower likelihood of recurrence, only 3.5%. Overall, this study showed that patients with thymomatous MG had a more severe disease course than nonthymomatous MG. They were less likely to achieve CSR following thymectomy.[20]

Following the surgery, the patient did well and became asymptomatic.

CASE 3: A WOMAN WHO BECAME WEAK WHILE SHE WAS PREGNANT

A 21-year-old woman presented to the emergency room for diplopia, weakness, and difficulty speaking. She had just given birth to her first child 2 weeks previously. She states that her pregnancy and delivery were uneventful except she noticed weakness in her arms and legs around her third trimester. She had difficulty lifting her arms over her head. She underwent CT spine imaging by her obstetrician, which was normal. Her symptoms worsened following her delivery. She reported dysarthria and diplopia in addition to her limb weakness.

Neurologic Examination

On cranial nerve examination, there was no ptosis. She noted horizontal, binocular diplopia immediately on lateral gaze. Limitation of bilateral ocular abduction was noted. She had weak bilateral orbicularis oculi and oris muscles. There was mild labial dysarthria.

Strength examination showed fatigable, proximal and symmetric weakness was worse in the upper extremities.

Diagnostic Testing

Serology for AChR antibodies was sent. EMG and nerve conduction studies with repetitive nerve stimulation were performed (**Fig. 5**).

Clinical Course

The patient was diagnosed with MG. She was started on prednisone and pyridostigmine. Serology for AChR antibodies was negative. She was subsequently positive for anti-MuSK antibodies. Her symptoms continued to deteriorate leading to dyspnea.

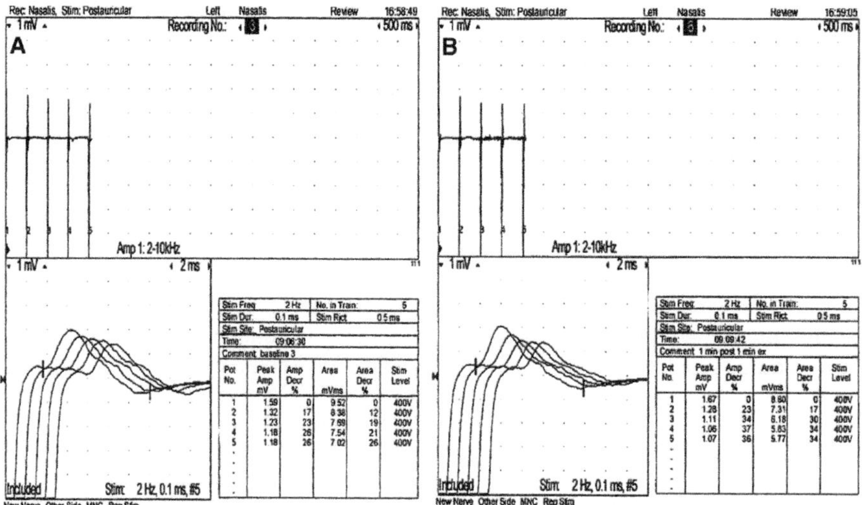

Fig. 5. (*A*) Repetitive nerve stimulation of the facial nerve was performed in trains of 5 stimuli at 2 Hz with the muscle at rest. On this baseline study, significant decrement of greater than 20% was noted. (*B*) After long exercise of 1 minute, the facial nerve and nasalis muscle nerve pair were again studied with trains of 5 stimuli at 2 HZ. Note the worsening decrement greater than 30% following long exercise, consistent with postexercise exhaustion.

She was hospitalized and required intubation for myasthenic crisis. She was treated with plasma exchange and improved after 5 courses of plasma exchange.

Question 1: which of the following statements are true regarding MG and pregnancy?

a. Prednisone should be discontinued in most patients with MG who become pregnant.
b. Patients with MG should undergo cesarean section because of the weakness of striated muscle that occurs during the second stage of labor.
c. Intravenous immunoglobulin (IVIG) is considered the treatment of choice during an acute myasthenic crisis in a pregnant woman.
d. The treatment of eclampsia is the same in pregnant women with or without MG.

Discussion

MG is bimodal in frequency and occurs in young women and older men. Given its frequency in women of childbearing age, neurologists will often encounter management issues in pregnant women with MG.

As in this case, patients can display initial symptoms of MG during pregnancy.[21] However, for most of them, the diagnosis is known before pregnancy.[21] During pregnancy, the course of MG varies significantly and is difficult to predict. Symptoms can deteriorate, improve, or remain unchanged.[22] MG exacerbations may be more likely in the post-partum state or first trimester. This may be due to the protective effects of alpha fetoprotein, which are highest in second and third trimesters.[22] Sleep deprivation and stress associated with caring for a newborn can also add additional risk for exacerbation.

Treatment decisions for pregnant patients with MG are made on a case-by-case basis, weighing the risks of worsening myasthenia symptoms and medication adverse effects. In general, prednisone and pyridostigmine should be continued at the lowest effective dose to avoid risk of exacerbation (**Table 1**). Although prednisone carries some risk of increased cleft palate with exposure during the first trimester, most clinicians believe the risk of myasthenic crisis due to sudden discontinuation is more concerning.[23] In optimal situations, women of childbearing age will not be on medications with known teratogenicity such as mycophenolate mofetil, methotrexate, cyclosporine, or cyclophosphamide. In general, these medications should be discontinued up to 6 months before planned conception.[24] If exacerbations occur despite treatment with prednisone, IVIG is considered the treatment of choice. Plasma exchange can be used if close maternal-fetal fluid monitoring occurs.[24,25]

Myasthenia can theoretically affect striated muscle during active labor. However, most obstetricians and neurologists agree that vaginal delivery is optimal and can be safely performed unless there is a specific obstetric indication.[24,25] However, retrospective data reveal a high rate of cesarean section in patients with MG, up to 66%.[26] Regional or spinal anesthesia is preferred during labor. General anesthesia and nondepolarizing muscle relaxants should be avoided if possible.

Magnesium should be avoided in treatment of eclampsia in myasthenic women. Magnesium inhibits presynaptic release of acetylcholine and can worsen MG symptoms. Phenytoin or barbiturates can be used to treat seizures.[24]

Table 1
Recommendations and management considerations at each stage of pregnancy

Stage	Recommendations
Planning for pregnancy	Discuss childbearing plans at every juncture of considering immunomodulators Stop teratogenic immunomodulators at least 3–6 mo in advance of conception[24] Counsel patients on double-barrier method of conception if on teratogenic immunomodulators. Avoid teratogenic immunomodulators in women with childbearing plans if possible. Treat MG with goal of complete remission, pharmacologic remission, or minimal manifestation state.
During pregnancy	Continue prednisone at the lowest effective dose. (The risks of MG worsening are considered greater than the risk of cleft palate from prednisone exposure in the first trimester).[23,24] Continue acetylcholinesterase inhibitors.[24] Close follow-up with counseling that MG can be highly variable during pregnancy but does not usually worsen in the second and third trimesters.[22]
Labor and delivery	Patients with MG can generally deliver via vaginal delivery.[21,22,25,27] Caesarean section is recommended if there are obstetric indications.[24,25] Regional and spinal anesthesia is preferred.[24,25] Magnesium should be avoided. Seizures can be treated with phenytoin or phenobarbital.[24] Pyridostigmine can be converted to IV form in a 1:30 ratio. (60 mg of oral pyridostigmine is 2 mg of intravenous pyridostigmine).
Post-partum	Prednisone can be continued if breastfeeding.[24] Pyridostigmine can be continued during breastfeeding, but watch for signs of neonatal gastrointestinal distress.[24] Neonates require close monitoring for signs of transient MG. Pregnancy-related MG exacerbations are more likely to happen in post-partum period.[22]

CASE 4: A YOUNG MAN WITH MYASTHENIA GRAVIS AND A COMPLEX COURSE OF TREATMENTS

Case: a 22-year-old man presents for continuing care and treatment of MG. He was diagnosed at age 19 years. His initial presentation was dysphagia, dysarthria, and dyspnea, which subsequently led to 2 intensive care unit (ICU) admissions in the first few months. In the first ICU admission, the patient was diagnosed with respiratory failure and aspiration pneumonia and discharged without a neuromuscular diagnosis. On the second ICU admission, he was diagnosed with MG based on clinical symptoms, bedside edrophonium test, and electrodiagnostic testing. His diagnosis was subsequently confirmed by the presence of high-titer AChR antibodies. He was treated with plasma exchange during his crisis with significant benefit. He was also started on acetylcholinesterase inhibitors.

He underwent transsternal thymectomy1 month subsequent to his diagnosis. This was complicated by lung collapse requiring chest tube. He then started high-dose prednisone up to 80 mg daily. Three months after initiation of high-dose steroids, he was diagnosed with cytomegalovirus hepatitis. He also had multiple intercurrent respiratory infections. He then started methotrexate as a steroid-sparing agent. Over the next 18 months azathioprine was titrated up to 3 mg per kilogram per day. He was unable to wean high-dose prednisone. He started to develop significant lower back pain. After 18 months of treatment with azathioprine medication was stopped due to lack of efficacy, as he continued to require high-dose steroids and did not tolerate attempts to wean prednisone. He subsequently started mycophenolate mofetil at goal dose of 1000 mg twice daily. He saw a spine specialist who found severe osteoporosis and multiple compression fractures. He now presents for a second opinion regarding treatment.

Examination

The patient displays significant labial, lingual, and guttural dysarthria. He did not have ptosis on sustained upgaze or subjective diplopia on lateral gaze. He had moderate, symmetric, proximal weakness with fatigability.

Question 1: what is considered the most common period to develop myasthenic crisis?

1. First 2 years after diagnosis
2. 3 to 4 years after diagnosis
3. 5 to 6 years after diagnosis
4. 7 to 8 years after diagnosis

Discussion

Based on epidemiologic studies, it is more common to develop myasthenic crisis in the first 2 years of the diagnosis.[28] Myasthenic crisis is defined as respiratory failure requiring artificial ventilation or difficulty swallowing leading to failure to protect the airway.[29]

Patient Course

Patient had a complicated course of MG although multiple mechanisms of treatment were trialed. There was an urgent need to reduce high-dose steroids, given severe osteoporosis and compression fractures at a young age. He underwent the following treatment modalities including serial plasma exchange, intravenous immunoglobulin, and rituximab treatment. Despite these treatment modalities, patient was unable to completely wean off prednisone.

The patient was deemed to have refractory MG. He was started on eculizumab after receiving meningococcal vaccinations. After 4 infusions, the patient started to notice a significant improvement in his MG symptoms. He was eventually able to wean off prednisone.

Discussion

An estimated 15% of patients may be categorized as refractory MG.[30] These patients develop significant adverse effects to immunotherapy or remain symptomatic despite adequate therapy and/or relapse when immunotherapy is weaned. Younger age of onset, female gender, and positive anti-MuSK antibodies have been identified as risk factors in developing refractory disease.[30]

The Food and Drug Administration) approved eculizumab as a treatment of patients with positive AChR MG in 2018. Eculizumab is a monoclonal, humanized antibody directed against C5 protein. It leads to reduced formation of C5b, which plays a role in membrane attack complex formation. This approval was based on a randomized, placebo-controlled, clinical trial studying eculizumab in a refractory, positive AChR MG population. The trial used a primary endpoint of improvement in the MG-ADL scale. This primary endpoint did not reach statistical significance. However, on post-hoc analysis, it was felt that this was an error of worst rank-ANCOVA analytical technique. Worst-rank ANCOVA assigns a worst rank to any patient who dropped out of the study regardless of clinical status. After analyzing the clinical outcome of 3 patients who dropped out of the study in the eculizumab arm, due to reasons unrelated to MG or treatment, eculizumab treatment met the outcome of clinical improvement. Improvement began at week 2, usually detected by week 12 and was sustained throughout the 26 week study.[31]

The patient did well on eculizumab and is currently continuing the medication. Overall, 45% of patients on eculizumab responded with an improvement of 5 points or more based on Quantitative Myasthenia Gravis score analysis. Cost and insurance coverage may limit widespread use. Further clinical trials are needed for effective management options in patients with refractory MG.

CASE 5: A WOMAN WITH ANTI-MUSCLE-SPECIFIC TYROSINE KINASE MYASTHENIA GRAVIS THAT DID NOT RESPOND TO CONVENTIONAL TREATMENT

A 40-year-old patient presents for continuation of care regarding her anti-MuSK MG. The patient presented at age 35 years with symptoms of diplopia, dyspnea, bulbar, and neck weakness. She was diagnosed with MG based on antibody testing and clinical examination. She reports improvement to high-dose prednisone, 60 mg daily, but does not like the side effects of weight gain. She also has concurrent psychiatric diagnoses of bipolar disorder, posttraumatic stress disorder, and anxiety. She developed an allergic reaction to azathioprine. She did not respond to intravenous immunoglobulin. This was previously administered during a myasthenia exacerbation. She responded well to plasma exchange during myasthenic exacerbations.

Examination

On cranial nerve examination, there is significant guttural and labial dysarthria. She has mild weakness of orbicularis oris. She reported binocular diplopia after 50 seconds of lateral gaze. There was no ptosis at baseline or after 1 minute of sustained upward gaze. She had neck flexion weakness of 4/5. Upper extremity testing showed proximal, symmetric deltoid and elbow flexion weakness of 4/5 with fatigability. Lower extremity strength was normal.

Course

The patient was started on rituximab intravenous infusions. Her initial dose was given at 1000 mg, and then a few weeks later she was received subsequent rituximab infusions at 1000 mg. Her symptoms subsequently improved at the next visit and she was beginning to taper off prednisone to every other day dosing.

Question: which of the following statements are true regarding positive anti-MuSK antibody MG?

1. Patients with MuSK MG have equal response to IVIG and plasma exchange for worsening symptoms
2. Eculizumab is a treatment option for patients with refractory MuSK MG
3. MuSK MG patients tend to have a predilection for bulbar, neck, and upper extremity proximal weakness
4. Anti-MuSK MG patients have a better prognosis in regard to their overall course of MG compared with patients with AChR MG

Discussion

Anti-MuSK antibodies can be found in up to 60% of patients with AChR antibody-negative MG.[32] These patients tend to be younger women. They often present with predilection of symptoms affecting bulbar, neck, and upper extremity proximal muscles. Overall, their disease course may be more refractory.[30]

They often differ from patients with positive AChR MG in regard to their response to treatments. They may report no improvement or worsening to acetylcholinesterase inhibitors.[33] In a retrospective case series, only 20% responded to treatment with IVIG, compared with 50% response to plasma exchange.[34] Patients with MuSK MG generally improve with prednisone and plasma exchange. In addition, patients with anti-MuSK MG have a very favorable response to rituximab, a chimeric, monoclonal antibody directed at CD20 cells. In a prospective chart review, 77 of 119 patients with MuSK were included. The rituximab-treated group was significantly more likely to reach a primary outcome of a favorable postintervention status and a low dose of immunomodulators. The number needed to treat for rituximab in MuSK MG was 2.4.[35] This is postulated to be primarily due to MuSK MG's IgG4-mediated autoimmune response.[36] MuSK-MG antibody status was an independent factor for predicting treatment response to rituximab.[37] Rituximab dosing is variable. Rituximab can be dosed at 1000 mg followed by an additional 1000 mg dose 2 weeks later. However, the most commonly used rituximab dosing is 375 mg per meters squared weekly for 4 weeks with variable schedules and methods for redosing.[37] Some physicians give a second rituximab regimen only at relapse. In an extended prospective trial of rituximab-treated patients with refractory MG (both AChR and MuSK), 10 of 22 patients had a clinical relapse after the induction regimen. The average time to relapse was 17 months, showing a sustained response to the initial rituximab treatment. Unfortunately, CD19 and CD20 cells did not prove to be a reliable surrogate marker of impending relapse. Six of ten patients who relapsed continued to show prolonged B-cell depletion with CD19 less than 1%. Others give a scheduled second rituximab induction regimen after 6 months regardless of clinical status. In a retrospective case series of 16 patients with AChR MG, 4 patients received 2 cycles. Those 4 patients had a mean time to relapse of 33 months.[38,39] However, a recent multicenter, randomized, double-blind, placebo-controlled phase II clinical trial of rituximab in patients with AChR MG has been completed. Although unpublished, data are available on clinicaltrials.gov. This study showed that rituximab was futile and did not achieve the primary outcome of reducing prednisone dose by 75%. Despite the disappointing results of this phase 2 trial, rituximab continues to be an effective drug in the armamentarium of physicians treating MuSK MG.

SUMMARY

MG is the most common neuromuscular condition encountered by practicing neurologists. Caring for patients with MG is gratifying, as many patients respond well to treatment. The mortality rate for MG was historically 40%. However, most recent census data show that MG mortality rate is now less than 5%. As a plethora of clinical trials are planned or underway in MG, practitioners will be able to provide patients' improved quality of life and offer more treatment choices.

DISCLOSURE

Dr C.L. Phan acts as an advisor for Biogen, Canada. Dr T. Nguyen has no relevant financial disclosures. Dr T. Nguyen receives royalties from Springer publishing. Dr E. Supsupin has no financial disclosures to report. Dr. Sheikh is supported by U.S. Department of Defense (DoD; Award#: W81XWH-18-1-0422) and National Institute of Neurological Disorders and Stroke (NINDS; grant R21NS107961).

REFERENCES

1. Rubin DI, Hentschel K. Is exercise necessary with repetitive nerve stimulation in evaluating patients with suspected myasthenia gravis? Muscle Nerve 2007;35(1): 103–6.
2. Costa J, Evangelista T, Conceicao I, et al. Repetitive nerve stimulation in myasthenia gravis–relative sensitivity of different muscles. ClinNeurophysiol 2004; 115(12):2776–82.
3. Sanders DB, Stalberg EV. AAEMminimonograph #25: single-fiber electromyography. Muscle Nerve 1996;19(9):1069–83.
4. C N Machado F, A Kouyoumdjian J, E Marchiori P. Diagnostic accuracy of concentric needle jitter in myasthenia: Prospective study. Muscle Nerve 2017; 55(2):190–4.
5. Benatar M, McDermott MP, Sanders DB, et al. Efficacy of prednisone for the treatment of ocular myasthenia (EPITOME): A randomized, controlled trial. Muscle Nerve 2016;53(3):363–9.
6. NORDIC Idiopathic Intracranial Hypertension Study Group Writing Committee, Wall M, McDermott MP, et al. Effect of acetazolamide on visual function in patients with idiopathic intracranial hypertension and mild visual loss: the idiopathic intracranial hypertension treatment trial. JAMA 2014;311(16):1641–51.
7. Higuchi O, Hamuro J, Motomura M, et al. Autoantibodies to low-density lipoprotein receptor-related protein 4 in myasthenia gravis. Ann Neurol 2011;69(2): 418–22.
8. Pevzner A, Schoser B, Peters K, et al. Anti-LRP4 autoantibodies in AChR- and MuSK-antibody-negative myasthenia gravis. J Neurol 2012;259(3):427–35.
9. Guo Z, Meng X, Wang Y, et al. Effects of temperature, mechanical motion and source positional jitter on the resolving power of beamline02B at the SSRF. J SynchrotronRadiat 2017;24(Pt 4):877–85.
10. Li Y, Zhang Y, Cai G, et al. Anti-LRP4 autoantibodies in Chinese patients with myasthenia gravis. Muscle Nerve 2017;56(5):938–42.

11. Zisimopoulou P, Evangelakou P, Tzartos J, et al. A comprehensive analysis of the epidemiology and clinical characteristics of anti-LRP4 in myasthenia gravis. J Autoimmun 2014;52:139–45.
12. Blalock A, Mason MF, Morgan HJ, et al. Myasthenia Gravis and Tumors of the Thymic Region: Report of a Case in Which the Tumor Was Removed. Ann Surg 1939;110(4):544–61.
13. Cavalcante P, Le Panse R, Berrih-Aknin S, et al. The thymus in myasthenia gravis: Site of "innate autoimmunity"? Muscle Nerve 2011;44(4):467–84.
14. Wolfe GI, Kaminski HJ, Aban IB, et al. Long-term effect of thymectomy plus prednisone versus prednisone alone in patients with non-thymomatous myasthenia gravis: 2-year extension of the MGTXrandomised trial. Lancet Neurol 2019; 18(3):259–68.
15. Wolfe GI, Kaminski HJ, Cutter GR. Randomized Trial of Thymectomy in Myasthenia Gravis. N Engl J Med 2016;375(20):2006–7.
16. Clifford KM, Hobson-Webb LD, Benatar M, et al. Thymectomy may not be associated with clinical improvement in MuSK myasthenia gravis. Muscle Nerve 2019; 59(4):404–10.
17. Uzawa A, Kawaguchi N, Kanai T, et al. Two-year outcome of thymectomy in non-thymomatous late-onset myasthenia gravis. J Neurol 2015;262(4):1019–23.
18. Hamedani AG, Pistilli M, Singhal S, et al. Outcomes after transcervicalthymectomy for ocular myasthenia gravis: a retrospective cohort study with inverse probability weighting. J Neuroophthalmol 2020;40(1):8–14.
19. Koneczny I, Rennspiess D, Marcuse F, et al. Characterization of the thymus in Lrp4 myasthenia gravis: Four cases. Autoimmun Rev 2019;18(1):50–5.
20. Maggi L, Andreetta F, Antozzi C, et al. Thymoma-associated myasthenia gravis: outcome, clinical and pathological correlations in 197 patients on a 20-year experience. J Neuroimmunol 2008;201-202:237–44.
21. Hoff JM, Daltveit AK, Gilhus NE. Myasthenia gravis in pregnancy and birth: identifying risk factors, optimising care. Eur J Neurol 2007;14(1):38–43.
22. Batocchi AP, Majolini L, Evoli A, et al. Course and treatment of myasthenia gravis during pregnancy. Neurology 1999;52(3):447–52.
23. Park-Wyllie L, Mazzotta P, Pastuszak A, et al. Birth defects after maternal exposure to corticosteroids: prospective cohort study and meta-analysis of epidemiological studies. Teratology 2000;62(6):385–92.
24. Hamel J, Ciafaloni E. An update: myasthenia gravis and pregnancy. NeurolClin 2018;36(2):355–65.
25. Toscano M, Thornburg LL. Neurological diseases in pregnancy. CurrOpinObstet Gynecol 2019;31(2):97–109.
26. Ducci RD, Lorenzoni PJ, Kay CS, et al. Clinical follow-up of pregnancy in myasthenia gravis patients. NeuromusculDisord 2017;27(4):352–7.
27. Wen JC, Liu TC, Chen YH, et al. No increased risk of adverse pregnancy outcomes for women with myasthenia gravis: a nationwide population-based study. Eur J Neurol 2009;16(8):889–94.
28. Phillips LH 2nd. The epidemiology of myasthenia gravis. NeurolClin 1994;12(2): 263–71.
29. Sanders DB, Wolfe GI, Benatar M, et al. International consensus guidance for management of myasthenia gravis: Executive summary. Neurology 2016;87(4): 419–25.
30. Suh J, Goldstein JM, Nowak RJ. Clinical characteristics of refractory myasthenia gravis patients. Yale J Biol Med 2013;86(2):255–60.

31. Howard JF Jr, Utsugisawa K, Benatar M, et al. Safety and efficacy of eculizumab in anti-acetylcholine receptor antibody-positive refractory generalised myasthenia gravis (REGAIN): a phase 3, randomised, double-blind, placebo-controlled, multicentre study. Lancet Neurol 2017;16(12):976–86.
32. Hoch W, McConville J, Helms S, et al. Auto-antibodies to the receptor tyrosine kinase MuSK in patients with myasthenia gravis without acetylcholine receptor antibodies. Nat Med 2001;7(3):365–8.
33. Guptill JT, Sanders DB, Evoli A. Anti-MuSK antibody myasthenia gravis: clinical findings and response to treatment in two large cohorts. Muscle Nerve 2011; 44(1):36–40.
34. Pasnoor M, Wolfe GI, Nations S, et al. Clinical findings in MuSK-antibody positive myasthenia gravis: a U.S. experience. Muscle Nerve 2010;41(3):370–4.
35. Hehir MK, Hobson-Webb LD, Benatar M, et al. Rituximab as treatment for anti-MuSK myasthenia gravis: Multicenter blinded prospective review. Neurology 2017;89(10):1069–77.
36. Binks S, Vincent A, Palace J. Myasthenia gravis: a clinical-immunological update. J Neurol 2016;263(4):826–34.
37. Tandan R, Hehir MK 2nd, Waheed W, et al. Rituximab treatment of myasthenia gravis: A systematic review. Muscle Nerve 2017;56(2):185–96.
38. Beecher G, Anderson D, Siddiqi ZA. Rituximab in refractory myasthenia gravis: Extended prospective study results. Muscle Nerve 2018;58(3):452–5.
39. Robeson KR, Kumar A, Keung B, et al. Durability of the rituximab response in acetylcholine receptor autoantibody-positive myasthenia gravis. JAMA Neurol 2017;74(1):60–6.

Refractory Chronic Immune-mediated Demyelinating Polyneuropathy

Aziz Shaibani, MD[a,b,*], Husam Al Sultani, MD[a]

KEYWORDS

• Neuropathy • Demyelinating • CIDP • Refractory • Conduction block • POEMS • NF-155 • MAG antibodies

KEY POINTS

- When a patient with chronic immune-mediated demyelinating polyneuropathy (CIDP) does not respond to first-line therapies (intravenous immunoglobulin [IVIG], plasma exchange [PLEX], and steroids), it is important to revise the diagnosis in light of published diagnostic criteria. The authors prefer European Federation of Neurological Societies and Peripheral Nerve Society criteria.
- If the diagnosis is confirmed, identifying features of resistant CIDP-like syndromes must be pursued, such as polyneuropathy, organomegaly, endocrinopathy, monoclonal protein, and skin changes syndrome (POEMS); neurofascin-155 (NF-155) antibodies; and myelin-associated glycoprotein (MAG) antibody–associated diseases, because those deserve different treatment approaches.
- If the cause of poor responsiveness is aggressive CIDP, it is recommended that IVIG frequency is increased to biweekly sessions before deemed ineffective. Sometimes a combination of IVIG, PLEX, and/or steroids is needed.
- Immunosuppressive agents, such as azathioprine and monoclonal antibodies such as rituximab are the next reasonable options.

Video content accompanies this article at http://www.neurologic.theclinics.com.

INTRODUCTION

Chronic immune-mediated demyelinating polyneuropathy (CIDP) is the most common treatable neuropathy. It is an autoimmune disorder of the peripheral nerves, which, on average, affects 5 per 100,000 population.[1] There are no universally accepted diagnostic criteria; 50% of those diagnosed by community practitioners and 18% of those

[a] Nerve and Muscle Center of Texas, 6624 Fannin Street Suite 1670, Houston, TX 77030, USA;
[b] Baylor College of Medicine, Houston, TX, USA
* Corresponding author. Nerve and Muscle Center of Texas, 6624 Fannin Street Suite 1670, Houston, TX 77030.
E-mail address: ather@aol.com

Neurol Clin 38 (2020) 591–605
https://doi.org/10.1016/j.ncl.2020.03.006

enrolled in clinical trials based on expert diagnosis received a different diagnosis after further evaluation.[2] There are more than 15 sets of diagnostic criteria that vary in specificity and sensitivity, leaving room for misdiagnosis, particularly in the absence of accurate diagnostic biological markers.[3] The authors prefer the European Federation of Neurological Societies and the Peripheral Nerve Society (EFNS/PNS) criteria for this purpose.[4]

Only 50% of patients meet the diagnostic criteria of typical CIDP. This may explain why 20% of patients are refractory to first-line treatments (steroids, gamma globulins, and/or plasmapheresis).[5] Approximately half of these patients received an alternative diagnosis with further evaluation.

The Most Common Causes of Treatment Failureof Chronic Immune-mediated Demyelinating Polyneuropathy Are

- Inadequate immunosuppression
- Alternative diagnoses, including amyotrophic lateral sclerosis; small fiber neuropathy; Charcot-Marie-Tooth disease; inclusion body myositis; amyloid neuropathy; diabetic polyneuropathy; POEMS and MAG neuropathy[2]

CIDP variants like multifocal motor neuropathy and NF-155 antibodies syndrome require more aggressive therapy. Some classic cases of CIDP are associated with a more aggressive and refractory immune attack. Usually, these are associated with axonal damage.

Common Sources of Misdiagnosis Are

- A liberal interpretation of electrodiagnostic findings
- Reliance on mild cytoalbuminemic dissociation (In most CIDP cases, the cerebrospinal fluid [CSF] protein level is >100 mg/dL, and elevation are as high as 10 times the upper limit of normal occasionally are seen.)
- Putting too much emphasis on patient-reported outcome measures[2]

Although a review of the diagnostic criteria is beyond the scope of this article, a review of the cardinal feature of CIDP is important.

Cardinal Features of Chronic Immune-mediated Demyelinating Polyneuropathy Are

Clinical features

- Slowly progressive course over more than 8 weeks of the proximal and distal weakness of the upper and lower extremities
- Large fiber loss more than small fiber loss (ataxia is more pronounced than pain or dysautonomia)
- Motor symptoms more than sensory symptoms
- Diffuse areflexia
- Demyelinating findings in nerve conduction study (NCS)
- Elevated CSF protein

Cardinal Neurophysiologic Findings Are

- Prolonged distal motor latencies
- Delayed F-wave
- Motor slowing
- Conduction block
- Temporal dispersion. Distal temporal dispersion seems to be the most specific of the demyelinating features[6]

Nerve Biopsy Findings

- Segmental and paranodal demyelination
- Inflammation is seen in less than 15% of cases

Usually, nerve biopsy is unnecessary for most patients with suspected CIDP, especially those with typical electroclinical findings.

Nerve Biopsy Is Indicated In The Following Scenarios

- When other studies fail to establish the diagnosis of CIDP clearly
- When electrophysiologic criteria for demyelination are not met
- There is high suspicion for an infiltrative or vasculitis process[7]

This article includes several videos of cases of refractory CIDP referred to a tertiary neuromuscular clinic. Each case is discussed, with emphasis of the diagnosis and misdiagnosis.

CASES

Case 1

Case presentation (Video 1)

A 70-year-old woman presented with:

- A 1-year history of progressive feet and hands numbness
- Loss of balance due to sensory ataxia
- Proximal legs and arms weakness
- Elevated CSF protein (180 mg/dL)
- Frank peripheral nerves demyelination with multiple conduction blocks, temporal dispersions, prolonged distal latencies, and delayed F-wave in multiple nerves
- She responded to IVIG for a year and then to plasma exchange (PLEX)
- She relapsed several times but responded to an increasing frequency of IVIG and/or PLEX
- The last relapse did not respond to IVIG, PLEX, and intravenous methylprednisolone(IVMP), and she progressed to respiratory failure and passed away

Clinical question

The most likely diagnoses

1 Severe CIDP
2 POEMS syndrome
3 Guillain-Barré syndrome
4 NF-155 antibody–associated CIDP
5 Distal acquired demyelinating symmetric (DADS) neuropathy

Discussion

- The case illustrates the fact that some CIDP cases follow a progressive and non-responsive course from the beginning or later on. There are no clear risk factors identified to explain or predict such a drastic course.
- A recent article has suggested the benefit of bortezomib in these cases[8]
- When treating a patient with CIDP, before considering IVIG as ineffective, a biweekly regiment is to be tried[6]

- Low compound muscle action potential amplitudes and active denervation of the weak muscles identified by electromyogram (EMG) suggest an axonal injury, which is a bad prognostic factor

Case 2

Case presentation

- A 76-year-old man with 5-year history of poor balance and feet numbness
- Examination showed
  - Mild weakness of the feet extensors (4/5 MRC); normal proximal strength
  - Proprioceptive loss in the feet
  - Absent deep tendon reflexes (DTR) in the legs and arms
- CSF protein, 140 mg/dL
- NCS revealed
  - Severe prolongation of the distal motor and distal sensory latencies and normal F-wave
  - Mild motor slowing; no conduction block or temporal dispersion
  - A 3-month course of IVIG was ineffective

Clinical question

The most likely positive test is

1 Elevated vascular endothelial growth factor (VEGF) serum level
2 Elevated NF-155 antibody titer
3 Elevated urinary lead level
4 Elevated MAG antibody titer and IgM spikes
5 Elevated GM1 antibody titer

Discussion

DADSAM neuropathy

- It is a demyelinating neuropathy with IgM monoclonal gammopathy (usually IgM kappa). It is the most common paraproteinemic neuropathy
- 50% to 70% of cases have MAG antibodies. These antibodies are considered pathogenic because IgM and complement are deposited on the myelin sheath, splitting the myelin lamellae, while the adoptive transfer of patients' IgM into susceptible host animals causes sensory ataxia and reproduces the human pathology[9]
- Predominantly distal weakness (foot extensor weakness) and large fiber sensory loss (ataxia) are characteristic features
- NCS shows severe prolongation of DML and DSL with no major slowing or proximal demyelinating features
- Responds poorly to treatment with IVIG and an immunosuppressive agent. Two clinical trials of rituximab failed to show statistically significant improvement compared with placebo.
- It is important to investigate and monitor the level of the M protein. Waldenström macroglobulinemia may result from malignant transformation of the IgM monoclonal gammopathy.
- Otherwise, it may be safer to just monitor the patient clinically than to take a risk of immunomodulation

Case 3

Case presentation (Video 2A)

- A 28-year-old woman with inability to get up from a chair and with frequent falls that evolved over days
  - Those symptoms were preceded a month earlier by acute feet numbness
  - Muscle pain, cramping, hoarseness, slurred speech, double vision, poor coordination, and fatigue also were reported
- Past medical history revealed controlled diabetes mellitus (DM) and gastric sleeve surgery a week before the symptoms started
- CSF protein level was 479 mg/dL with no pleocytosis
- NCS revealed severe prolongation of distal motor latencies, severe motor slowing, temporal dispersion, and prolonged F-wave in multiple nerves and absent sensory responses in the limbs
- Brain magnetic resonance imaging (MRI) was normal
- The patient was diagnosed with CIDP
- Unfortunately, she responded only slightly and transiently to IVIG and developed severe hemolytic anemia
- Later, she mildly and transiently responded to a 5-day course of intravenous methylprednisolone, followed by a monthly booster for 3 months
- Normal immunofixation protein electrophoresis and VEGF level
- MAG antibodies were negative
- There was a noticeable improvement in function after plasmapheresis treatment, as shown in Video 2B

Case 4

Case presentation (Video 3A)

A 53-year-old man with a history of DM presented

- With progressive ataxia developed over weeks
- Ascending numbness in the hands and feet
- Weakness of the handgrips and hip flexor weakness
- Lost 10 kg
- Diffuse areflexia
- CSF protein level was 420 mg/dL
- Normal brain MRI
- NCS is shown in **Table 1**
- There was a noticeable improvement in function after rituximab treatment, as shown in Video 3B

Table 1
Nerve conduction study for case 4 showing onset, amplitude, and conduction velocity for multiple nerves of the upper and lower limbs

Nerve	Distal Latency	Amplitude	Conduction Velocity
Left peroneal motor	11.34 ms	2.2 mV	33 m/s
Left tibial motor	11.39 ms	1.8 mV	27 m/s
Left median motor	10.3 ms	5.5/2.2 mV	21 m/s
Left ulnar motor	7.47 ms	3.1 mV	34 m/s
Left sural nerve	3.55 ms	23 mV	
Right sural nerve	3.58 ms	24 mV	

Courtesy of Aziz Shaibani, MD, Nerve and Muscle Center of Texas, Houston, TX.

Clinical question

Regarding cases 3 and 4, the following tests are likely abnormal and diagnostically useful:

1 MAG antibody titer
2 NF-155 antibody titer
3 IgM level
4 VEGF level
5 IgG level

Discussion

- The electrodiagnostic findings showed demyelinating motor neuropathy. The proximal median motor conduction block is significant because this is not a conventional site for focal slowing.
- NF-155 IgG4 antibody titer was elevated, confirming the diagnosis of NF-155 antibody–associated CIDP.

Features of NF-155 antibody–associated CIDP:[10]

- NF-155 antibodies were recovered from 7% of 533 sera from CIDP patients.
- Earlier age of onset
- Cerebellar signs are common. In this case, the ataxia is much more cerebellar than sensory.
- Severe peripheral demyelination
- Very high CSF protein
- Central nervous system demyelination
- Responds less frequently to IVIG
- NF-155 is a member of the L1 family of adhesion molecules
- It is expressed at the paranodes by the terminal loops of myelin.
- It is associated with the axonal cell adhesion molecules contactin 1 and contactin-associated protein 1 (Caspr1).
- Antibodies to NF-155 block neurofascin and inhibit interaction with contactin 1/ Caspr1.
- Specifically, IgG4 binding to NF-155 causes paranode dismantling and conduction defects, surprisingly without inflammatory cell infiltration.
- Patients with neurofascin antibody–mediated CIDP have distinct pathologic features compared with patients with typical CIDP
  - Lack of macrophage infiltrates
  - Selective loss of the transverse bands at the paranodal loops
  - This kind of CIDP is strongly related to HLA-DRB1*15, which is reported in 10 of 13 patients with CIDP who were positive for anti–NF-155 compared with only 5 of 35 patients with CIDP who were negative for anti–NF-155 antibodies.
- Genetic studies showed that NF-155 glycoprotein is encoded by NFASC. Inactivation of NFASC in adult mouse cerebellar Purkinje cells causes a rapid loss of NFASC glycoproteins, which might explain the predominant cerebellar signs and symptoms associated with anti–NF-155–associated CIDP variant.
- Other causes of refractory CIPD, such as multiple myeloma, POEMS syndrome, MAG antibody syndrome, and Castleman disease, are not associated with cerebellar abnormalities.
- Take-home message: check antibodies to NF-155 in refractory CIDP, especially with cerebellar tremor.

- The best therapeutic approach to this kind of CIDP is not known but there are case reports of good response to rituximab or PLEX. The first patient responded to PLEX initially then to rituximab and the second patient responded to rituximab.

Case 5

Case presentation

A 55-year-old man with a 4-month history of

- Progressive distal numbness and proximal weakness
- Diffuse areflexia
- CSF protein level was 155 mg/mL
- The patient responded to IVSM and PLEX partially and temporarily
- He gradually needed more frequent treatments
- He developed the changes shown in Video 4

Clinical question

The most likely abnormal and diagnostically useful test:

1 VEGF level
2 MAG antibody titer
3 NF-155 antibody titer
4 Serum IgM level
5 Serum lead level

Discussion

- The video shows brownish discoloration and thickening of the skin of the hands and feet. The patient developed ascites, and computed tomography of the abdomen showed splenomegaly.
- Further testing revealed VEGF level of 486 (normal values: 31–86).
- Monoclonal gammopathy of IgA lambda-type also was found.
- He used to report to the emergency room almost weekly for abdominal paracentesis and he stopped responding to PLEX.
- The patient made full recovery after auto–peripheral blood stem cell transplantation (PBSCT)

POLYNEUROPATHY, ORGANOMEGALY, ENDOCRINOPATHY, MONOCLONAL PROTEIN, AND SKIN CHANGES SYNDROME

POEMS syndrome is a paraneoplastic neuropathy associated with osteosclerotic myeloma and is characterized by

- Peripheral neuropathy: the most prominent feature
- Organomegaly
- Endocrinopathy
- M protein (monoclonal gammopathy)
- Skin changes: hyperpigmentation, hypertrichosis, plethora, hemangiomata, and white nails

Diagnostic Criteria of Polyneuropathy, Organomegaly, Endocrinopathy, Monoclonal Protein, and Skin Changes Syndrome

A diagnosis requires meeting both mandatory major criteria (neuropathy and monoclonal gammopathy), 1 major criterion, and 1 minor criterion.[11]

- Mandatory major criteria
  1 Polyneuropathy, typically demyelinating
  2 Monoclonal plasma cell proliferative disorder
- Other major criteria
  3 Castleman disease
  4 Sclerotic bone lesions
  5 VEGF elevation
- Minor criteria
  1 Organomegaly (hepatomegaly, splenomegaly, lymphadenopathy)
  2 Extravascular volume overload (ascites, edema, pleural effusion)
  3 Endocrinopathy
  4 Skin changes
  5 Papilledema
  6 Thrombocytopenia

Compared with CIDP, POEMS syndrome is characterized by

- Affecting older patients with average age in mid-50s (CIDP affects patients in mid-40s)
- Less cranial nerve involvement (2% vs 18%)
- More muscle atrophy
- More distal weakness
- More pain (76% vs 7%): usually starts with feet pain
- More positive neuropathic sensory symptoms
- More uniform demyelination and axonal loss
- Not responding to traditional therapy
- VEGF increased—68% sensitive and 95% specific
- Thrombocytosis occurring in 50% of cases (vs 2% in CIDP)
- Auto-PBSCT is an effective treatment.[12]

Case 6

Case presentation (Video 5)

- The patient was referred because the insurance denied more IVIG despite the reported improvement by the patient
- NCS is shown in **Table 2**

Table 2
Nerve conduction study for case 6 showing onset, amplitude, and conduction velocity for multiple nerves of the upper and lower limbs

Site	Onset (ms)	Normal Onset (ms)	amplitude (mV)	Conduction Velocity (m/s)	Normal Conduction Velocity (m/s)
Left peroneal motor	Nonce recordable				
Right peroneal motor	Nonce recordable				
Right median motor	9.09	<4.6	8.06	23.57	>50
Left median motor	8.36	<4.6	9.8	21.34	>50
Left ulnar motor	7.00	<3.6	8.13	23.37	>50

Courtesy of Aziz Shaibani, MD, Nerve and Muscle Center of Texas, Houston, TX.

Clinical question
The most appropriate next steps

1. Nerve biopsy to look for demyelination/inflammation
2. Testing for hereditary demyelinating neuropathy
3. Continuing IVIG as findings are consistent with CIDP
4. Repeating EMG/NCS in 6 months
5. Testing for serum MAG antibodies

Discussion

- The NCS showed uniform severe demyelinating neuropathy. Temporal dispersion and conduction block are important for diagnosis of CIDP. Acquired demyelinating neuropathy mostly is asymmetric and patchy and the weakness is due to conduction block rather than to demyelination. On the other hand, in hereditary demyelinating polyneuropathy, the failure of the formation of myelin is diffuse and does not cause severe weakness despite severe motor slowing.
- Objective measures are important to monitor outcome of therapy. Allen and Lewis[2] studied 59 patients referred with a diagnosis of CIDP; 47% turned out to have a different diagnosis, such as amyotrophic lateral sclerosis (ALS), small fiber neuropathy, fibromyalgia, and so forth. When the outcome measure relied on patient-reported subjected symptoms, 89% of CIDP patients and 85% of non-CIDP patients reported improvement. Subjective improvement is caused by the placebo effect, the wish of the patient and physician to see improvement, and by other nonspecific factors. Grip dynamometer and Rasch-built Overall Disability Scale are recommended to measure response to treatment and to avoid unnecessary prolonged and expensive courses of treatments that are not risk-free.
- Nerve biopsy no longer is indicated for diagnosis of the hereditary or acquired demyelinating neuropathies.

Case 7

Case presentation (Video 6)
A 42-year-old woman of a mixed African American and Latin American ancestry was referred to Nerve and Muscle Center of Texas to confirm a diagnosis of Miller Fisher syndrome. The following clinical features were noted:

- A nonambulatory, cachectic, deaf woman
- Abdominal bloating, nausea, and chronic diarrhea
- Profound external ophthalmoplegia, and ptosis
- Dysarthria
- Profound hypotonia, areflexia, and muscle atrophy of the lower extremities
- Sensation was intact
- Fundoscopic examination—no pigmentary retinopathy
- NCS: demyelinating sensorimotor polyneuropathy
- MRI: enhancing lesions in the basal ganglia and diffuse white matter changes
- CSF studies
    - Protein: 101 mg/dL (15–45 mg/dL)
    - Resting serum lactate: 4 mmol/L (1.1–2.2 mmol/L)
    - Resting serum pyruvate: 2 mmol/L (0.04–0.1 mmol/L)
- Normal creatine phosphokinase

Clinical question:
The most likely diagnosis is:

1 Miller Fisher syndrome
2 Guillain-Barré syndrome
3 CIDP
4 Mitochondrial demyelinating neuropathy
5 DADSAM neuropathy

Discussion

- Muscle biopsy revealed many ragged red fibers and cytochrome oxidase (COX)-negative, succinate dehydrogenase–positive fibers highly suggestive of mitochondrial dysfunction (**Figs. 1 and 2**).
- Ptosis, ophthalmoplegia, gastrointestinal dysmotility, cachexia, demyelinating neuropathy, and leukoencephalopathy are symptoms of mitochondrial neurogastrointestinal encephalopathy (MNGIE)
- Onset usually is between the first and fifth decades; in approximately 60% of individuals, symptoms begin before age 20 years.
- All cases of MNGIE are associated with demyelinating neuropathy.[13] The presence of multifocal manifestations, especially encephalopathy, seizures, and deafness, should raise the possibility of mitochondrial disease and lead to screening measurement of resting serum lactate and pyruvate. Muscle biopsy rarely is needed because a diagnosis easily can be made by genetic testing on white blood cell count to study the nuclear mitochondrial genes. In other mitochondrial disorders that are due to mutations of the mitochondrial DNA itself, muscle tissue is more sensitive than white blood cells.
- Acute exacerbation of different clinical manifestations of MNGIE may be caused by infections or other sources of stress.
- Classic MNGIE is caused by thymidine phosphorylase (endothelial cell growth factor 1, platelet-derived) deficiency and is associated with increased plasma thymidine level. Pathogenic mutations of TYMP gene (nuclear gene) are typical. It is an autosomal recessive condition.
- RRM2B mutations also are reported to cause MNGIE.[14]

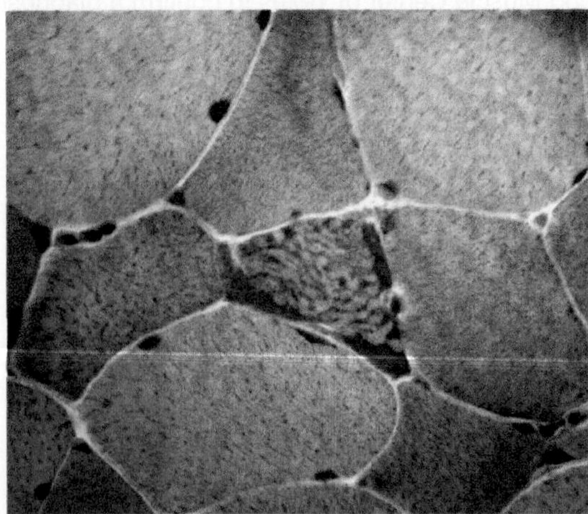

Fig. 1. Left biceps muscle fibers for case 7 stained with modification of the Gomori trichrome (400X), showing a ragged red fiber. (*Courtesy of* Aziz Shaibani, MD, Nerve and Muscle Center of Texas, Houston, TX.)

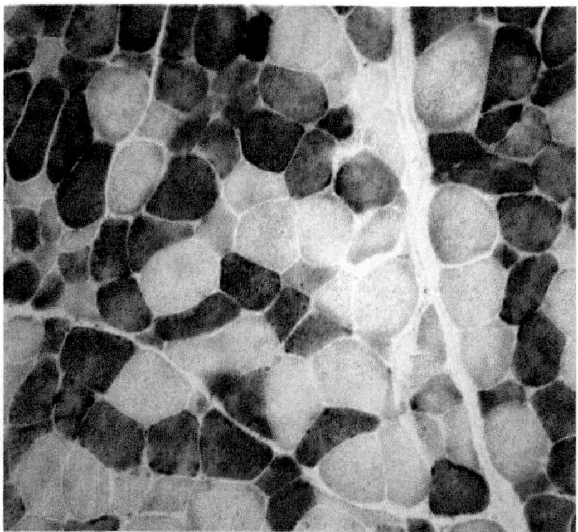

Fig. 2. Left biceps muscle fibers for case 7 stained with COX (100X) showing COX-negative fibers. (*Courtesy of* Aziz Shaibani, MD, Nerve and Muscle Center of Texas, Houston, TX.)

Case 8

Case presentation (Video 7)

- The patient disclosed a history of monoclonal gammopathy of undetermined significance (MGUS)
- The patient responded to IVIG for several years but his response decreased with time
- He developed severe lower back pain
- He developed anemia
- Serum protein electrophoresis: M protein increased to 3 g/dL over a year

Clinical question:

The most likely causes of refractory CIDP is:

1 POEMS syndrome
2 Multiple myeloma
3 MAG antibodies
4 NF-155 antibodies
5 Waldenström macroglobulinemia

Discussion

- This patient had typical CIDP for years, responding well to therapy, and then he progressed and became less responsive
- This case illustrates the importance of serial measurement of IFPE in patients with MGUS to detect malignant transformation early, which can cause loss of response to therapy
- A skeletal survey revealed multiple osteolytic lesions in the skull. Bone marrow biopsy revealed increased clonal plasma cells to 60%. Treatment of the multiple myeloma leads to remission of the CIDP.
- MGUS occurs in 4% of individuals above age 50 years.[15] The rate of transformation of MGUS to malignant myeloma is 1% per year.[16]

- MGUS requires the presence of
  - Serum M protein at a concentration less than 3 g/dL
  - Bone marrow with less than 10% monoclonal plasma cells
  - Absence of end-organ damage (lytic bone lesions, anemia, hypercalcemia, renal insufficiency, or hyperviscosity) related to the proliferative process

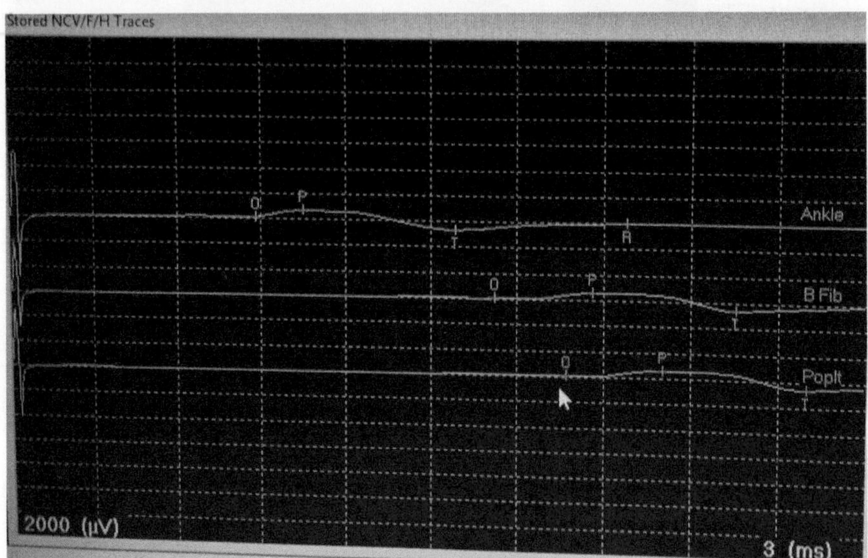

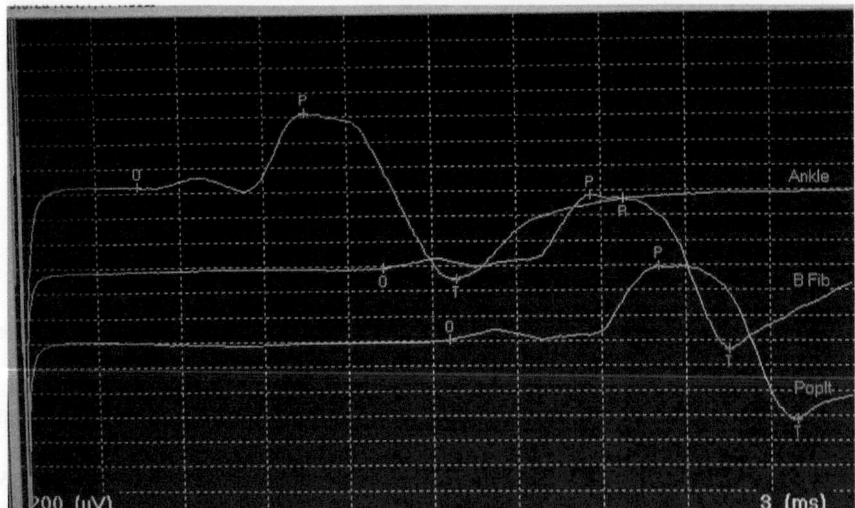

Fig. 3. (*A*) NCS for case 9, at 2000 μV, showing motor unit action potential before the gain change. (*B*) NCS for case 9, at 200 μV, showing motor unit action potential after the gain change. (*Courtesy of* Aziz Shaibani, MD, Nerve and Muscle Center of Texas, Houston, TX.)

- The appearance of anemia, hypercalcemia, bone pain, and renal impairment in a patient with MGUS always should raise suspicion of malignant transformation

Case 9

Case presentation
A 66-year-old man with:

- Progressive painless pure motor weakness of the arms and legs proximally and distally
- Absent DTR
- Normal sensation
- Mild CSF protein elevation
- Failed adequate IVIG therapy for 3 months
- NCS: motor nerves were in 30-s range and slightly prolonged distal latencies; normal sural responses (**Figure 3** A and B)
- EMG: widespread denervation, including fasciculations

Clinical question:
The most likely diagnosis is:

1 CIDP
2 ALS
3 Amyloid neuropathy
4 POEMS
5 Spinal muscular atrophy

Discussion

- ALS may be confused with CIDP mostly due to associated motor slowing and areflexia in the progressive muscular atrophy variant.[17]
- Mild slowing of motor nerves is seen in motor neuron diseases due to the loss of large motor neurons, which contribute to nerve conduction velocity.
- Diagnosis of CIDP should not rely on soft neurophysiologic findings but on validated diagnostic criteria.
- Another source of mistake is the measurement of the distance of a motor unit action potential (MUAP) from atrophied muscles. As **Fig. 3** shows, when the gain was changed (B), the onset of the MUAP was earlier and the conduction velocity was closer to normal.

SUMMARY

- Causes of non-responsiveness of CIDP
  - Wrong diagnosis
  - Severe disease with secondary axonal damage
  - Inadequate immunosuppression
  - Transformation to malignancy
- CIDP rarely is a straightforward diagnosis, and different sets of diagnostic criteria have different sensitivities and specificities.
- Diagnosis should not be made based on soft findings in isolation, such as mild elevation of CSF protein, mild demyelinating changes, or subjective response to treatment.
- Failure to respond to first-line therapies should prompt revision of the diagnosis before subjecting the patient to more aggressive treatment.

- Some causes are not responsive to immunotherapy like Charcot-Marie-Tooth disease, ALS, and DADSAM neuropathy.
- Other causes require more aggressive or specific therapies, such as POEMS syndrome, multiple myeloma, and NF-155–associated CIDP (nodopathy).
- If no cause is found and a diagnosis is confirmed, more aggressive treatment with 1 or more modalities, including IVIG, intravenous steroids, and PLEX, would be warranted. Some patients require weekly or biweekly IVIG or PLEX. Rituximab and cyclophosphamide are used as a second line of therapy.
- Physical therapy is an important adjunct to immunomodulatory therapy.

DISCLOSURE

The authors disclose no financial interests in subject matter or materials discussed in the article or with a company making a competing product.

SUPPLEMENTARY DATA

Supplementary data to this article can be found online at https://doi.org/10.1016/j.ncl.2020.03.006.

REFERENCES

1. Laughlin R, Dyck P, Melton L, et al. Incidence and prevalence of CIDP and the association of diabetes mellitus. Neurology 2009;73(1):39–45.
2. Allen J, Lewis R. CIDP diagnostic pitfalls and perception of treatment benefit. Neurology 2015;85(6):498–504.
3. Breiner A, Brannagan T. Comparison of sensitivity and specificity among 15 criteria for chronic inflammatory demyelinating polyneuropathy. Muscle Nerve 2013;50(1):40–6.
4. European Federation of Neurological Societies/Peripheral Nerve Society Guideline on management of chronic inflammatory demyelinating polyradiculoneuropathy: Report of a joint task force of the European Federation of Neurological Societies and the Peripheral Nerve Society - First Revision. J Peripher Nerv Syst 2010;15(1):1–9.
5. Cocito D, Paolasso I, Antonini G, et al. A nationwide retrospective analysis on the effect of immune therapies in patients with chronic inflammatory demyelinating polyradiculoneuropathy. Eur J Neurol 2009;17(2):289–94.
6. Kaplan A, Brannagan T. Evaluation of patients with refractory chronic inflammatory demyelinating polyneuropathy. Muscle Nerve 2016;55(4):476–82.
7. Molenaar D, Vermeulen M, Haan R. Diagnostic value of sural nerve biopsy in chronic inflammatory demyelinating polyneuropathy. Neurol Neurosurg Psychiatry 1998;64(1):84–9.
8. Pitarokoili K, Yoon M, Kröger I, et al. Severe refractory CIDP: a case series of 10 patients treated with bortezomib. Neurology 2017;264(9):2010–20.
9. Dalakas M. Advances in the diagnosis, immunopathogenesis and therapies of IgM-anti-MAG antibody-mediated neuropathies. Ther Adv Neurol Disord 2018; 11. 175628561774664.
10. Devaux J, Miura Y, Fukami Y, et al. Neurofascin-155 IgG4 in chronic inflammatory demyelinating polyneuropathy. Neurology 2016;86(9):800–7.
11. Dispenzieri A. POEMS syndrome: update on diagnosis, risk-stratification, and management. Am J Hematol 2015;90(10):951–62.

12. Dispenzieri A, Lacy M, Hayman S, et al. Peripheral blood stem cell transplant for POEMS syndrome is associated with high rates of engraftment syndrome. Eur J Haematol 2008;80(5):397–406.
13. Bedlack RS, Vu T, Hammans S, et al. MNGIE neuropathy: five cases mimicking chronic inflammatory demyelinating polyneuropathy. Muscle Nerve 2004;29(3): 364–8.
14. Shaibani A, Shchelochkov O, Zhang S, et al. Mitochondrial neurogastrointestinal encephalopathy due to mutations in RRM2B. Arch Neurol 2009;66(8):1028–32.
15. Chaudhry H, Mauermann M, Rajkumar S. Monoclonal gammopathy–associated peripheral neuropathy: diagnosis and management. Mayo Clinic Proc 2017; 92(5):838–50.
16. Zingone A, Kuehl W. Pathogenesis of monoclonal gammopathy of undetermined significance and progression to multiple myeloma. Semin Hematol 2011; 48(1):4–12.
17. Rajabally Y, Jacob S. Chronic inflammatory demyelinating polyneuropathy–like disorder associated with amyotrophic lateral sclerosis. Muscle Nerve 2008; 38(1):855–60.

Small Fiber Neuropathy

David S. Saperstein, MD

KEYWORDS

- Small fiber neuropathy • Length-dependent symptoms
- Intraepidermal nerve fiber density • Fibromyalgia

KEY POINTS

- Small fiber neuropathy can have a broad array of presentations.
- Length-dependent symptoms and findings present little diagnostic difficulty, but non–length-dependent or multifocal symptoms can be challenging, especially if sensory examination is normal.
- The role of intraepidermal nerve fiber density (IENFD) testing in apparent fibromyalgia warrants further study, but, based on currently available data, skin biopsy testing of this patient population is reasonable.
- Avoidance of IENFD testing in situations where diagnosis of neuropathy is already clear (such as in the case of a mixed-fiber neuropathy) or where neuropathy is clearly not the cause of symptoms helps to prevent incorrect diagnostic and therapeutic conclusions.
- Careful history and physical examination coupled with a reasoned appreciation of pretest probability are important factors to consider when assessing the results of an IENFD test report.

INTRODUCTION

The entity of neuropathy affecting small nerve fibers (small fiber neuropathy) has been understood for some time. However, before the ready availability of intraepidermal nerve fiber density (IENFD) testing via skin punch biopsy, diagnosis was difficult and largely rested on clinical suspicion. Having an objective test proved valuable, especially in cases where the presentation is not typical. IENFD testing has allowed an appreciation of how much more diverse the range of symptoms in small fiber neuropathy (SFN) can be. The cases presented in this article represent actual patients seen by the author in referral. It is hoped that these cases and questions will allow an enhanced understanding of the spectrum of clinical ministrations that can be seen in SFN and the benefits and pitfalls of IENFD testing.

CASE 1

Case 1 is a 42-year-old woman with gradual onset of numbness and tingling in both feet 2 years ago. The symptoms have been slowly progressive. She also describes

Center for Complex Neurology, EDS & POTS, University of Arizona College of Medicine, 1010 East McDowell Road, Suite 101, Phoenix, AZ 85006, USA
E-mail address: drsaperstein@complexneurology.com

Neurol Clin 38 (2020) 607–618
https://doi.org/10.1016/j.ncl.2020.04.001

a burning sensation in the same areas. This sensation is moderately uncomfortable. Examination reveals decreased light-touch and pinprick sensation to bilateral ankles. Vibration and joint position sense are normal. Deep tendon reflexes are normal. Nerve conduction studies and electromyogram (EMG) show no abnormalities.

Question 1. What is the most likely cause of this patient's symptoms?

1. SFN
2. Mixed-fiber neuropathy
3. Multiple sclerosis
4. Conversion disorder

Correct answer is (1).

This patient most likely has an SFN. Although most polyneuropathies involve small and large fibers (a so-called mixed-fiber neuropathy), there are some patients in whom only small myelinated A-delta and unmyelinated C fibers are affected. It is not known why.

The small fibers are involved in pain and temperature sensation. Therefore, symptoms of SFN typically involve pain, which most commonly has characteristics of burning, stabbing, shooting, or prickling (**Table 1**).[1,2] It is often thought that SFN is always painful. However, patients can experience only numbness and tingling, and not pain. Among 110 patients diagnosed with SFN, Devigili and colleagues[3] found 12% to be without pain; SFN diagnosis was based on at least 2 of the following being abnormal: sensory examination, quantitative sensory testing (QST), or IENFD. In other studies, the percentage of patients with SFN and no pain symptoms has ranged from 15% to 30%.[2,4,5]

Neurologic examination usually shows a length-dependent stocking or stocking/glove decrease in light-touch or pinprick sensation. Other components of the sensory examination, such as vibration and position sense, deep tendon reflexes, and Romberg testing, are normal because these assess functioning of large nerves.

Because of their slow rate of conduction, small nerve fibers do not contribute to sensory nerve action potentials. Therefore, nerve conduction studies (NCSs) are normal in patients with purely SFN.

Usually the diagnosis of SFN is strongly suspected by history and examination. However, with routine electrodiagnostic testing for neuropathy being normal, the diagnosis cannot be solidified beyond this. A central nervous disorder could potentially produce similar clinical and examination features. A further stumbling block to diagnosis is that up to a third of patients with SFN may have an entirely normal sensory examination.[3] In such a setting, some patients may be suspected of having a nonorganic cause for their symptoms. For all of these reasons, it can valuable to have an objective laboratory test that can support a diagnosis of SFN.

Question 2. Which of the following tests could help with diagnosis?

1. Skin biopsy for determination of IENFD.
2. Quantitative sudomotor axon reflex testing (QSART)?

Table 1
Symptoms observed in patients with confirmed small fiber neuropathy

Symptom	%
Pain	76%
Numbness	75%
Tingling	61%
Burning	30%
Cramping	15%

3. (1) and (2).
4. None of the above.
Correct answer is (3).

For some time, tests of autonomic function had been used to support a diagnosis of SFN.[6,7] Because small nerve fibers comprise autonomic nerves, it is not surprising that autonomic dysfunction can occur in patients with SFN. Sometimes there are symptoms of autonomic dysfunction, but, even in patients with SFN and no symptoms of autonomic dysfunction, autonomic testing can be abnormal.[8] Autonomic testing includes evaluation of sudomotor function such as sympathetic skin response, QSART, cardiovagal function (heart rate response to deep breathing, Valsalva ratio), and orthostatic vital signs or tilt-table testing. Autonomic testing is often not easily performed. Furthermore, the test with the highest yield, QSART, is not widely available to most clinicians.

Small nerve fibers can be assessed in a conventional cutaneous nerve biopsy. However, this is invasive, and evaluation of small nerve fibers is not routinely done. Therefore, it was a significant advance when investigators at University of Minnesota and Johns Hopkins University devised reliable means to measure small nerve fibers in a skin punch biopsy.[9,10] Although originally a research tool, over the last decade this became a readily available commercial test. The number of small nerve fibers in the epidermis is assessed, yielding the IENFD.

Skin punch biopsy is a minimally invasive test that can be easily and quickly performed by a physician or midlevel provider in the office or clinic. Proficiency can attained quickly, allowing testing to be easily completed in less than 15 minutes. The procedure does not require sutures. Most patients experience little to no pain. Complications are rare and include bleeding and infection.

It is important that IENFD testing be performed at a laboratory proficient in this testing. It is a complex process that takes several days. Skin specimens are initially placed in a fixative (usually Zamboni solution). They are then transferred to cryoprotectant solution and frozen and sectioned. Tissue is cut more thickly than is done for most histopathologic studies. For IENFD testing, sections are cut to 50 μm, compared with less than 10 μm for standard nerve or muscle biopsies. The thicker sections are more difficult to handle. Furthermore, staining is done manually. Tissue is immunostained with antibodies against protein gene product (PGP) 9.5, an antigen found on all neurons. After staining, the intraepidermal nerve fibers must be carefully counted (**Fig. 1**). This process

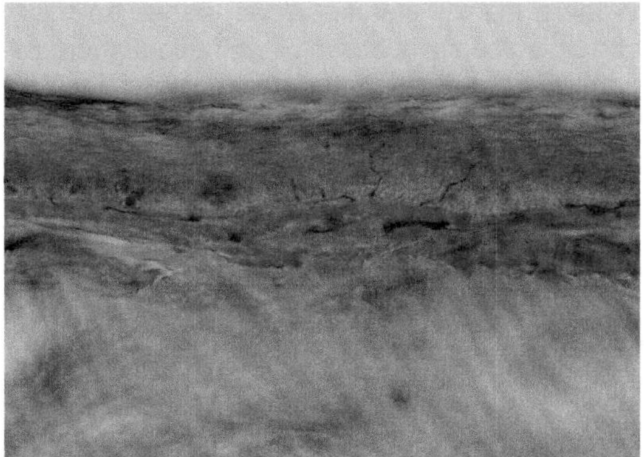

Fig. 1. Normal skin biopsy stained with PGP 9.5 immunostain and counterstained with eosin. Horizontal fibers are intraepidermal nerves. Thicker horizontal fibers are subdermal nerves (original magnification X 40x).

is also manual and time consuming. At present, most histopathology for other purposes is done in an automated fashion. Therefore, this antiquated and time-consuming hands-on approach is foreign and undesirable to most pathology laboratories.

Normative values have been determined for several sites. Age and gender affect normal values, so ideally normal values should be age and gender specific. Normal values are available for foot (over the extensor digitorum brevis muscle), distal leg (10 cm above lateral malleolus), distal thigh (10 cm above lateral edge of patella), proximal thigh (10 cm below iliac crest), wrist (4 cm proximal to wrist crease at dorsal midline), and over the deltoid. Age-specific and gender-specific normal values have been published only for the distal leg.[11]

By convention, IENFD is considered abnormal if it is less than the fifth percentile of normal. Certain morphologic features, such as an increased number of axonal swellings or excessive branching of fibers, may suggest SFN, but how to define this remains uncertain.[12]

Question 3. To further assess the patient presented in the first case, it is decided to obtain skin biopsies to assess intraepidermal small nerve fibers. Which of the following choices represents the best strategy for testing?

1. Right distal leg, distal thigh. and proximal thigh
2. Bilateral foot
3. Bilateral distal leg and proximal thigh
4. Left distal leg, proximal thigh, and wrist

Correct answer is (1).

It is advised that IENFD testing be performed on at least 2 sites with the sites representing a distal and proximal area.[12] This method allows for an assessment of whether an SFN is length dependent or non–length dependent. In a length-dependent SFN, IENFD is abnormal in distal sites and normal or less abnormal in skin taken from proximal sites. In contrast, in a non–length-dependent SFN, IENFD is more abnormal in proximal sites than distal. Approximately a third of patients tested for SFN have a non–length-dependent pattern.[2,13] A non–length-dependent pattern is not by itself diagnostic; however, patients with this pattern are more likely to be female, younger, and have an immune-mediated cause for their neuropathy.[13] Non–length-dependent SFN is suspected to represent a ganglionopathy.[14]

To best determine length dependency, taking a biopsy from 2 or 3 sites is recommended. Biopsying more than 3 sites is seldom necessary. Taking biopsies from only 1 side of the body is usually sufficient. A situation where bilateral testing can be helpful is when there are symptoms unilaterally in a part of the body for which normal values are not available (eg, the back). Biopsies can be taken bilaterally, from the affected side and the contralateral unaffected side.[12,15]

Although there are normative data for the foot (over the extensor digitorum brevis muscle), there are concerns about sampling this area. There is the potential for trauma to the foot to artifactually decrease IENFD. At least 1 study suggests that measuring IENFD from the foot can be sensitive and specific.[16] The diagnostic yield from the distal leg site is high, even in patients who have distal symptoms,[13] and this is the site recommended by international guidelines.[12]

Normal values have been determined for sites in the upper extremity. However, these have not been investigated anywhere near as thoroughly as have sites from the lower extremity. In the author's experience, IENFD is most often abnormal in sites from the lower extremity, even in patients with symptoms predominately in the upper extremity.

Question 4. Potential causes of SFN include which of the following?
1. Impaired glucose metabolism
2. Genetic disorders
3. Autoimmune disorders
4. All of the above.
Correct answer is (4).

No cause for SFN is identified in approximately 50% of cases, so idiopathic is the most common cause.[2,13] As is the case for mixed-fiber neuropathy, several causes need to be considered (**Table 2**). As discussed earlier, an immune-mediated cause is more likely among patients with a non–length-dependent pattern. However, the laboratory work-up is generally similar for both groups. The most important features that help point toward a potential cause are rate of symptom onset (abrupt onset favors immune mediated or toxic), age of patient, past medical history, and family history. Autonomic neuropathy can coexist with small fiber sensory neuropathy because both involve small nerve fibers. The presence of autonomic symptoms or findings should lead to greater consideration of amyloidosis or an immune-mediated process.

In addition to PGP 9.5 staining to identify the intraepidermal nerve fibers, skin biopsies processed for IENFD testing are usually also stained with hematoxylin and eosin (H&E) and Congo red stains. H&E staining can identify inflammatory cells, as has been reported in conventional skin biopsies from patients with mixed-fiber neuropathy caused by vasculitis.[17] However, this has not been observed in more than 50,000 skin biopsies submitted for IENFD testing (Saperstein, unpublished

Table 2
Potential causes of small fiber neuropathy and testing

Condition	Test
Diabetes, impaired glucose tolerance	Fasting glucose, oral glucose tolerance test or fasting insulin
Vitamin B abnormalities	Vitamin B_1, B_6, B_{12}, methylmalonic acid, homocysteine
Kidney, liver disease	Complete metabolic profile
Thyroid dysfunction	TSH, T4
Connective tissue disorder	CRP, ANA, SS-A, SS-B
Sarcoidosis	ACE level, chest CT
Paraprotein, amyloidosis	Serum immune fixation electrophoresis
Celiac disease	Gliadin antibodies, tissue transglutaminase
Infectious	Hepatitis C, HIV
Inherited	
Familial amyloid	TTR gene sequencing
Sodium channel mutations	SCN9A, SCN10A gene sequencing
Fabry disease	Alpha-galactosidase assay or gene sequencing
Immune mediated	Increased CSF protein, antinerve antibodies, paraneoplastic antibodies
Toxin	History for exposure to ethanol, chemotherapy, statins, organic solvents

Abbreviations: ACE, angiotensin-converting enzyme; ANA, antinuclear antibody; CSF, cerebrospinal fluid; CT, computed tomography; HIV, human immunodeficiency virus; SCN, sodium channe; T4, thyroxine; TSH, thyroid-stimulating hormone; TTR, transthyretein.

observations, 2019). Congo red stain can show amyloid,[18] although this, too, is uncommon in routine clinical practice (author's unpublished observations).

There has been enthusiasm about the role of antibodies against the nerve components fibroblast growth factor-3 or trisulfated heparin disaccharide as indicators of immune-mediated SFN.[19] Although these antibodies can be obtained from at least once commercial laboratory, their significance is unclear[20] and further study is needed.

CASE 2

A 35-year-old man presents with a 1-year history of painful numbness and tingling. Symptoms come and go and involve different parts of his body at different times: face, chest, hands, or feet. Neurologic examination is normal, as are NCS/EMG and MRI of the brain and cervical spine.

Skin biopsies were taken from the right distal leg, distal thigh, and proximal thigh (**Table 3**).

Question 5. What is the most likely interpretation of these IENFD testing results?

1. The findings are spurious because this patient does not have an SFN.
2. The test vials were mislabeled.
3. The patient has a non–length-dependent SFN.
4. Testing should be repeated.

Correct answer is (4).

The clinical picture is consistent with a non–length-dependent SFN and the skin biopsy findings support this. As already discussed, sensory examination can be normal in SFN. A small percentage of patients experience intermittent sensory symptoms. In 1 series, this occurred in 10% of patients.[4]

In the setting of a normal neurologic examination and unusual clinical manifestations, some patients with SFN can be suspected of having a nonorganic disorder. IENFD testing can be very useful in such cases.

As already discussed, a non–length-dependent pattern of decreased IENFD occurs in a significant percentage of cases of SFN. Therefore, the findings in this case should not prompt consideration of mislabeling of specimen vials. Nevertheless, it is always of utmost importance that care is taken by the clinician performing the biopsy and the laboratory processing the specimens so that such errors do not occur.

If IENFD testing is performed at a laboratory adept at such analysis, there is no reason to believe that repeat testing would provide different results. Good reproducibility of IENFD determinations has been shown when the same sections were processed at several different laboratories and read by different readers.[21]

IENFD testing can be useful in predicting response to symptomatic therapy for neuropathic pain. Patients with abnormal skin biopsy results are twice as likely to respond to such treatment compared with those with similar symptoms but normal IENFD.[4] Furthermore, patients with non–length-dependent SFN are less likely to

Table 3
Skin biopsy results for case

Biopsy Site	Patient's IENFD (Fibers/mm)	Normal Value (Fibers/mm)
Right distal leg	6.6	5.2
Right distal thigh	4.2	6.0
Right proximal thigh	3.8	7.0

respond to treatment of neuropathic pain compared with patients with length-dependent SFN.[13]

CASE 3

A 28-year-old woman presents with a 6-month history of slowly progressive numbness and tingling in both of her feet. There is no past medical history. She is on no medications. Neurologic examination and NCS/EMG testing are normal. Routine chemistry, vitamin B_{12}, thyroid function tests, antinuclear antibody (ANA) level, and erythrocyte sedimentation rate are normal. Skin biopsies of the left distal leg and proximal thigh showed normal IENFD at both sites.

Question 6. Possible reasons for normal IENFD in this case include:

1. False-negative testing in a patient with SFN.
2. The patient has a central nervous system lesion producing her symptoms.
3. The wrong sites for biopsy were tested.
4. All of the above.

Correct answer is (4).

The sensitivity of IENFD testing for SFN is approximately 90%. Therefore, there is a 10% false-negative rate, so a normal skin biopsy does not exclude SFN. Other tests may be abnormal in patients with SFN and normal IENFD.[8] QSART has shown sensitivities ranging from 60% to 80%.[1,8] QST has shown similar sensitivity.[1] In 1 study IENFD, QST and QSART were all abnormal in only 36% of 68 patients with SFN.[5]

It is clear that patients with suspected SFN but normal IENFD can show abnormal QST or QSART.[3,5] However, these studies do not clearly indicate how often QST or QSART are abnormal when IENFD is normal. Nevertheless, it is clear that these different tests have additional value for diagnosing SFN: if IENFD testing is normal, an alternative test of small nerve fiber function can be of diagnostic value.

The usefulness of QST and QSART is limited because they are not readily available to most clinicians. Other tests that can identify SFN include confocal microscopy of the cornea, laser evoked potentials, and contact heat evoked potentials.[22] These are even less accessible.

A central nervous system lesion could produce the symptoms and findings described in this case. Neuroimaging would be a reasonable next step. IENFD is not expected to be abnormal in patients with a central nervous system cause for their sensory symptoms.[23]

As discussed earlier, it is possible that a biopsy from a more distal site, such as the foot, could have a decreased IENFD while the distal leg shows normal results. However, the potential for false-positive results from biopsy of the foot likely outweighs any gains in sensitivity it might provide. The yield of the distal leg for detecting SFN is extremely good.

Question 7. The patient from case 3 asks whether her SFN is likely to affect her balance. How likely is an SFN to progress to a mixed-fiber neuropathy?

1. SFN never progress to a mixed-fiber neuropathy.
2. Less than 15% chance.
3. More than a 50% chance.
4. All patients with SFN progress to a mixed-fiber neuropathy.

Correct answer is (2).

A recent study found that 12% of patients progressed to a mixed-fiber neuropathy.[24] All patients with a non–length-dependent pattern remained purely small fiber. Patients with diabetes or impaired glucose tolerance are more likely to progress.

CASE 4

A 41-year-old woman has diffuse muscle aching. There are no sensory symptoms. She fulfills diagnostic criteria for fibromyalgia. Neurologic examination and NCS/EMG are normal. Serum creatine kinase levels are normal.

Question 8. What is the likelihood that skin biopsy would show abnormal IENFD?
1. Less than 5%
2. 10% to 20%
3. 30% to 50%
4. Greater than 70%

Correct answer is (3).

Several studies have found that patients meeting criteria for fibromyalgia, when tested with skin biopsy, have abnormal IENFD consistent with SFN in 30% to 50% of cases.[25–27] Two of these studies included age-matched and gender-matched healthy controls.[25,26] The percentage of controls having decreased IENFD was 3% in both studies. Based on how the normal values are constructed, 3% is the expected rate of normal individuals having IENFD below the lower limit of normal. These studies show that the false-positive rate for IENFD testing is extremely low, at least under research conditions.

It is not exactly clear what the findings of these studies mean. There is a lot of research showing that central abnormalities are present in patients with fibromyalgia.[27] It remains to be determined whether the patients with abnormal skin biopsies represent SFN incorrectly diagnosed as fibromyalgia or whether IENFD can become decreased secondary to central nervous system processes. However, the percentage of such patients having decreased IENFD is strikingly high and is not simply the result of false-positive testing.

CASE 5

A 70-year-old man has a 15-year history of non–insulin-dependent diabetes mellitus and a 10-year history of progressive numbness and dysesthesias in a stocking/glove distribution. Examination reveals normal strength, markedly decreased light-touch and pinprick sensation to the knees and wrists, absent vibratory sensation in the toes, and absent deep tendon reflexes in the legs. NCSs show absent sensory and motor responses in the legs. Skin biopsies taken from the right distal leg, distal thigh, and proximal thigh show IENFD of zero at all sites.

Question 9. How does the information from the skin biopsies help with this case?
1. Because the patient has an SFN, there is a strong likelihood that the cause is immune mediated and he may benefit from treatment with intravenous immunoglobulin (IVIg).
2. The skin biopsies show a severe neuropathy. The patient needs to be informed of how this new information will change the management of his neuropathy.
3. The skin biopsies reveal a length-dependent neuropathy, which has ramifications for further work-up and management.
4. The skin biopsies add no helpful information and should not have been performed.

Correct answer is (4).

However, this case represents a too-common occurrence. There is a misunderstanding among many clinicians regarding the use and value of IENFD testing. Most patients with sensory or sensorimotor polyneuropathies have a mixed-fiber neuropathy. Therefore, tests of IENFD are usually abnormal. However, given that neurologic examination and, usually, NCS are abnormal, there is arguably no useful information that IENFD testing could provide. In the case presented here, the patient has an obviously severe length-dependent polyneuropathy. Given the presence of neuropathic pain, small fibers would be expected to affected. This patient's examination and NCS indicate that medium and large fibers are involved. The severity of the neuropathy is already readily apparent; IENFD testing adds no additional information in this regard.

There are many clinicians who mistakenly believe that the presence of abnormal IENFD on skin biopsy suggests a strong likelihood of an immune-mediated neuropathy. It is not clear where this idea comes from. As presented earlier, there are many potential causes for SFN. Clinical features and laboratory tests are the way to identify patients with potentially immune-mediated neuropathies.

Question 10. What are the potential reasons why a skin biopsy might show decreased IENFD?

1. SFN
2. Mixed-fiber neuropathy
3. False-positive result
4. All of the above

Correct answer is (4).

As case 5 showed, most patients with a mixed-fiber neuropathy have abnormal IENFD. Looking at a skin biopsy report without knowing the results of the patient's neurologic examination and NCS does not allow the clinician to conclude whether the patient has a purely SFN or a mixed-fiber neuropathy.

A small percentage of individuals without neuropathy have abnormally decreased IENFD. If the skin tissue is not handled carefully by the personnel performing the biopsy or processing the tissue, then the chance for false-positive results is increased. Leaving the tissue in fixative too long before transferring to cryoprotectant can cause a decrease in IENFD.

As with any test, be it NCS or MRI, if it is not performed and interpreted with the utmost care, and with a watchful eye for artifacts, results and interpretation can be compromised.

CASE 6

A 48-year-old man is referred by another neurologist for evaluation of numbness and tingling in his feet and hands. This condition has been slowly progressive over the last 6 to 8 months. He notes trouble with balance, especially in the dark, and he often drops things. Past medical history is notable for impaired glucose tolerance with a mildly increased glycosylated hemoglobin level. He is on no medication for this.

Neurologic examination reveals normal strength. Light-touch and pinprick sensation are decreased in the feet. Joint position sense is decreased at the great toe bilaterally. Vibration is absent at the toes. Romberg sign is present. Deep tendon reflexes are brisk throughout with no clonus or Hoffman signs. Plantar responses are extensor bilaterally.

NCS/EMG were normal. Skin biopsies performed from the right distal leg, distal thigh, and proximal thigh revealed decreased IENFD in the distal leg with normal findings at the other sites.

Question 11. Which is the best next step?

1. Obtain MRI of the cervical spine.
2. Treat with gabapentin.

Table 4 Skin biopsy results for case 7		
Biopsy Site	**Baseline IENFD (Fibers/mm)**	**Repeat IENFD at 6 mo**
Right distal leg	6.0	7.2
Right proximal thigh	1.6	9.2

3. Treat with IVIg.
4. Obtain skin biopsies from the left leg.

Correct answer is (1).

Cervical spine MRI showed a herniated disc at C5-6 moderately compressing the cord and causing increased signal at that level. These findings are not surprising because the patient's examination showed brisk reflexes and extensor plantar responses. These findings would not be explained by a peripheral neuropathy, either small fiber or mixed fiber. In addition, his balance problems and hand symptoms are not explained by SFN. The abnormal IENFD at the distal leg is likely caused by the patient's impaired glucose tolerance.

This case is another example of how inappropriate ordering of skin biopsy led to an incorrect diagnosis of SFN as the cause for all the patient's symptoms. This case underscores the importance of the basics: history and physical examination, which clearly indicated the patient did not have just an SFN and pointed to a myelopathy as the likely primary problem. The patient was referred to a spine surgeon and made an excellent recovery after appropriate surgery. Mild distal lower extremity sensory symptoms and light-touch/pinprick deficits remained.

CASE 7

A 52-year-old woman presents for evaluation of numbness and pain. Symptoms came on abruptly 2 years earlier and have been progressive. There is stinging pain in her hands, feet, and face. Her pain has been refractory to appropriate trials of multiple medications to include gabapentin, pregabalin, duloxetine, and amitriptyline. She has dry eyes and dry mouth. Neurologic examination, NCS, and brain MRI were normal. Laboratory testing revealed positive ANA, SS-A and SS-B antibodies. Skin biopsies taken from the right calf and proximal thigh showed a non–length-dependent SFN (**Table 4**). She was treated with intravenous methylprednisolone (1000 mg/d for 3 days followed by 1000 mg weekly) for presumed Sjögren syndrome–associated SFN. Her pain improved significantly. Repeat skin biopsies at 6 months showed a significant increase in IENFD at both sites (see **Table 4**). The second set of skin biopsies were taken several millimeters from the initial biopsies.

This case shows the potential for serial skin biopsies to serve as biomarkers for response to immunomodulating therapy in patients with suspected immune-mediated neuropathies.[19,28,29] This potential is important for cases where subjective outcomes, such as pain and numbness, are being followed. There have been no placebo-controlled studies assessing this. However, the natural history in patients with SFN is continued decrease of IENFD. Spontaneous improvement has not been observed.[30]

SUMMARY

It is hoped that these cases show the broad array of presentations that SFN can have. Length-dependent symptoms and findings present few diagnostic difficulties, but non–length-dependent or multifocal symptoms can be challenging, especially if sensory examination is normal. Well-performed skin biopsies can be especially useful in this situation. The role of IENFD testing in apparent fibromyalgia warrants further study, but, based on currently available data, skin biopsy testing of this patient population is reasonable.

Avoidance of IENFD testing in situations where diagnosis of neuropathy is already clear (such as in the case of a mixed-fiber neuropathy) or where neuropathy is clearly not the cause of symptoms helps to prevent incorrect diagnostic and therapeutic conclusions.

As with any diagnostic test, skin biopsies have potential false-positive and false-negative results. Careful history and physical examination coupled with a reasoned appreciation of pretest probability are important factors to consider when assessing the results of an IENFD test report.

DISCLOSURE

Dr D.S. Saperstein is Chief Medical Officer of Neuropath Diagnostics laboratory, Houston, TX; he is a speaker or consultant for CSL Behring, Diplomate Specialty Pharmacy, Grifols, and RE Pharmacy.

REFERENCES

1. Lacomis D. Small-fiber neuropathy. Muscle Nerve 2002;26:173–88.
2. Saperstein DS, Levine T, Lopate G, et al. Characteristics of patients evaluated for small fiber neuropathy with skin biopsy. Neurology 2014;P4:117.
3. Devigili G, Tugnoli V, Penza P, et al. The diagnostic criteria for small fibre neuropathy: from symptoms to neuropathology. Brain 2008;131:1912–25.
4. Saperstein DS, Levine TD, Levine M, et al. Usefulness of skin biopsies in the evaluation and management of patients with suspected small fiber neuropathy. Int J Neurosci 2013;123:38–41.
5. Thaisetthawatkul P, Fernandes Filho JA, Herrmann DN. Autonomic evaluation is independent of somatic evaluation for small fiber neuropathy. Neurol Sci 2014;344(1–2):51–4.
6. Stewart JD, Low PA, Fealey RD. Distal small fiber neuropathy: results of tests of sweating and autonomic cardiovascular reflexes. Muscle Nerve 1992;15:661–5.
7. Low VA, Sandroni P, Fealey RD, et al. Detection of small-fiber neuropathy by sudomotor testing. Muscle Nerve 2006;34:57–61.
8. Thaisetthawatkul P, Fernandes Filho JA, Herrmann DN. Contribution of QSART to the diagnosis of small fiber neuropathy. Muscle Nerve 2013;48:883–8.
9. McCarthy BG, Hsieh ST, Stocks A, et al. Cutaneous innervation in sensory neuropathies: evaluation by skin biopsy. Neurology 1995;45:1848–55.
10. Kennedy WR, Nolano M, Wendelschafer-Crabb G, et al. A skin blister method to study epidermal nerves in peripheral nerve disease. Muscle Nerve 1999;22:360–71.
11. Lauria G, Bakkers M, Schmitz C, et al. Intraepidermal nerve fiber density at the distal leg: a worldwide normative reference study. J Peripher Nerv Syst 2010;15:202–7.
12. Lauria G, Hsieh ST, Johansson O, et al. European federation of neurological societies/peripheral nerve society guideline on the use of skin biopsy in the diagnosis of small fiber neuropathy. report of a joint task force of the European Federation of Neurological Societies and the Peripheral Nerve Society. Eur J Neurol 2010;17:903–12.

13. Chan AC, Wilder-Smith EP. Small fiber neuropathy: Getting bigger! Muscle Nerve 2016;53:671–82.
14. Gorson KC, Herrmann DN, Thiagarajan R, et al. Non-length dependent small fibre neuropathy/ganglionopathy. J Neurol Neurosurg Psychiatry 2008;79:163–9.
15. Lauria G, McArthur JC, Hauer PE, et al. Neuropathological alterations in diabetic truncal neuropathy: evaluation by skin biopsy. J Neurol Neurosurg Psychiatry 1998;65:762–6.
16. Walk D, Wendelschafer-Crabb G, Davey C, et al. Concordance between epidermal nerve fiber density and sensory examination in patients with symptoms of idiopathic small fiber neuropathy. J Neurol Sci 2007;255:23–6.
17. Uçeyler N, Devigili G, Toyka KV, et al. Skin biopsy as an additional diagnostic tool in non-systemic vasculitic neuropathy. Acta Neuropathol 2010;120:109–16.
18. Ebenezer GJ, Liu Y, Judge DP, et al. Cutaneous nerve biomarkers in transthyretin familial amyloid polyneuropathy. Ann Neurol 2017;82:44–56, enezer. Hopkins amyloid.
19. Levine T, Saperstein D, Pestronk A, et al. Identification of a novel immune mediated cause for small fiber neuropathy. Neurology 2017;P4:137.
20. Samara V, Sampson J, Muppidi S. FGFR3 antibodies in neuropathy: what to do with them? J Clin Neuromuscul Dis 2018;20:35–40.
21. Smith AG, Howard JR, Kroll R, et al. The reliability of skin biopsy with measurement of intraepidermal nerve fiber density. J Neurol Sci 2005;228:65–9.
22. Astrid J Terkelsen AJ, Karlsson P, Lauria G, et al. The diagnostic challenge of small fibre neuropathy: clinical presentations, evaluations, and causes. Lancet Neurol 2017;16:934–44.
23. Herrmann DN, O'Connor AB, Schwid SR, et al. Broadening the spectrum of controls for skin biopsy in painful neuropathies. Muscle Nerve 2010;42:436–8.
24. MacDonald S, Sharma TL, Li J, et al. Longitudinal follow-up of biopsy-proven small fiber neuropathy. Muscle Nerve 2019;60:376–81.
25. Oaklander AL, Herzog ZD, Downs HM, et al. Objective evidence that small-fiber polyneuropathy underlies some illnesses currently labeled as fibromyalgia. Pain 2013;154:2310–6.
26. Kosmidis ML, Koutsogeorgopoulou L, Alexopoulos H, et al. Reduction of Intraepidermal Nerve Fiber Density (IENFD) in the skin biopsies of patients with fibromyalgia: a controlled study. J Neurol Sci 2014;347:143–7.
27. Levine TD, Saperstein DS. Routine use of punch biopsy to diagnose small fiber neuropathy in fibromyalgia patients. Clin Rheumatol 2015;34:413–7.
28. Nodera H, Barbano RL, Henderson D, et al. Epidermal reinnervation concomitant with symptomatic improvement in a sensory neuropathy. Muscle Nerve 2003;27: 507–9.
29. Levine T, Saperstein D. Improvement in small fiber neuropathies following immunomodulatory therapy. Neurology 2011;76(Suppl 4):A109.
30. Khoshnoodi MA, Truelove S, Burakgazi A, et al. Longitudinal assessment of small fiber neuropathy: evidence of a non-length-dependent distal axonopathy. JAMA Neurol 2016;73:684–90.

Other Myopathies

Yessar Hussain, MD[a,b,*], Samantha Miller, MD[a]

KEYWORDS

• Toxic myopathy • Drug-induced myopathy • Statin myopathy
• Necrotizing myopathy • Myalgia • Progressive weakness • Metabolic myopathy
• Pompe disease

KEY POINTS

- Toxic myopathies have a variable presentation and most resolve with discontinuation of the offending agent.
- Metabolic myopathies are genetic disorders that typically present with exercise-induced symptoms.
- Mitochondrial disorders are multisystemic disorders caused by impaired oxidative phosphorylation.
- Congenital myopathies usually present in early childhood with static or slowly progressive muscle weakness and hypotonia.
- Genetic testing/next-generation sequencing is becoming an integral part of the workup.

Video content accompanies this article at http://www.neurologic.theclinics.com.

TOXIC MYOPATHIES

Case Report

Title: proximal weakness and myalgia

Case presentation A 58-year-old man presented with progressive muscle weakness. His symptoms started 1 year before presentation, noted first at lower extremities with difficulty climbing stairs and standing from sitting position. It later progressed to his upper extremities with diffuse muscle pain. His weakness progressed to more severe and diffuse with worsening pain, leading to admission to inpatient due to severe weakness. He has been on chronic statin therapy (atorvastatin). His statin was held at the hospital and presented at an outpatient clinic 2 months later.

His examination (Video 1) showed proximal upper and lower extremity weakness including mild facial involvement and neck flexion weakness with sensory sparing and normal reflexes. He had no skin rash.

[a] UT Austin/Dell Medical School, Austin, TX, USA; [b] Austin Neuromuscular Center, 3901 Medical Parkway, Suite 300, Austin, TX 78756, USA
* Corresponding author. 3901 Medical Parkway, Suite 300, Austin, TX 78756.
E-mail address: yessar@austinneuromuscle.com

Neurol Clin 38 (2020) 619–635
https://doi.org/10.1016/j.ncl.2020.04.002

His workup showed creatine kinase (CK) at 10,000 range during his admission to the hospital, and currently at 3000. Anti–signal recognition particle (anti-SRP) and HMGCR (3-hydroxy-3-methylglutaryl-coenzyme A reductase) antibodies were negative. Electromyogram (EMG) showed irritable myopathic changes. Muscle biopsy showed (**Fig. 1**) myopathic changes with necrotic muscle fibers and no lymphocytic infiltration.

He continued to be off of statin therapy and started having gradual improvement over time. He was back to baseline after a year from ceasing statin therapy.

Clinical question

- Are progressive muscle weakness and myalgia related to direct statin toxicity or a related inflammatory/autoimmune pathology?
- What are the pathologic findings that are suggestive of the final diagnosis?
- What circumstances should lead to starting immune therapy?

Discussion

The proximal weakness with diffuse myalgia and elevated CK were suggestive of underlying myopathic pathology, supported by EMG. Chronic statin therapy and myofiber necrosis with minimal lymphocytic inflammatory changes on muscle pathology lead to the diagnosis of non–immune-mediated necrotizing myopathy, likely statin induced. Usually recovery starts after holding statin therapy, but continuous progression or lack of recovery should raise the possibility of immune-mediated pathology and considering immune therapy. For further details see Toxic Myopathy review below.

Toxic Myopathy

A thorough medication history is integral in the workup of myopathy, as several commonly prescribed medications are known to cause muscle toxicity.[1–3] Early identification of toxic myopathy is important, as in many cases symptoms resolve simply with cessation of the offending agent.[4] This article reviews causes of medication-induced toxic myopathy with a focus on necrotizing myopathy.

A thorough medication history includes the following:

- Current medications
- Past medications
- Date started
- Dose
- Date of dose adjustment
- Alcohol and drug use
- Toxin exposure

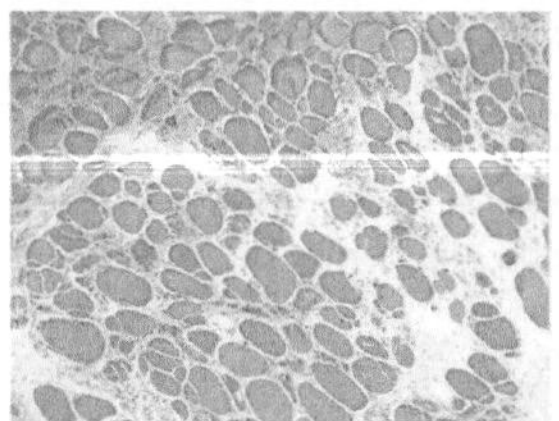

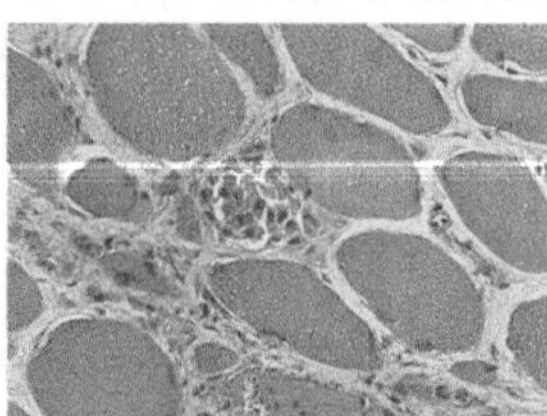

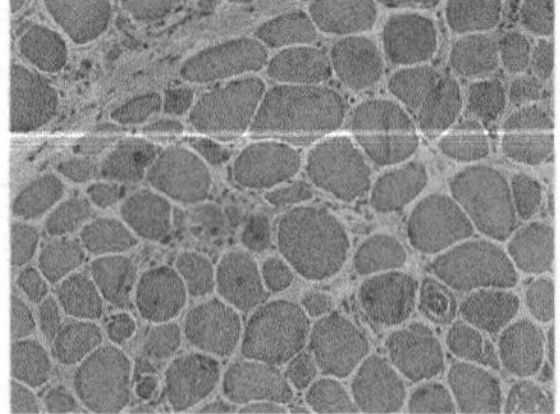

Fig. 1. Hematoxylin-eosin stain (Original magnification x 10x [right]; Original magnification × 10x [left]; Original magnification × 40x [middle]) shows myopathic changed with necrotic muscle fiber and no lymphocytic infiltration.

There are a number of recognized myotoxic medications. It is useful to group these medications by their implicated pathogenic mechanism of muscle injury (**Fig. 2**), as this directly influences the associated clinical presentation and histopathology.[3]

Clinical Presentation

Fig. 2 illustrates why toxic myopathies have a variety of clinical presentations depending on pathogenic mechanism, and why they can mimic the presentation of other myopathies. For example,[4]

- Hypokalemic myopathies can present with triggered episodes of flaccid paralysis separated by periods of normal strength.
- Mitochondrial myopathies can present with exercise intolerance.
- Amphiphilic drugs (ie, amiodarone, chloroquine, hydroxychloroquine) can cause a neuromyopathy, so patients may present with complaints of numbness, tingling, and/or paresthesias in addition to myopathic symptoms.
- Necrotizing myopathies usually present with myalgia, proximal weakness, and elevated creatinine kinase. Statin medication can cause a necrotizing myopathy, as seen in the case discussed previously. We discuss this type of toxic myopathy in more depth.

Necrotizing Myopathy

Necrotizing myopathy is defined by the classic histologic finding of myofiber necrosis without significant lymphocytic inflammatory infiltrate.[5,6] Causes of necrotizing myopathy can be grouped into immune-mediated (IMNM) and non–immune-mediated (NIMNM).

- IMNM can be triggered by myositis-specific antibodies, connective tissue disease, malignancies, viral illness, and statin medications.
- NIMNM is caused by a toxin or a drug exposure. A number of commonly prescribed medications can cause a toxic necrotizing myopathy. Cholesterol-

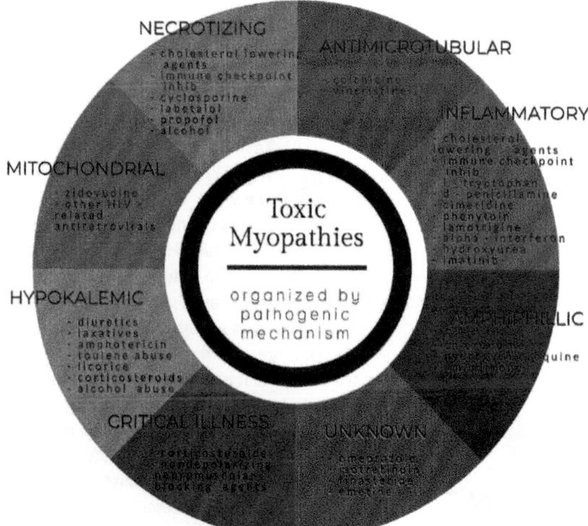

Fig. 2. There are a number of recognized myotoxic medications. It is useful to group these medications by their implicated pathogenic mechanism of muscle injury as this directly influences the associated clinical presentation and histnna1-hnlnev.

lowering drugs are a commonly identified cause; however, other culprits include immunophilins (cyclosporine and tacrolimus), labetalol, and propofol.[4] Organophosphate poisoning, recreational drugs (cocaine, heroin), and acute or chronic alcohol exposure can also cause a necrotizing myopathy.[7,8]

Refer to **Fig. 3** for the workup and treatment of necrotizing myopathy.

Statin Myopathy

Statin myalgia

Myalgia is the most common symptom associated with statin medications; however, it is also a common complaint in the general population, making it difficult to determine if a myalgia is truly statin-related in a given patient. The STOMP trial found that 9% of patients taking atorvastatin experienced true statin-associated myalgia[9] and shared the following characteristics[5]:

- Symptom onset soon after initiation or uptitration of statin medication
- Limb-girdle pattern of weakness/pain (rather than generalized myalgia, as seen in patients receiving a placebo)
- Symptom resolution with discontinuation of statin medication

When managing a patient with mild myalgia and no weakness, consider checking vitamin D, as low levels have been associated with a generalized myalgia that resolves with vitamin D repletion. In addition, CK level should be checked. However, keep in

Necrotizing Myopathy

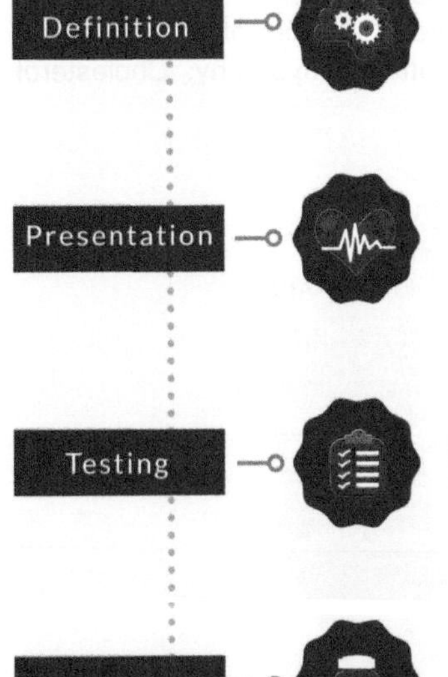

Defined by necrosis of myofibers without lymphocytic inflammatory infiltrates

- Two categories: immune mediated (IMNM) and nonimmune mediated (NIMNM) necrotizing myopathy
- IMNM etiologies: myositis specific Ab, connective tissue disease, viral illness, malignancy, statin medication
- NIMNM etiologies: myotoxic medication / toxin

Most common presentation is proximal muscle weakness with myalgia

- Presentation can range from mild myalgias with or without weakness to profound weakness and rhabdomyolysis
- Patients exposed to more than one myotoxic medication / toxin generally have a more severe clinical presentation

Workup of acute onset proximal weakness: Serum CK level, EMG and muscle biopsy

- Moderately elevated CK and myopathic changes on EMG narrow the differential to acquired muscle diseases: dermatomyositis, polymyositis, inclusion body myositis and necrotizing myopathy
- Prominent myofiber necrosis and lack of inflammatory cell infiltrates on muscle biopsy is indicative of necrotizing myopathy
- NIMNM is diagnosed when there is clinical improvement after discontinuation of myotoxic medication / toxin

NIMNM should be ruled out prior to diagnosis and/or treatment of IMNM

- NIMNM treatment: discontinue myotoxic medication / toxin
- IMNM treatment: high dose prednisone followed by a steroid sparing agent. IVIG can be used as rescue or maintenance therapy.

Fig. 3. The definition, presentation, testing, and treatment of necrotizing myopathies. IVIG, intravenous immunoglobulin. Ab, Anti body.

mind that if a baseline CK was not assessed before initiation of statin medication, it is difficult to say with certainty that an elevated level is due to statin use. If the patient has a very elevated CK or develops proximal muscle weakness, consider further workup for immune-mediated necrotizing myopathy (see later in this article). Refer to **Fig. 4** for the workup and treatment of statin myalgia.[9]

Statin-associated rhabdomyolysis

Statin-associated rhabdomyolysis is estimated to occur in 1 of every 7428 patients treated.[8] It is relatively rare, but given the large number of patients taking statin medications, it is not uncommonly seen. As shown in **Fig. 5**, one study found that statin medications accounted for almost 18% of patients hospitalized with a medication-induced rhabdomyolysis.[8] Of note, statin medications (except pravastatin) are metabolized by the CYP 450 enzyme system; therefore, serum concentration can iatrogenically increase due to drug or food interactions that inhibit statin breakdown, such as grape juice consumption.[9] The 2 main triggers for statin-associated rhabdomyolysis are

- High-dose statin
- Elevated serum statin concentration due to drug interactions (ie, concurrent use of amiodarone, calcium channel blockers, cyclosporine, fibrates, ezetimibe, niacin, "azole" antifungals, colchicine).

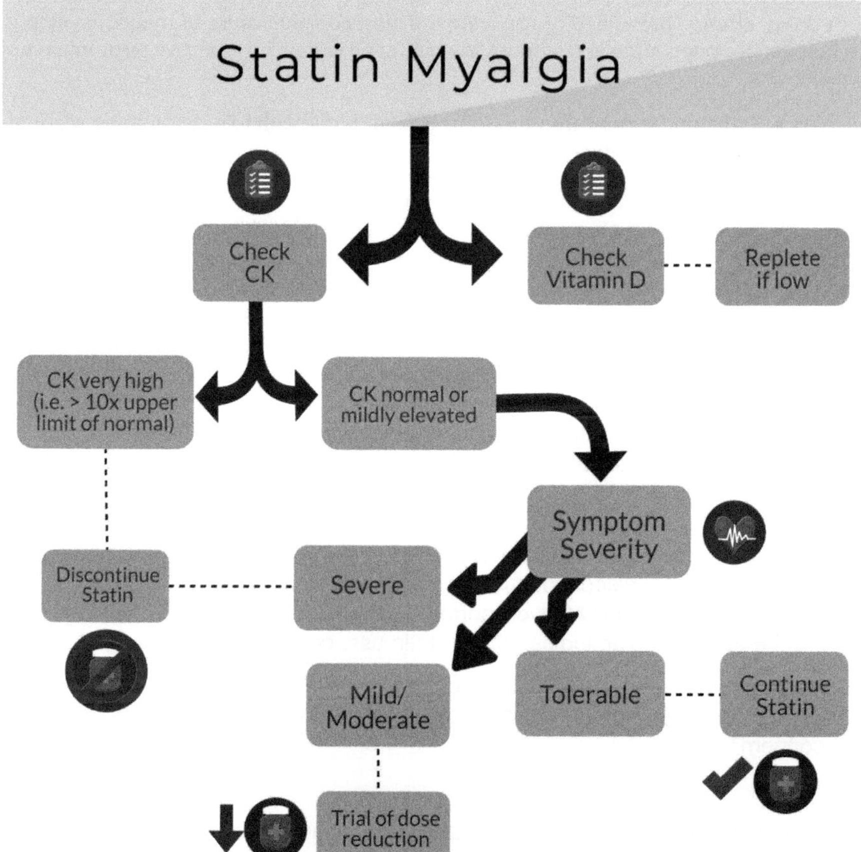

Fig. 4. Workup and treatment of statin myalgia.

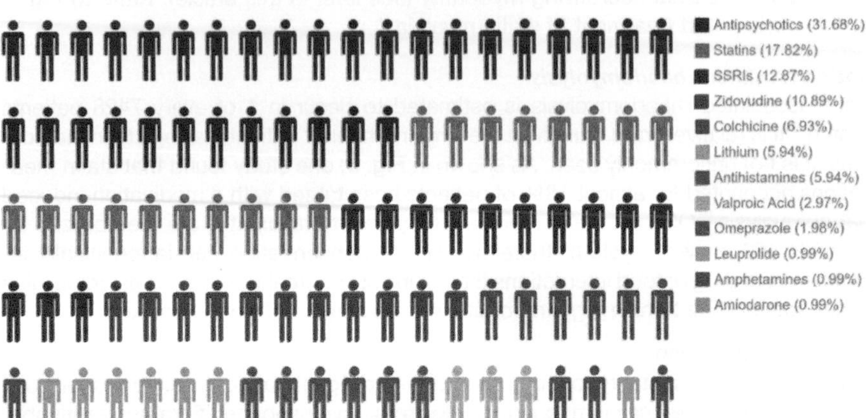

Fig. 5. Causes of drug-induced rhabdomyolysis in hospitalized patients at Johns Hopkins Hospital based on inpatient records from January 1993 to December 2001. Exogenous toxins (illicit drugs, alcohol, prescribed drugs) were the most common cause of rhabdomyolysis in this hospitalized population and account for 46% of all cases. SSRI, selective serotonin reuptake inhibitor.

Treatment of statin-associated rhabdomyolysis is discontinuation of statin medication and supportive treatment.

Statin-associated necrotizing autoimmune myopathy

Statin-associated necrotizing autoimmune myopathy (SANAM) classically causes severe and isolated proximal muscle weakness with markedly elevated CK. In these patients, discontinue statin medication and check for anti–HMG-CoA reductase and anti-SRP antibodies. A seronegative patient with persistent symptoms and elevated CK can undergo further evaluation with muscle biopsy, which classically shows myofiber necrosis without lymphocytic infiltration; however, this is seen in both toxic and immune-mediated necrotizing myopathy. Increased expression of MHC-1 on healthy myofibers is suggestive of autoimmune necrotizing myopathy. Treatment is discontinuation of statin medication and immunotherapy (ie, intravenous immunoglobulin).

Monitoring

Patients should be followed to ensure resolution of symptoms and normalization of CK level after reduction or discontinuation of statin medication.

If symptoms resolve and CK levels normalize after discontinuation of statin medication and the patient has an indication for statin use, consider the following:

- Restarting the same statin medication at a lower dosage; continue to monitor CK
- Trial of an alternate statin; consider pravastatin if drug interactions are of concern[9]

Red flags:

- Symptoms persist 2 to 3 months after discontinuation of statin medication or progress. This should raise concern for SANAM and requires further workup and treatment with immunosuppression.

- Persistently elevated CK after discontinuation of statin medication should raise concern for presence of CK elevation before initiation of statin and prompt further workup for alternate diagnosis.

SUMMARY

Toxic myopathies can present in a number of ways and can even mimic other myopathies. Clinicians should maintain a high index of suspicion and be sure to thoroughly examine the medication history of all patients presenting with myalgia and/or weakness, as simply discontinuing the myotoxic agent can resolve symptoms and avoid unnecessary testing and treatment. Statin-associated myalgia occurs in approximately 9% of patients and does not necessitate statin discontinuation if symptoms are mild. Failure of symptoms or elevated CK to improve after statin discontinuation or development of proximal weakness should raise concern for an alternate diagnosis and prompt further workup.

METABOLIC MYOPATHIES

Case Report

Title: progressive axial and proximal weakness with orthopnea

Case presentation A 48-year-old woman presented with upper and lower extremity weakness. Her symptoms started in her early 40s, with lower extremity myalgia and frequent falls. She noted having trouble standing from sitting and climbing stairs. Her myalgia and weakness progressed to her upper extremities and she started noting difficulty breathing when lying down. As a result, she started sleeping in a more upright position. Her ambulation deteriorated, and she ended up using a wheelchair. She has been evaluated initially by an outside facility, diagnosed with polymyositis, and placed on prednisone 60 mg daily. Her weakness did not improve, but myalgia showed some improvement. She had no significant family history.

Her examination (Video 2) showed severe proximal weakness, including thighs, adductors, neck flexion, and mild facial involvement with distal muscle groups sparing and Trendelenburg gait. Sensory examination was normal and showed relatively spared reflexes.

Her workup showed normal CK; EMG showed irritable myopathic changes in proximal muscle groups and pseudomyotonic discharges in the axial muscles. Her supine forced vital capacity (FVC) was 1.4 L (45% of predicted) and sitting FVC was 2.1 L (61% predicted).

Muscle pathology (**Fig. 6**) showed vacuolar myopathy (subsarcolemmal and internal), increased cytoplasmic lysosomes staining (acid phosphatase), and normal to

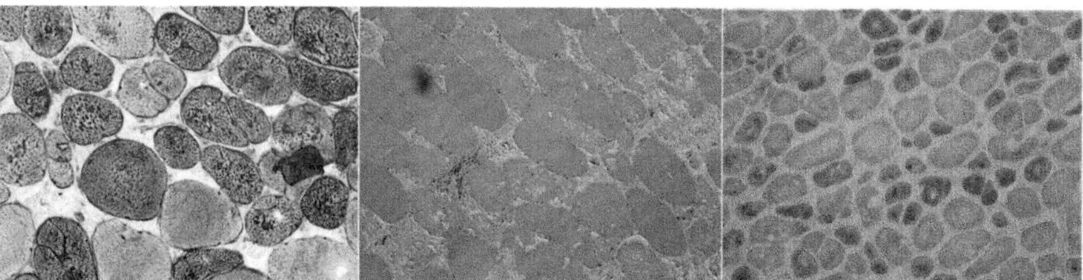

Fig. 6. Vacuolar myopathy (subsarcolemmal and internal), increased cytoplasmic lysosomes staining, and normal to slightly patchy increased glycogen in periodic acid–Schiff (PAS) stain. Left to right: hematoxylin-eosin (Original magnification x 20x), PAS (Original magnification x 20x), nonspecific esterase.

slightly patchy increased glycogen in periodic acid–Schiff stain. Blood alpha glucosidase was low at 2.0 (Nl >3.88 pmol/punch per hour). GAA gene sequencing showed 2 heterozygous variants (splicing mutation at first intron and deletion at axon 18).

Alpha-glucosidase 20 mg/kg every 2 weeks was started, and the patient showed gradual improvement over the following 2 years with respiratory function, and started ambulating with a walker.

Clinical question

- What were the signs and symptoms at presentation that were suggestive of the final diagnosis?
- Was muscle biopsy needed?
- What is the best screening test for the final diagnosis?

Discussion The proximal weakness at presentation is not specific, but the relatively more severe thigh adductors and axial involvement with significant orthopnea are suggestive of acid maltase deficiency. Pseudomyotonia on EMG of the axial muscles is another clue and should have promoted screening for acid maltase deficiency (blood alpha-glucosidase level) before proceeding with muscle biopsy. For further details, refer to Glycogen Storage Disease review below.

Metabolic Myopathy

Metabolic myopathies are genetic disorders that impair intermediary metabolism in skeletal muscle. Most fall into 1 of 3 categories: glycogen storage diseases, fatty acid oxidation defects, and mitochondrial myopathies.[10] Metabolic myopathies typically present with exercise-induced muscle cramps, pain, and/or myoglobinuria. Symptoms can also be provoked by fasting, cold, and metabolic stress. Some metabolic myopathies present with progressive proximal muscle weakness and can resemble limb-girdle muscular dystrophies.[11] The different metabolic myopathies can be described as either dynamic (symptomatic with exertion) or static (nonexertional symptoms).

All metabolic myopathies are autosomal recessive (AR) and cause CK elevation. Most can be diagnosed via muscle biopsy or genetic testing.

Glycogen Storage Diseases

Presenting during brief periods of high-intensity exercise, glycogen storage diseases cause muscle cramps within seconds to minutes of exercise. Many people with glycogen storage disease also have pigmenturia (dark or red urine from myoglobin caused by rhabdomyolysis during exercise). Most glycogen storage diseases are AR with no family history. Neurologic examination is typically normal between episodes.

Myophosphorylase deficiency (glycogen storage disease V, McArdle disease), a disorder of glycolysis, is the most common metabolic myopathy affecting 1 in 100,000 people. It is an AR disorder due to mutations in the muscle isoform of phosphorylase (muscle glycogen phosphorylase, *PYGM*) Many individuals may have a second-wind phenomenon, unique to McArdle disease, in which pain resolves after initial onset of exertional myalgias or cramps, allowing the individual to resume exercising.

In glycogen storage diseases, CK can be, but is not always, elevated, and EMG and nerve conduction studies are often normal and not of diagnostic value with the exception of Pompe disease.

Pompe disease (glycogen storage disease II, acid maltase deficiency) is an AR disease caused by mutations in the gene encoding lysosomal acid alpha-1,4-glucosidase (GAA).

Pompe disease has a classic infantile form presenting with hypertrophic cardiomyopathy and a late-onset juvenile/adult form without cardiomyopathy. The late-onset form should be suspected in people with progressive proximal weakness in a limb-girdle distribution with or without respiratory involvement. In Pompe disease, EMG and nerve conduction study results show characteristic myotonic and complex repetitive discharges. In mild forms of the disease these findings may be present only in the paraspinal muscles.[12] The classic histopathological finding is myofibers with glycogen-filled vacuoles that intensely stain for acid phosphatase; however, in late-onset disease, there may be only nonspecific changes. Gene sequencing is the preferred test for diagnosis.[13] Early diagnosis of Pompe disease is important, as it is the only metabolic myopathy that is treatable. Intravenous recombinant alpha-glucosidase enzyme can treat infantile Pompe disease but may have only a modest effect in late-onset disease.[12]

The classic diagnostic test for glycogen storage myopathies is the forearm exercise test in which a blood pressure cuff is inflated beyond arterial pressure while isometric rhythmic exercises are performed for 1 minute, followed by release of the cuff. Lactate and ammonia values collected before inflating and immediately after deflation are collected and compared. In glycolytic and glycogenolytic diseases, ammonia is elevated threefold, but lactate shows no significant rise.[14] Genetic testing can be done with next-generation sequencing or targeted analysis of a known genetic mutation. Muscle biopsy is not necessary after these steps, but can show high glycogen, absent phosphorylase, or absent phosphofructokinase.

Fatty Acid Oxidation Defects

Fatty acid oxidation defects present during long-duration or short-intensity activities, fasting, or stressful events (eg, surgery, fever, or flu). In fatty acid oxidation defects, CK levels may be elevated during acute rhabdomyolysis, and EMG and nerve conduction study results are often normal. The most sensitive and specific diagnostic test is a serum acylcarnitine profile, performed under fasting conditions.[14] Next-generation sequencing panels or target analysis of the known genetic mutation based on the serum acylcarnitine profile can be done afterward. Muscle biopsy is not necessary after genetic testing; when done, it may show nonspecific increase in neutral lipid.

Mitochondrial Myopathies

A heterogeneous group of disorders with a range of phenotypes and genotypes, mitochondrial myopathies also present during long-duration or short-intensity exercise, fasting, or stressful events. Rhabdomyolysis and pigmenturia are uncommon, and findings on the neurologic examination are variable owing to the multisystem involvement of the disease (eg, ptosis, ophthalmoplegia, or deafness, encephalopathy). The resting serum lactate level is elevated in 65% of patients with mitochondrial myopathies, and EMG and nerve conduction study results are often normal or nonspecific.[13] Muscle biopsy is more helpful than in the glycogen storage diseases and fatty acid oxidation defects with characteristic histologic features of ragged red fibers on the modified Gomori-trichrome stain. As with the other myopathies, next-generation sequencing or target analysis of the known genetic mutation or of the mitochondrial genome is available for diagnosis.

MITOCHONDRIAL MYOPATHIES

Case Report

Title: slowly progressive proximal weakness with ophthalmoplegia

Clinical presentation A 37-year-old man presented with 3 years' history of progressive fixed bilateral ptosis, occasional blurry vision, and chronic exercise intolerance for the past 7 years. His symptoms progressed to muscle weakness as well as difficulty climbing stairs and reaching over his head. He had no shortness of breath or dysphagia, and no significant family history.

His examination (Video 3) showed ophthalmoplegia at all directions, with ptosis, mild bulbar weakness, and proximal upper and lower extremity weakness. His ice pack test showed no ptosis improvement.

Laboratory work showed elevated CK at 400s, normal aldolase, and negative acetyl choline receptors binding antibodies. Carnitine and acylcarnitine panels were negative. EMG showed nonirritable myopathic changes from proximal muscle groups and no decrement on slow repetitive nerve stimulation (RNS). Pyridostigmine trial failed.

Muscle pathology (**Fig. 7**) showed evidence of chronic myopathy with mitochondrial changes (positive succinic dehydrogenase and negative cytochrome oxidase [COX], and ragged red fiber). Mitochondrial assay showed reduced complex I and complex II/III activities.

Cardiac Evaluation Showed Normal Electrocardiogram and 2Dcho

Clinical question

- What is the differential diagnosis of proximal muscle weakness with ocular involvement?
- What are the signs and symptoms at presentation that are suggestive of the final diagnosis?
- What is the diagnostic test for the final diagnosis?

Discussion The slowly progressive proximal weakness at presentation is not specific, but the nonfluctuating ptosis and progressive ophthalmoplegia with no diplopia are suggestive of mitochondrial myopathy. Myasthenia gravis needs to be considered, but the lack of diplopia, dysphagia, shortness of breath, and symptom fluctuation makes it unlikely. Muscle biopsy and mitochondrial assay are necessary to establish final diagnosis, and genetic testing is helpful to further classify the underlying pathology. For further details refer to the review below.

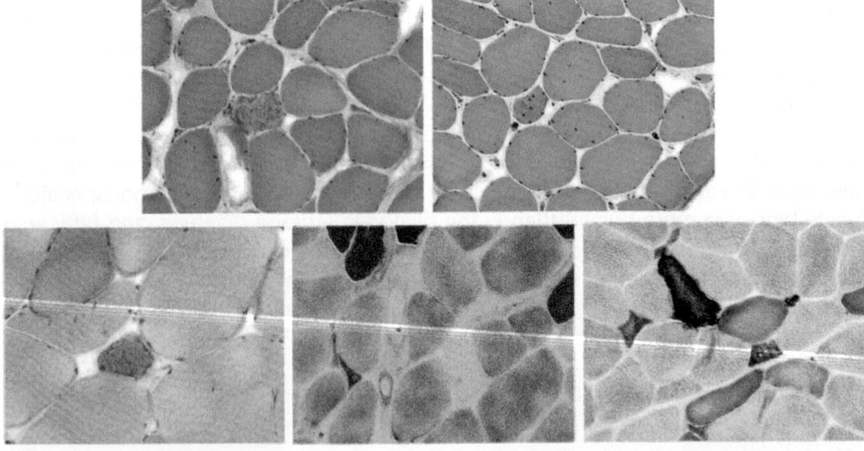

Fig. 7. Chronic myopathic pathology with mitochondrial changes (positive succinic dehydrogenase and negative COX, and ragged red fiber). Top: hematoxylin-eosin (Original magnification x 20x) bottom: Gomori trichrome (Original magnification x 20x).

Mitochondrial Myopathy

Mitochondrial myopathy refers to a group of clinically highly variable progressive muscle conditions that are caused by impaired oxidative phosphorylation related to mitochondrial enzyme deficits.[15] This group of conditions can be thought of as a myopathic manifestation of a mitochondrial cytopathy. Mitochondrial function is controlled by both mitochondrial and nuclear DNA; genetic variation in either can cause dysfunction. This results in multiple possible inheritance patterns.

There are several mitochondrial disorders associated with myopathy:

- Myoclonic epilepsy with ragged red fibers (MERRF)
- Mitochondrial encephalopathy, lactic acidosis, and stroke-like episodes (MELAS)
- Mitochondrial myopathies associated with recurrent myoglobinuria
- Kearns-Sayre syndrome
- Progressive external ophthalmoplegia
- Mitochondrial DNA depletion syndrome

Clinical Presentation

It is important to obtain a thorough family history in patients with suspected mitochondrial myopathy, as the identification of inheritance pattern will help to guide genetic testing. Because of the high energy requirement of skeletal muscle, exercise intolerance is a common feature among patients with these conditions.

In severe forms, ATP production is insufficient to meet metabolic demands at rest, and there is an overreliance on anaerobic metabolism, producing high baseline lactate concentrations.[15] Understandably, these patients also can be tachycardic, tachypneic, and diaphoretic at rest. Less severely affected patients will be asymptomatic at rest but exercise testing can cause tachycardia and increased oxygen consumption despite a low level of work.[16] Other common symptoms include proximal myopathy and fatigue.

However, mitochondrial diseases are multisystemic disorders that can affect several organ systems, including the eyes, heart, liver, and nervous systems, among others. The most common clinical presentation is in fact a combination of symptoms.[15] Specifically, myopathic symptoms co-occurring with external ophthalmoplegia, heart conduction block, short stature, deafness, diabetes, or epilepsy are suggestive of mitochondrial disease.[17]

Workup

When mitochondrial myopathy is suspected, diagnostic tools include the following[15,17,18]:

- Resting serum CK, lactate, and pyruvate levels.
- Cerebrospinal fluid lactate and pyruvate levels.
- Histologic and immunohistochemical studies: ragged red fibers (in modified Gomori Trichrome stain), although not specific, are the classic histopathological muscle biopsy finding in mitochondrial disease; however, muscle biopsy also can appear normal in these patients. It remains an important tool in the workup of mitochondrial disease and can help guide genetic testing.
- Enzymatic analysis of oxidative phosphorylation complexes: COX (complex IV of the mitochondrial respiratory chain) negative fibers are another classic finding in mitochondrial diseases.

- Genetic analysis of mitochondrial DNA: performed when mitochondrial mutation is suspected. DNA analysis on muscle tissue is more sensitive than blood in mitochondrial DNA mutations due to the phenomenon of heteroplasmy.
- Targeted nuclear DNA sequencing: performed when nuclear mutation is suspected.
- Whole genome/whole exome screens: becoming increasingly popular in the setting of next-generation sequencing. Functional testing must be done when new genetic variants of unclear significance are found to verify pathogenicity.

Treatment

Treatment is largely focused on symptom management but also includes ensuring patients receive proper screening based on their syndrome or genetic deficit. For example, annual cardiac screening is recommended for patients with MELAS or MERRF.[19] Exercise programs are shown to be beneficial to patients with mitochondrial myopathy both biochemically and chemically. There are no effective or disease-modifying therapies at this time; however, there are several ongoing studies and clinical trials. In addition, there are reproductive options for patients that decrease the risk of transmission of the pathologic genetic mutation.[15]

CONGENITAL MYOPATHIES

Case Report

Title: a young man with long-standing history of slowly progressive proximal weakness

Clinical presentation A 30-year-old man presented with slowly progressive proximal weakness since his teens, having exercise intolerance as well as trouble climbing stairs and reaching over his head with minimal myalgia, mainly induced by exercise. He showed no dysphagia or shortness of breath and no ocular symptoms and had no significant family history.

His examination showed proximal upper and lower extremity weakness with facial involvement, no bulbar weakness, and no scapular winging or clinical myotonia. His sensory examination and reflexes were normal.

CK level was 500 IU/L and EMG showed proximal nonirritable myopathy with normal RNS.

Cardiology workup was negative.

His muscle biopsy (**Fig. 8**) showed chronic myopathic changes with type I predominance, and many fibers with central nuclei, no inflammatory or mitochondrial pathology.

Genetic testing showed novel X-linked SRPKs gene mutation.

Clinical questions

- What is the differential diagnosis of slowly progressive proximal muscle weakness since childhood with no scapular winging or ocular involvement?
- What are the signs and symptoms at presentation that are suggestive of the final diagnosis?
- What is the diagnostic test of the final diagnosis?

Discussion The long-standing history of proximal myopathy and with minimal and slow progression raise the possibility of congenital myopathy rather dystrophic myopathy. Mitochondrial myopathy and congenital myasthenia gravis are less likely given the lack of ocular involvement and the workup findings (elevated CK and normal slow RNS). Muscle pathology and genetic testing will establish the final diagnosis. For further details refer to the review below.

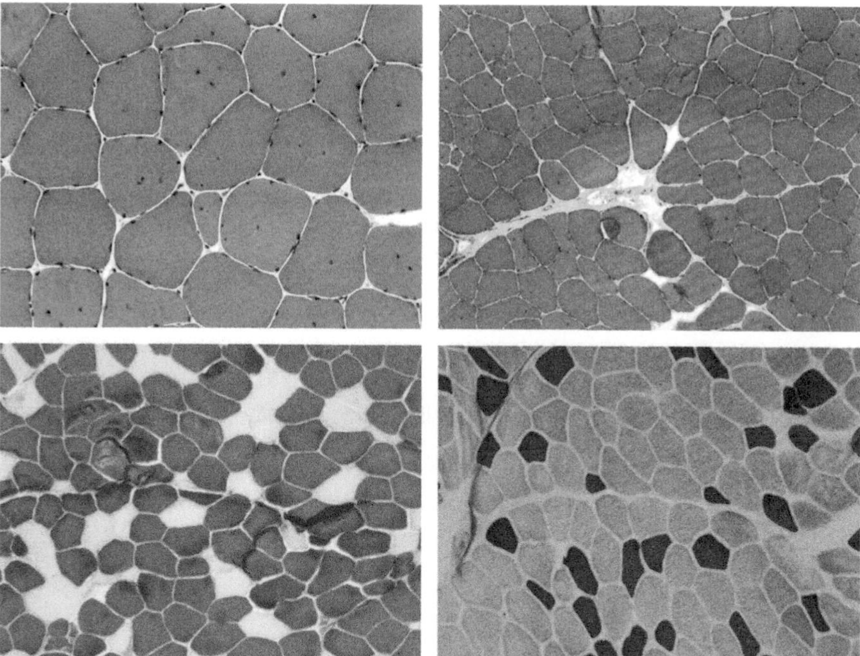

Fig. 8. Chronic myopathic changes with type I predominance, and many fibers with central nuclei, no inflammatory or mitochondrial pathology. Top: hematoxylin-eosin (Original magnification x 20x [upper left]; Original magnification x 10x [upper right]) Bottom: ATPase (Original magnification x 10x[lower]).

Congenital Myopathy

Classically, congenital myopathies present in infancy or childhood with static or slowly progressive muscle weakness and hypotonia.[20] They are rare conditions; estimated prevalence is 0.6 to 2 per 100,000 individuals.[21] Rarely, congenital myopathies can present or progress in adulthood. This is important because these patients will present for evaluation in the adult neurology clinic where congenital myopathies are less commonly seen. This article reviews the basics of congenital myopathies with a focus on adult-onset disease.

Overview

Congenital myopathies are defined by their histologic appearance on muscle biopsy, which classically includes local myofibrillar disorganization, nuclear centralization, and protein aggregation.[20]

Congenital myopathies have been subdivided into groups based on classically shared myopathologic features. The following are identified groups[20]:

1. Core myopathy: Characterized by the absence of oxidative enzyme activity in the center of the myofiber due to mitochondrial depletion. There are 2 recognized subgroups:
   - Central core myopathy
   - Multiminicore myopathy
2. Centronuclear/myotubular myopathy: characterized pathologically by the presence of abundant centrally located nuclei. Most associated gene mutations encode proteins implicated in membrane trafficking.[22]

3. Nemaline myopathies: characterized by the classic finding of numerous nemaline rod bodies on muscle biopsy.
4. Congenital fiber-type disproportion myopathy.

Clinical History

Diagnosis of congenital myopathy is challenging, as patients can present in a variety of ways. It is important to include a thorough familial history in the workup of these patients to identify if a pattern of inheritance is present. Family members may be brought into the clinic for evaluation, as clinical findings may be subtle and otherwise go unnoticed.

Common clinical features of congenital myopathy include the follwoing[22]:

- Pronounced truncal weakness
- Pronounced proximal weakness
- Orthopedic manifestations: scoliosis, ligamentous laxity

Clinical features suggestive of underlying genetic defect include the following[22]:

- Extraocular muscle involvement
- Distal muscle involvement
- Respiratory muscle involvement
- Cardiac involvement

Adult-Onset Congenital Myopathy

Adult-onset congenital myopathy (**Table 1**) can occur with central core myopathy, centronuclear myopathy, and nemaline myopathy, and is associated with genetic mutations in RYR1 (autosomal dominant [AD] > AR), DNM2, BIN1 (AD), KBTD13, ACTA1, and MYH7.[21,22] In adult-onset congenital myopathies, muscle weakness may not present until adulthood, but some patients will retrospectively report difficulty with sports in childhood.[22]

One retrospective study of congenital myopathies diagnosed in adulthood (>18 years old) at the Mayo Clinic over a 10-year period identified 18 patients with pediatric onset and 26 patients with adult-onset congenital myopathy. Pediatric-onset patients were diagnosed at a median age of 40 years, whereas in adult-onset disease the median age of symptom onset was 47 years. The following were the most frequently identified reasons for a delay in diagnosis[21]:

- Absence of prior neurologic workup due to symptoms that were considered benign or were attributed to a non-neurologic condition
- Not knowing that nonspecific changes on muscle biopsy can still represent a congenital myopathy

The most common misdiagnosis that patients received were the following:

- Non-neurologic disorders (ie, rheumatologic and orthopedic disorders)
- Statin-induced myopathy
- Neuropathy
- Mitochondrial myopathy
- Limb-girdle muscular dystrophy

Note that a couple of patients underwent immunosuppressive treatment due to a misdiagnosis.

This retrospective analysis highlights some key features of adult-onset congenital myopathy:

Table 1
Clinical and genetic characteristics of congenital myopathies

	Late-Onset Centronuclear	Late-Onset Nemaline Myopathy	Multi/Minicore Myopathy	Central Core Myopathy
Inheritance	AD	AD/AR/Sporadic	AR/Spontaneous/AD	AD
Clinical findings	Variable pattern of weakness. Some patients may have only proximal or only distal weakness.	Myopathy presenting after age 40. Proximal, distal, and generalized weakness. Dysphagia, cardiomyopathy. Isolated neck extensor weakness possible.	Infant or adult onset. Generalized weakness and atrophy Proximal >> Distal. Subset with distal hand weakness.	Proximal weakness. Mild face/neck extensor weakness.
Facial/EOM involvement	May be present	None or mild	Rare	Spares EOM
Progression	Mild, slowly progressive	Fast onset with slow progression	Stable/slowly progressive	
Contractures	None	None	Common	Rare
CK	Normal/mild elevation	Normal	Normal/mild elevation	Normal/mild elevation
Gene	DNM2 on 19p13.	Sporadic	Classic form: SEPN1 1p36	RYR1 on 19q13
Histopathology	Central nuclei often forming chains/clusters. Lack of ATPase staining around the nuclei. Type 1 fiber predominance and atrophy. Normal Type 2 fiber morphology	Nemaline rods best seen on EM.	Disorganized myofibrils form minicores (lack of NADH staining) in both Type1 and Type 2 muscles. Type 1 predominance and atrophy and fiber size variation.	Cores in Type 1 muscle fibers only (lack of NADH-TR staining) extend longitudinally throughout the muscle fiber. Fiber size variation, internalized nuclei.
Other	DNM2 mutation is known to be associated with some forms of CMT, may have abnormal NCS.	Respiratory weakness. Dysphagia. Cardiomyopathy. May be associated with MGUS.	High arched palate. Club feet. Cardiomyopathy. Respiratory weakness particularly during sleep	Risk of malignant hyperthermia.

Abbreviations: AD, autosomal dominant; AR, autosomal recessive; CK, creatine kinase; CMT, Charcot–Marie–Tooth disease; EM, electron microscopy; EOM, extraocular muscles; MGUS, monoclonal gammopathy of unknown significance; NADH, nicotinamide adenine dinucleotide; NCS, nerve conduction study; TR, tetrazolium reductase.

- A progressive rather than static disease course
- Decreased sensitivity of muscle biopsy due to lack of classic histopathological findings

The results indicate that there is a need for a classification system of congenital myopathies that does not rely so heavily on histopathological findings, especially when it comes to adult-onset variants. It also supports the use of next-generation sequencing (NGS) of associated genes in the diagnostic workup of these conditions.

Workup

Laboratory tests

- Serum CK: typically normal or slightly elevated.[23] Significantly elevated CK (ie, >10 times upper limit of normal) suggests an alternate diagnosis.[20]
- Acetylcholine receptor antibody assay: excludes autoimmune myasthenic conditions
- Analysis of multiple congenital myopathy–associated genes via NGS: preferred diagnostic approach

Neurophysiological studies

- Nerve conduction study (NCS)/EMG: exclude congenital neuropathies, myotonic disorders, and congenital myasthenic syndromes

Muscle biopsy followed by standard panel of histologic, histochemical, and immunohistochemical stains will confirm a specific congenital myopathy and exclude conditions with overlapping pathologic features, that is, congenital muscular dystrophies and mitochondrial conditions.

Muscle imaging (MRI, ultrasound) can identify specific patterns of muscle weakness associated with specific genetic myopathies.

Note that Nemaline rods are also commonly associated with nongenetic causes of myopathy, many of which present in adulthood and are referred to as sporadic late-onset Nemaline myopathy (SLONM). The most common etiologies are monoclonal gammopathy, human immunodeficiency virus (HIV), and autoimmune disorders. Clinically, SLONM presents with the following:

- Absence of weakness in childhood/adolescence
- Fast rate of progression (patients can develop severe limb-girdle, axial, and respiratory weakness within a few years)

It is important to recognize SLONM, as it can be treatable. Workup of rapidly progressive muscle weakness in an adult should include screening for M-protein and HIV.

Treatment

The treatment of congenital myopathies is mainly supportive at this time; however, there are ongoing clinical trials that are looking at genetic therapies, enzyme replacement therapies, and pharmacologic therapies as potential treatment options.[23]

DISCLOSURE

The authors have nothing to disclose.

SUPPLEMENTARY DATA

Supplementary data related to this article can be found online at https://doi.org/10.1016/j.ncl.2020.04.002.

REFERENCES

1. Mamman AL. Toxic myopathies. Continuum (Minneap Minn) 2013;19(6 Muscle Disease):1634–49.
2. Kuncl RW. Agents and mechanisms of toxic myopathy. Curr Opin Neurol 2009; 22(5):506–15.
3. Pasnoor M, et al. Toxic myopathies. Curr Opin Neurol 2018;31:575–82.
4. Pasnoor M, et al. Toxic myopathies. Neurol Clin 2014;32(3):647–viii.
5. Katzberg HD, et al. Toxic and endocrine myopathies. Continuum (Minneap Minn) 2016;22(6):1815–28.
6. Quinn C, et al. Necrotizing myopathies: an update. J Clin Neuromuscul Dis 2015; 16:131–40.
7. Allenbach Y, et al. Acquired necrotizing myopathies. Curr Opin Neurol 2013;26: 554–60.
8. Melli G, et al. Rhabdomyolysis, an evaluation of 475 hospitalized patients. Medicine 2005;84:377–85.
9. Hilton-Jones D. Statin myopathies. Pract Neurol 2018;18:97–105.
10. Haller RG. Treatment of McArdle disease. Arch Neurol 2000;57(7):923–4.
11. Berkowitz AL. Diseases of muscle. Clinical Neurology and Neuroanatomy 2017; 30:304–6.
12. Daroff RB, et al. Disorders of carbohydrate metabolism. Bradley's Neurology in Clinical Practice 2016;7(110):1941–2.
13. Hobson-Webb DD, Dearmey S, Kishnani PS. The clinical and electrodiagnostic characeristics of Pompe disease with post-enzyme replacement therapy findings. Clin Neurophysiol 2011;122(11):2312–7.
14. Tanopolsky MA. Metabolic myopathies. Continuum (Minneap Minn) 2016;22(6): 1829–51.
15. Ahmed ST, et al. Diagnosis and treatment of mitochondrial myopathies. Neurotherapeutics 2018;15:943–53.
16. Daroff RB, et al. Mitochondrial myopathies. Bradley's Neurol Clin Pract 2016; 7(110):1941–6.
17. Gray F, et al. Pathology of skeletal muscle. Basic Neuropatholohy 6(12):325–7.
18. Phadke R. Myopathology of adult and paediatric mitochondrial diseases. J Clin Med 2017;6(7):64.
19. Quadir A, et al. Systematic review and meta-analysis of cardiac involvement in mitochondrial myopathy. Neurol Genet 2019;5:339.
20. Mah JK. An overview of congenital myopathies. Continuum (Minneap Minn) 2016; 22(6):1932–53.
21. Nicolau S, et al. Congenital myopathies in the adult neuromuscular clinic. Neurol Genet 2019;5:e341.
22. Jungbluth H, et al. Congenital myopathies: not only a pediatric topic. Curr Opin Neurol 2016;29:642–50.
23. Jungbluth H, et al. Congenital myopathies: disorders of excitation-contraction coupling and muscle contraction. Nat Rev Neurol 2018;14:151–67.

Distal Myopathies

Kevin J. Felice, DO[a,b,*]

KEYWORDS

- Distal myopathy • Myofibrillar myopathy • Congenital myopathy
- Muscular dystrophy • Genetic myopathy

KEY POINTS

- The distal myopathies are a rare and heterogeneous group of disorders causing myopathic weakness at onset of the muscles of the hands, feet, or both.
- In addition to the classic distal myopathies, distal-onset or distal-prominent weakness is sometimes encountered in other genetic disorders including the myofibrillar, congenital, and dystrophic myopathies.
- The list of genetic disorders associated with distal-onset weakness is the ever-expanding and further complicated by pronounced genetic heterogeneity, phenotypic variability, and complex multisystem involvement.
- There are no known effective disease-modifying treatments for the distal myopathies.
- Evaluation, symptomatic management, and periodic monitoring of patients in a multidisciplinary neuromuscular center are the mainstays of care.

INTRODUCTION

The distal myopathies are a rare and heterogeneous group of disorders causing myopathic weakness at onset of the hands, feet, or both.[1] The term distal myopathy is usually reserved for genetic disorders; however, weakness of the distal muscles is sometimes present in the acquired muscle diseases.[2] In addition, prominent distal muscle weakness is also a feature of several of the most common inherited myopathies including myotonic muscular dystrophy type 1 and facioscapulohumeral muscular dystrophy (FSHD).[2,3] The first description of a distal myopathy was provided by the Russian neurologist, Dr Vladimir Roth, in a series of case studies from 1885 through 1893.[4] Detailed clinicopathologic study of these cases documented distal muscular atrophy—or "peripheral muscular tabes"—in the absence of nervous system involvement. The term distal myopathy was first mentioned by Gowers in 1902 in a patient with concurrent facial weakness—possibly an early description of myotonic dystrophy type 1.[5] In 1951, Welander reported the clinicopathologic findings of 249

[a] The Charles H. Kaman Foundation Neuromuscular and Muscular Dystrophy Association Care Center, Hospital for Special Care, 2150 Corbin Avenue, New Britain, CT 06053, USA; [b] University of Connecticut School of Medicine, Farmington, CT, USA
* Hospital for Special Care, 2150 Corbin Avenue, New Britain, CT 06053.
E-mail address: felicek@hfsc.org

Neurol Clin 38 (2020) 637–659
https://doi.org/10.1016/j.ncl.2020.03.007

patients from 72 Swedish families in an autosomal-dominant disorder presenting in adulthood with weakness of the long extensors of the hands.[6] The molecular genetic era for the distal myopathies began in 1995 with the mapping of Laing distal myopathy to chromosome 14 and the later discovery of *MYH7* gene mutations as the molecular etiology.[7,8] Since that time, the field of genetic distal myopathies has blossomed. The Gene Table of Neuromuscular Disorders lists 19 gene disorders under the heading of distal myopathies and a recent comprehensive review of the topic has added an additional 7 gene disorders.[9,10] **Table 1** summarizes the major distal myopathy types. This case-based review highlights the classic distal myopathies, including genetic and clinicopathologic aspects; discusses several other categories of genetic myopathies associated with distal weakness including the myofibrillar myopathies, congenital myopathies, muscular dystrophies, and other inherited myopathies; and provides a brief review on the evaluation and care of patients with these disorders.

EVALUATION

Clinical experience and a systematic approach are important skills in the evaluation of a new patient with distal myopathy given the ever-expanding list of disorders, pronounced genetic heterogeneity and phenotypic variability, and complex multisystem involvement in many of the disorders under consideration. As with all neurologic and neuromuscular evaluations, the history and clinical examination are the most important initial steps. Identifying the onset of symptoms, family history, and pattern of muscle involvement are key components in guiding further diagnostic studies (**Fig. 1**). In clinical practice, distal limb weakness of myopathic origin is uncommon and, therefore, initial consideration must be given to other neuromuscular disorders including motor neuron diseases and polyneuropathies. Hereditary motor neuropathies and Charcot–Marie–Tooth neuropathies are particularly important disorders to consider in familial cases presenting with bilateral foot drop, hand weakness, or both. Clinical clues—including preservation of foot muscle bulk in the setting of bilateral foot drop, preservation of intrinsic hand muscle function in the setting of prominent finger extensor weakness, and concurrent neck or proximal limb muscle weakness—are points in favor of primary muscle disease rather than neuropathy. For most cases, electroneuromyography (EMG) will be an important initial test in differentiating myopathy from other causes of weakness. In addition, EMG may uncover other important clues—for example, myotonic discharges would implicate a myotonic dystrophy or, possibly, Pompe disease; and the finding of fibrillation potentials and positive sharp waves would focus further testing on the dystrophic myopathies. Creatine kinase values are also helpful and may be normal or mildly elevated in most of the disorders, but highly elevated in the dysferlinopathies and other muscular dystrophies. MRI of the limbs and truncal muscles provides valuable insight on patterns of involvement, especially when the clinical examination is limited (eg, obese patient) and when muscle groups are difficult to assess clinically (eg, paraspinal muscles).[11] MRI is also useful in differentiating edema from fatty degeneration, muscle loss from normal aging (sarcopenia) versus neuromyopathic-induced atrophy, and true hypertrophy from pseudohypertrophy. In the author's experience, MRI evaluation of myopathy is sometimes limited by insurance carriers who impede or deny authorization for this testing. Muscle biopsy findings in the distal myopathies vary widely—and may provide valuable diagnostic clues in certain disorders, or show only nonspecific or nondiagnostic myopathic changes. Some of the characteristic findings include dystrophic and inflammatory changes (eg, Miyoshi myopathy, *ANO5*-related myopathy), rimmed vacuoles (eg, *GNE*-related myopathy, myofibrillar myopathies), and fiber type

Table 1
Distal myopathies

Gene	Name	Locus	Inheritance	Age at Onset (y)	Distal Weakness	Other	CK	Pathology	Allelic
ADSSL1		14q32–33	AR	5–17	Anterior foreleg	Facial weakness	2–3X	Myopathic, rimmed vacuoles	
ANO5	Miyoshi type 3	11 p14–12	AR	20–25	Posterior foreleg	Calf hypertrophy	10–50X	Myopathic, dystrophic	LGMD2L
CAV3	Tateyama	3p25	AD	12–45	Hand and foot	Calf hypertrophy	3–30X	Myopathy, dystrophic	LGMD1C, RMD, CM
DNAJB6		7q36	AD	16–55	Anterior and posterior foreleg Proximal weakness	1–6X	Rimmed vacuoles	LGMD1D	
DNM2	Centronuclear type 1	19p13.2	AD	0–50	Hand and foreleg	Facial and EOM weakness	1–2X	Central nuclei, type 1 atrophy	CMT2M
DYSF	Miyoshi	2p12–14	AR	15–30	Posterior foreleg	Calf atrophy	20–150X	dystrophic	LGMD2B
FLNC		7q32	AD	20–50	Hand and foreleg	Thenar atrophy	2–6X	Myopathic, dystrophic	MFM5, CM
GNE	Nonaka	9p13.3	AR	15–30	Anterior foreleg	Quadriceps sparing	3–5X	Rimmed vacuoles	Sialuria
KLHL9		9p21.2-p22.3	AD	8–16	Anterior foreleg	Sensory symptoms	1–5X	Myopathic, dystrophic	
LDB3	Markesbery-Griggs	10q22	AD	40–50	Anterior foreleg	Proximal weakness	1–4X	Myofibrillar	CM
MATR3	VCPDM	5q31	AD	35–57	Anterior foreleg	Bulbar symptoms	1–8X	Rimmed vacuoles	FALS
MYH7	Laing	14q12	AD	3–25	Anterior foreleg	Neck flexors, finger extensors	1–3X	Myopathic, type 1 atrophy	MSM, CM
MYOT	Myofibrillar type 3	5q31	AD	45–60	Anterior foreleg	Dysarthria	1–15X	Myofibrillar	LGMD1A

(*continued on next page*)

Table 1 (*continued*)

Gene	Name	Locus	Inheritance	Age at Onset (y)	Distal Weakness	Other	CK	Pathology	Allelic
NEB	Nemaline type 2	2q22	AR	0–6	Anterior foreleg	Facial and neck weakness	1–2X	Nemaline rods	
SQSTM1		5q35.3	AD	40–60	Anterior foreleg	Facial and shoulder weakness	1–2X	Rimmed vacuoles	PD
TIA1	Welander	2p13	AD	40–60	Wrist and finger extensors	Sensory symptoms	1–3X	Myopathic, rimmed vacuoles	FALS, FTD
TTN	Udd	2q31	AD	35–50	Anterior foreleg	Upper limb muscle sparing	1–4X	Myopathic, rimmed vacuoles	LGMD2J, HMERF, CM
VCP		9p13-p12	AD	5–60	Anterior foreleg	Finger flexor and extensors	1–3X	Rimmed vacuoles	FALS, FTD, CMT2Y, IBMPFD

Abbreviations: CK, creatine kinase; CM, cardiomyopathy; CMT, Charcot–Marie–Tooth neuropathy; FALS, familial amyotrophic lateral sclerosis; FTD, frontotemporal dementia; HMERF, hereditary myopathy with early respiratory failure; IBMPFD, inclusion body myopathy with Paget disease and FTD; LGMD, limb girdle muscular dystrophy; MFM, myofibrillar myopathy; MSM, myosin storage myopathy; PD, Paget disease; RMD, rippling muscle disease; VCPDM, vocal cord and pharyngeal distal myopathy.

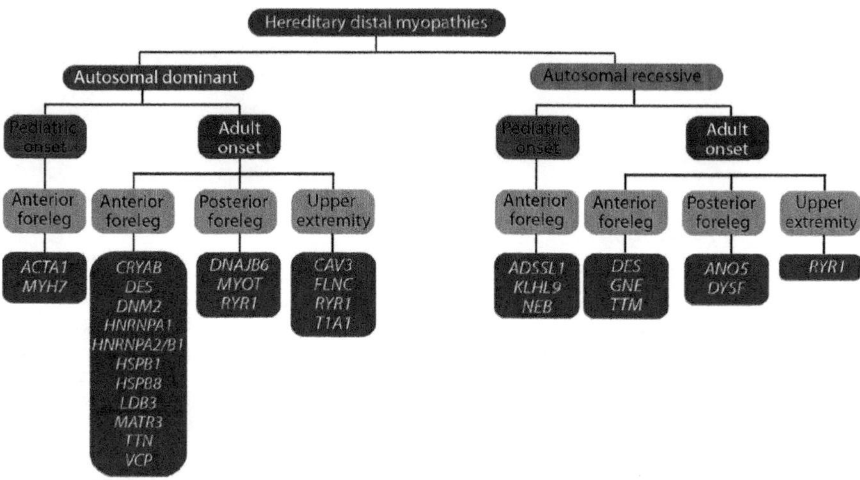

Fig. 1. Distal myopathy gene disorders based on inheritance patterns, age of onset, and presenting muscle involvement. (*Reproduced with permission from* Felice KJ. Differential diagnosis of distal myopathies. Practical Neurology 2019;18(6):82–85,91.)

disproportion (eg, Laing myopathy, congenital myopathies).[12] Muscle immunohistochemistry is often helpful in identifying deficient structural proteins in the recessive dystrophies (eg, Miyoshi myopathy) or abnormal protein accumulation in the myofibrillar myopathies (eg, *DES*-related myopathy). Muscle biopsy is not always a necessary step in the diagnostic evaluation given the availability of comprehensive and relatively inexpensive next-generation DNA testing panels, but may be important in cases in which DNA testing is negative or reports only variants of uncertain significance.

CASE 1

Clinical Presentation

A 23-year-old man presented with a 2-year history of progressive calf muscle weakness and atrophy. He first noted difficulty jumping and standing on tiptoes. He did not complain of back or leg pain, hand or arm weakness, or sensory symptoms. He was previously fit and athletic, and was able to participate on his high school basketball team. Past medical history was otherwise unremarkable. There was no known family history of neuromuscular disease. A right vastus lateralis muscle biopsy performed at another medical center diagnosed inflammatory myopathy. A 3-month course of prednisone did not improve his leg weakness. Examination revealed mild difficulties arising from a chair. Gait was slow and exhibited weak step-off bilaterally. There was calf muscle weakness (Medical Research Council [MRC] grade 3) and atrophy (**Fig. 2**). Other weak muscles included elbow flexors, elbow extensors, and hip flexors (all MRC 4). Cranial nerve examination was normal. Ankle reflexes were depressed. Sensory examination was normal.

Diagnostic Studies

An MRI of the lumbosacral spine was normal. Creatine kinase was 15,505 U/L. Nerve conduction studies were normal. Concentric needle electromyography showed fibrillation potentials and positive sharp waves in the lateral gastrocnemius and iliacus, increased (early) recruitment of small polyphasic motor unit action potentials in a

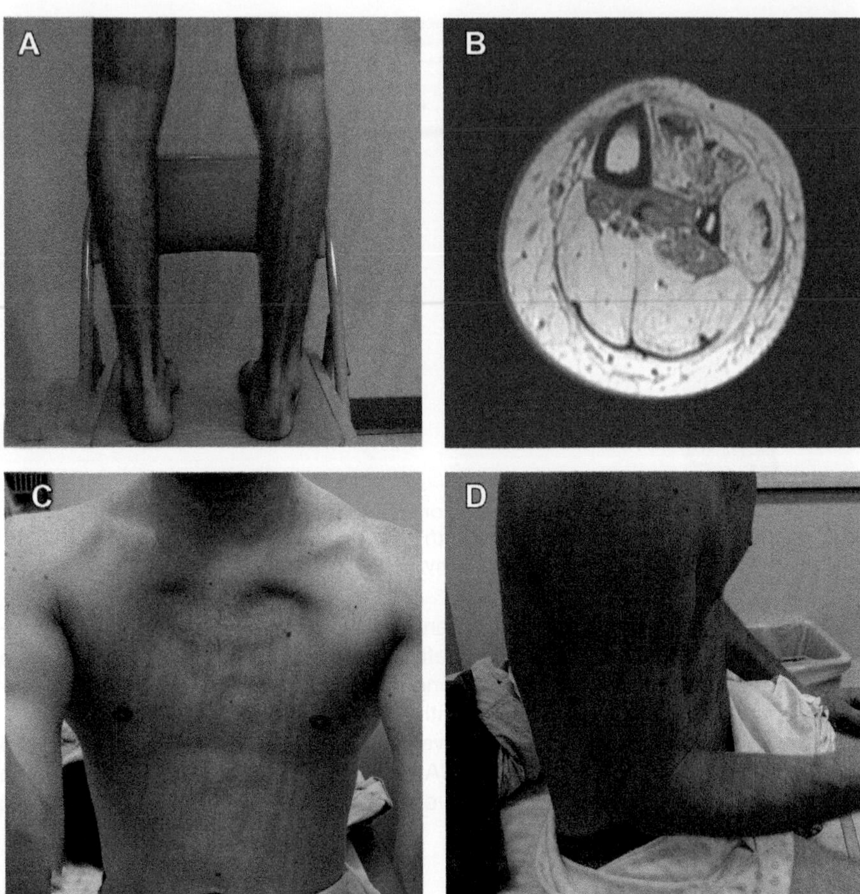

Fig. 2. Photographs and MRI findings in case 1 showing calf muscle atrophy (*A*), T1-weighted sequence of foreleg showing fatty replacement of gastrocnemius muscles (*B*), medial pectoralis muscle atrophy (*C*), and distal biceps brachii muscle atrophy (*D*).

diffuse pattern. Our review of the muscle biopsy showed increased variation in myofiber size, connective tissue, and internalized nuclei along with scattered muscle fiber necrosis and myophagocytosis (**Fig. 3**).

Clinical Questions

The patient's clinical presentation is highly suggestive of which disorder?

1. Becker muscular dystrophy
2. Autoimmune necrotizing myopathy
3. *Miyoshi myopathy*
4. Myofibrillar myopathy

All of the following studies would be helpful in determining the specific diagnosis except?

1. Muscle immunostaining for dysferlin
2. Monocyte test for dysferlin
3. Inherited myopathy next-generation DNA panel

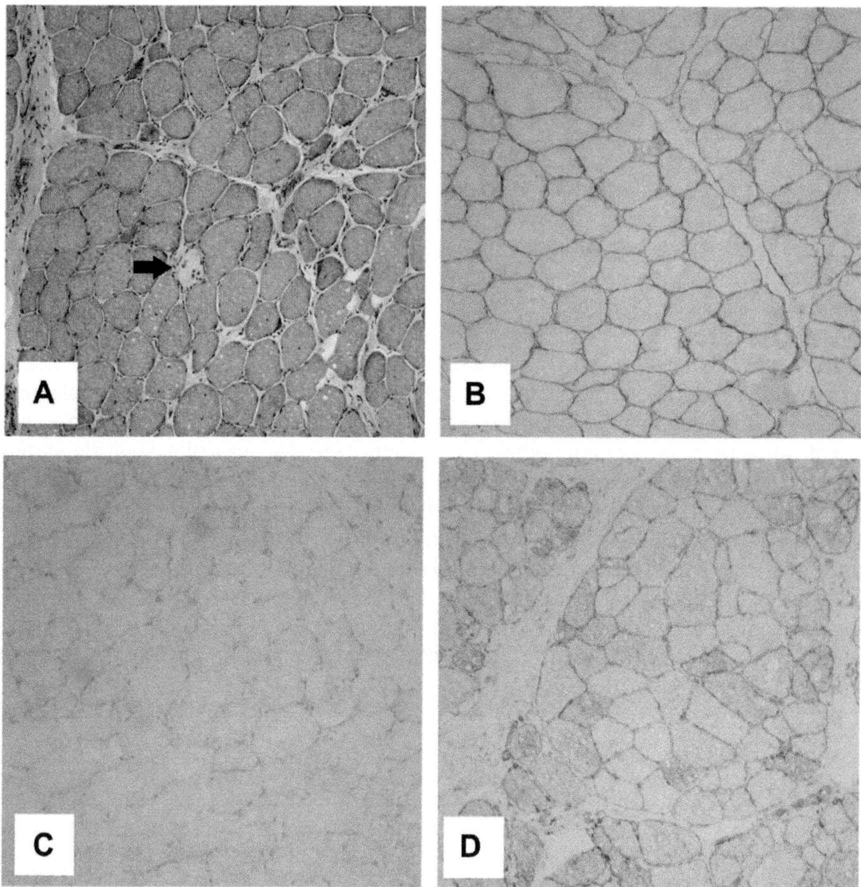

Fig. 3. Muscle histopathology in case 1 showing increased variation in myofiber size and scattered necrotic fibers (*arrow*) (H&E, x100) (*A*), normal immunoreactivity for dystrophin (*B*), and absent immunoreactivity for dysferlin in patient (*C*) compared with normal dysferlin immunoreactivity in control subject (*D*).

4. *Myositis-specific antibody panel*

Additional immunohistochemistry studies on remaining frozen muscle tissue revealed absent dysferlin staining. Next-generation DNA panel covering 35 hereditary myopathy genes disclosed a pathogenic heterozygous mutation (c.5979dupA) in the *DYSF* gene. A second *DYSF* gene variant was not identified. No sequence variants were found in other genes including *ANO5*, *MYOT*, *RYR1*, and *DNAJB6.*

Discussion

This patient's age of onset, pattern of clinical involvement, and markedly elevated creatine kinase were highly consistent with the diagnosis of Miyoshi myopathy.[13] Previous athleticism—uncommon in most inherited disorders of muscle—has been reported in the dysferlinopathies. Absent dysferlin staining on muscle immunohistochemistry was diagnostic for this disorder. Genetic testing was supportive, disclosing a known pathogenic mutation in the *DYSF* gene. The absence of a second identifiable gene variant is not uncommon—observed in approximately 22% of dysferlinopathy patients—and likely results from limitations in current DNA testing.[14] Mutations eluding molecular detection include those causing large rearrangements or those located in intronic DNA. Ultimately, RNA sequencing and/or protein-based studies (eg, Western blot, muscle immunohistochemistry) are required in such cases to secure a specific genetic diagnosis—thus allowing for appropriate genetic counseling and inclusion of patients in therapeutic clinical trials.

Miyoshi myopathy is a primary disorder of skeletal muscle usually presenting with the triad of onset before age 30 years, early involvement of posterior foreleg muscles, and markedly elevated creatine kinase values.[13] Progression is slow but relentless, eventually involving the proximal muscles and leading to wheelchair dependency 10 to 20 years after symptom onset. Creatine kinase values are elevated to 20 to 150 times the upper normal limit. In addition to myopathic recruitment patterns, electromyography shows fibrillations and positive sharp waves in resting muscle. Muscle biopsy shows varying degrees of dystrophic change, including myofiber necrosis and increased connective tissue. Inflammation is commonly observed, but vacuoles are absent. Muscle immunohistochemistry and monocyte Western blot analysis shows absent dysferlin. Miyoshi myopathy is due to mutations in the *DYSF* gene.[15] Diagnosis is confirmed with DNA testing, which shows homozygous or compound heterozygous mutations in the *DYSF* gene. To date, 611 mutations have been reported in the *DYSF* gene.[16] Other allelic disorders include limb girdle muscular dystrophy type 2B, proximodistal myopathy, distal myopathy with anterior foreleg-onset weakness, pseudometabolic myopathy, and asymptomatic hyperCKemia.[17,18] *DYSF* encodes the protein, dysferlin, which is located in the muscle membrane and plays a major role in sarcolemmal repair.[19]

CASE 2

Case Presentation

A 64-year-old woman presented with bilateral foot drop. Symptoms were present since early childhood and initially diagnosed as Charcot–Marie–Tooth neuropathies. In addition to leg weakness, she recalled weakness of neck flexion while performing sit-ups in gym class. Other medical problems included hypertension, osteoarthritis, hyperlipidemia, and glaucoma. Her deceased mother and maternal grandmother had leg weakness. Her brother had severe generalized weakness and was diagnosed with an unspecified muscular dystrophy. Examination showed a steppage pattern gait for which she wore bilateral ankle-foot orthoses. There were mild heel cord contractures, but no hand or foot deformities, scoliosis, scapular winging, or muscle hypertrophy. Cranial nerve examination showed mild facial weakness. She had full eye closure but was unable to bury eyelashes. She was able to perform a deep knee bend and stand on tiptoes, but was unable to stand on heels. In the supine position, neck flexor weakness was prominent (MRC 2). Limb weakness was restricted to the foot/toe extensors (MRC 0) and finger extensors (MRC 4) (**Fig. 4**). Reflexes and sensory examination were normal. Examination of her brother revealed more generalized weakness with bilateral wrist, finger, and foot drop.

Diagnostic Studies

Creatine kinase was 156 U/L (reference value, <143 U/L). Pulmonary function tests showed a forced vital capacity of 2.13 L (68% of predicted). Her electrocardiogram and echocardiogram were normal. Left ventricular ejection fraction was 65%. Nerve conduction studies showed normal right median, ulnar, superficial peroneal, and sural sensory nerve action potentials (SNAPs). Motor nerve conduction studies showed

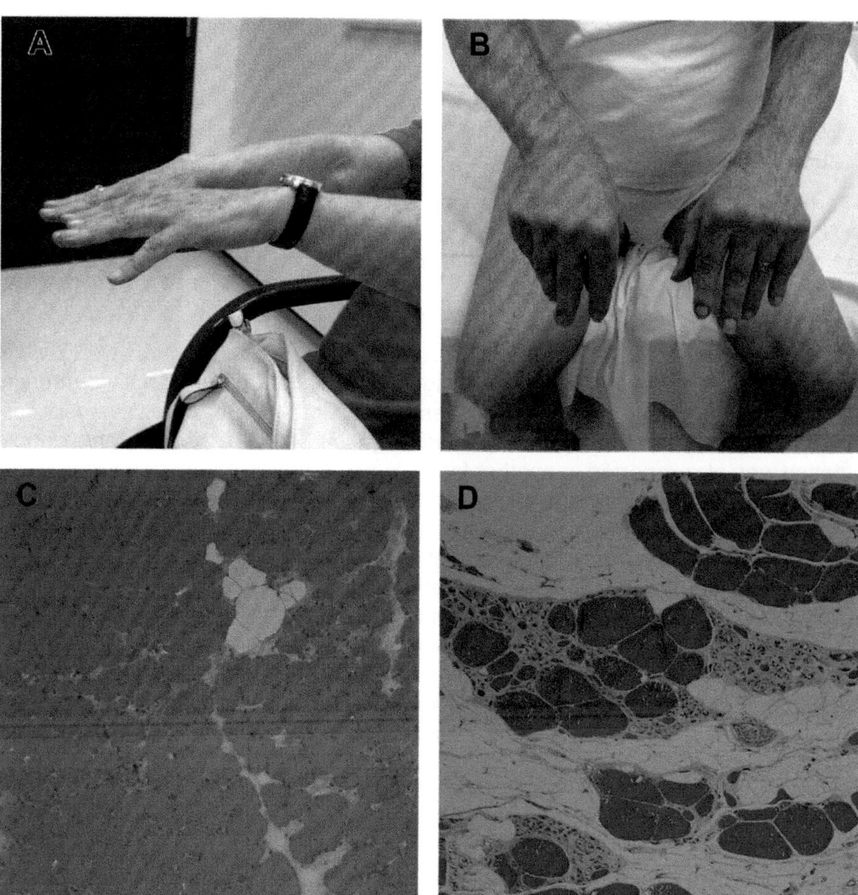

Fig. 4. Photographs and muscle histopathology in case 2 (*A*) and affected brother (*B–D*) showing weakness of fingers extensors (*A*, *B*), marked variation in myofiber size (H&E, x100) (*C*), and increased connective tissue and fat deposition (Gomori trichrome, x200) (*D*).

low-amplitude peroneal and tibial compound muscle action potentials, normal median and ulnar compound muscle action potential amplitudes, and normal motor conduction velocities. Concentric needle electromyography showed increased (early) recruitment of small polyphasic motor unit action potentials in a diffuse pattern—abnormalities were particularly prominent in clinically weak muscles. There were no fibrillations, positive sharp waves, or myotonic discharges. Muscle biopsy of her brother showed dystrophic changes (see **Fig. 4**).

Clinical Questions

The history and clinical findings in this patient are most consistent with which disorder?

1. *Laing myopathy*
2. Myofibrillar myopathy
3. ANO5 myopathy
4. Vocal cord and pharyngeal myopathy

All of the following are consistent with Laing myopathy except?

1. Pediatric onset
2. Finger extensor weakness
3. *Vacuolar myopathy*
4. Autosomal-dominant inheritance

Targeted DNA testing in the patient and her brother identified 2 mutations in the *MYH7* gene including V39 M (c.115 G > A) and K1617del (c.4850_4852delAGA)—both previously documented as causative for hypertrophic cardiomyopathy and Laing myopathy, respectively.[8,20]

Discussion

In this case, the pattern of inheritance, age of onset, and clinical findings strongly implicated Laing myopathy. After EMG testing secured a myopathy diagnosis, targeted DNA testing confirmed the suspected diagnosis. Interestingly, the same double mutation was also reported in another family in abstract form.[21]

Laing myopathy is an early-onset disorder beginning with selective weakness of foot dorsiflexors and great toe extensors, followed by weakness of neck flexors and finger extensors, and, in some affected individuals, progression to facial and proximal limb muscle weakness.[22] Creatine kinase values are normal or mildly elevated. Muscle histopathology varies widely to include mild nonspecific changes, congenital fiber type disproportion, cores and minicores, and dystrophic changes. Laing myopathy is an autosomal-dominant disorder owing to mutations in the *MYH7* gene, which encodes the beta heavy chain of myosin.[8] Other *MYH7*-allelic disorders include both skeletal myopathies (congenital myopathies, late-onset myopathies, myosin storage myopathy, scapuloperoneal myopathies) and cardiomyopathies (dilated, hypertrophic, and left ventricular noncompaction).[23] To date, 1049 *MYH7* gene mutations have been documented—spanning the globular head region and rod domains.[16] Mutations in the *MYH7* gene are likely to impair the development of a normal coiled structure impacting myosin dimerization, which is required to form the thick filament.[23,24]

CASE 3

Case Presentation

A 67-year-old man presented with generalized weakness and shortness of breath with exertion. He noted bilateral foot drop at age 30 years. Over time, he developed generalized limb and axial weakness, wheelchair dependency, and respiratory insufficiency requiring noninvasive nocturnal ventilation. Initially, the quadriceps muscles were spared—later, he developed right quadriceps muscle atrophy and weakness. His past medical history was remarkable for hypertension and osteoarthritis. There was no known family history of neuromuscular disease. Examination was remarkable for diffuse limb muscle weakness and atrophy with involvement of distal and proximal muscles and relative sparing of the left quadriceps. Cranial nerve, reflex, and sensory examinations were normal.

Diagnostic Studies

Forced vital capacity was 1.65 L (41% of predicted). A right gastrocnemius muscle biopsy performed at age 30 years showed increased variation in myofiber size, increased endomysial connective tissue and internalized nuclei, scattered muscle fiber necrosis and myophagocytosis, and diffuse vacuolar changes (**Fig. 5**).

Clinical Questions

Myopathies associated with vacuolar changes include all of the following except?

1. Sporadic inclusion body myositis
2. Myofibrillar myopathy
3. GNE myopathy
4. *Laing myopathy*

The patient's clinical presentation is highly suggestive of which disorder?

1. *GNE myopathy*
2. Becker muscular dystrophy
3. ANO5 myopathy
4. ACTA1 myopathy

Next-generation DNA panel disclosed compound heterozygous missense mutations, A662 V (c.1985C > T) and S730 L (c.2189 C > T), in the *GNE* gene.

Discussion

This patient developed anterior foreleg weakness at age 30 years that, over time, progressed into a severe generalized myopathy. The combined early phenotype and muscle histopathology implicated an inclusion body myopathy. The specific diagnosis was delayed for many years as the initial evaluation and muscle biopsy in 1979 predated the discovery of the *GNE* gene by more than 20 years.[25]

GNE-related myopathy (Nonaka myopathy, distal myopathy with rimmed vacuoles, hereditary inclusion myopathy type 2) is a primary skeletal myopathy usually presenting in late teenage and early adulthood with bilateral foot drop and steppage pattern gait owing to weakness of anterior tibialis muscles.[26] Progression of weakness is relentless, leading to generalized muscle weakness and wheelchair dependency usually 20 years after disease onset. For most patients, the quadriceps will be spared even in the advance stages of the disease. However, severe quadriceps weakness and atrophy have been reported.[27] Facial, oropharyngeal, cardiac, and respiratory muscles are usually spared, with rare exceptions.[27,28] Creatine kinase values are mildly elevated, usually less than 5 times the upper normal limit. Characteristic muscle histopathology features include rimmed vacuoles and filamentous inclusions. GNE myopathy is an autosomal recessive disorder owing to mutations in the *GNE* gene which encodes UDP-N-acetylglucosamine 2-epimerase/N-acetylmannosamine kinase. To date, 224 mutations have been reported in the *GNE* gene with founder mutations in

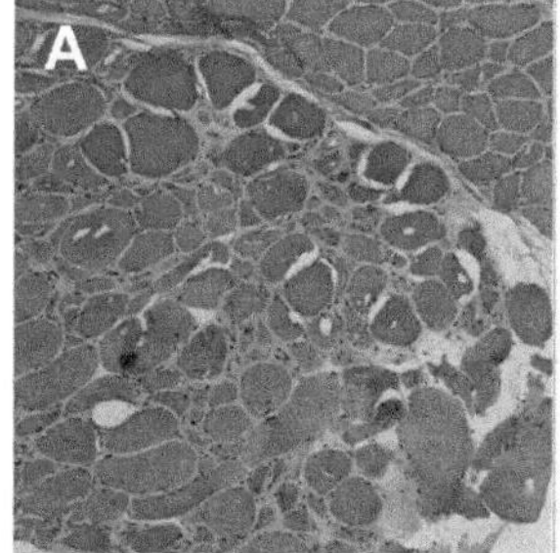

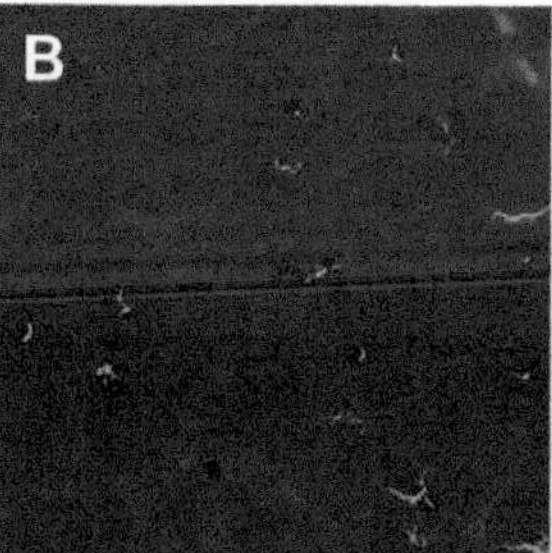

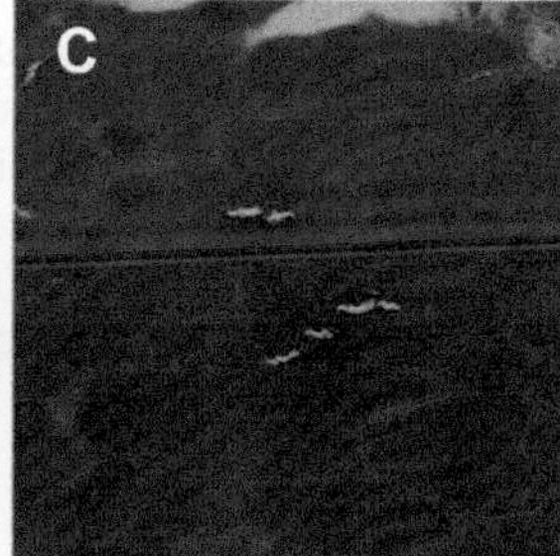

Fig. 5. Muscle histopathology in case 3 showing marked variation in myofiber size (H&E, x100) (*A*) and rimmed vacuoles (Gomori trichrome, x100, x200) (*B, C*).

patients of Japanese and Middle Eastern ancestry.[16] The pathophysiology is not entirely known, but hyposialylation of muscle glycans is believed to play a major role.[29] A recent phase III trial using sialic acid extended-release showed no benefit over placebo in improving muscle strength or function in patients with GNE myopathy.[30]

CASE 4

Case Presentation

A 53-year-old man presented with progressive bilateral foot drop and gait difficulties. Twelve years prior, he was found to have restrictive lung disease during a screening pulmonary function test that was required for his employment as a volunteer firefighter. Five years prior, he began to notice increasing shortness of breath with exertion and gait difficulties with occasional falls. He also noted mild numbness and tingling in his toes and feet. Gait problems progressed to the point that he required bilateral ankle-foot orthoses for severe foot drop. Other medical problems included prediabetes, hypertension, nephrolithiasis, and seborrheic dermatitis. Family history was remarkable for late-onset weakness and gait difficulties in his deceased father and older sister. Examination was remarkable for a steppage pattern gait. He was unable to stand on heels or tiptoes. He needed to push-off with both hands to arise from a chair. There were mild pes cavus foot deformities and tight heel cords, and prominent atrophy of foot and anterior foreleg muscles. Weakness was restricted to the lower extremities, affecting hip flexors (MRC grade 3), knee extensors and flexors (MRC grade 4), and foot and toe extensors (MRC grade 2). There was no myotonia. Ankle jerks were absent, although other myotatic reflexes were normal. Sensory examination revealed mildly decreased perception of vibration and pin prick sensations in the toes and feet. Toe position sensation was intact.

Diagnostic Studies

Creatine kinase was 422 U/L (reference value, <175 U/L). A complete blood count, chemistry panel, fasting blood glucose, thyroid function studies, serum protein electrophoresis, immunofixation, and vitamin B_{12} level were normal. Pulmonary function testing revealed a forced vital capacity of 1.81 L (35% of predicted). Chest radiograph was normal. Electrocardiogram and echocardiogram were normal. Nerve conduction studies showed low-amplitude sural SNAPs. Other sensory and motor nerve conduction studies were normal. Concentric needle electromyography showed increased insertional activity, sustained fibrillation potentials and positive sharp waves, and increased (early) recruitment of small polyphasic motor unit action potentials in a diffuse pattern; these abnormalities were particularly prominent in the tibialis anterior. Electromyography was consistent with a diffuse myopathy and concurrent length-dependent sensory neuropathy. Muscle biopsy of the right gastrocnemius showed marked variability in myofiber size, occasional necrosis and myophagocytosis, increased internalized nuclei, rare pyknotic nuclear clumps, increased endomysial fibrosis, sarcoplasmic masses on hematoxylin-eosin and Gomori trichrome stains, core-like lesions on NADH-TR stains, desmin-positive aggregates on immunostains, and granulofilamentous material on electron microscopy (**Fig. 6**).

Clinical Questions

Respiratory muscle weakness is observed in which of the following myopathies?

1. Laing myopathy
2. FSHD

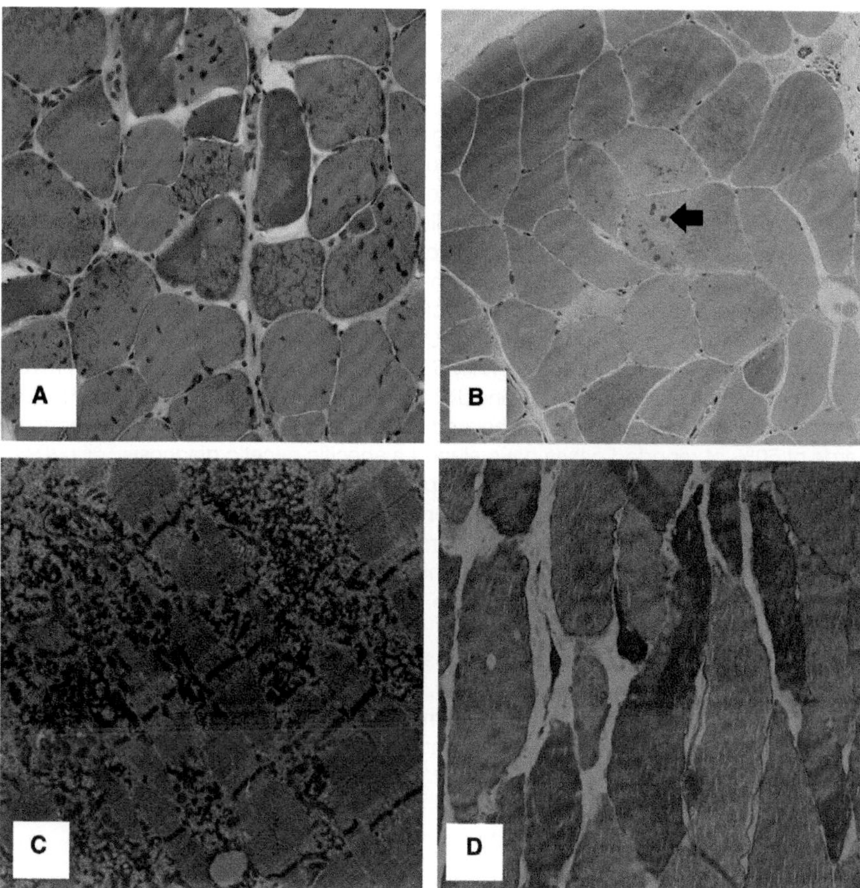

Fig. 6. Muscle histopathology in case 4 showing myofibrillar changes (H&E, x200) (*A*), inclusions (*arrow*) (epoxy-embedded semi-thin section stained with toluidine blue, x200) (*B*), granulofilamentous aggregates (electron microscopy, x8000) (*C*), and increased immunoreactivity for desmin (x200) (*D*).

3. GNE myopathy
4. *Myofibrillar myopathy*

All of the following gene disorders are associated with myofibrillar myopathy except?

1. DES
2. CRYAB
3. *MYH7*
4. MYOT

Genetic testing disclosed a heterozygous R415 W mutation (c.1243 C > T) in exon 6 of the *DES* gene.

Discussion

This patient developed late-onset respiratory insufficiency and lower extremity weakness. Symptoms in his deceased father and clinical findings in his sister implicated an autosomal-dominant disorder. Ultimately, the diagnosis was supported by the muscle histopathologic findings and proven by subsequent DNA testing. The concurrent neuropathy symptoms may have resulted from a primary desmin-related neuromyopathy, prediabetes, or both.

The myofibrillar myopathies are a heterogeneous group of genetic disorders characterized pathologically by disruption of myofibrils and accumulation of degradation products in intracellular inclusions.[31] Most patients present with progressive limb muscle weakness—distal, proximal, or both. Cardiomyopathy—dilated or hypertrophic—can be an isolated feature or may develop concurrently with the skeletal myopathy. Other common phenotypic features include length-dependent sensorimotor axonal polyneuropathy and chest wall/diaphragmatic muscle weakness leading to chronic respiratory insufficiency. Thus far, 11 genes—*DES*, *CRYAB*, *MYOT*, *LDB3*, *FLNC*, *BAG3*, *KY*, *PYROXD1*, *SELENON*, *TRIM54*, and *TRIM63*—have been implicated in causing myofibrillar myopathy. In addition, other gene disorders—*PLEC*, *TTN*, *FHL1*, *ACTA1*, *HSPB8*, and *DNAJB6*—have also been associated with myofibrillar histopathology, and upwards of 50% of reported cases have eluded a specific genetic diagnosis.[9,32]

Mutations in the *DES* gene account for approximately 7% of genetically determined myofibrillar myopathies.[33] *DES* encodes for the intermediate filament protein desmin, which is an essential component of the extrasarcomeric cytoskeleton in cardiac, skeletal, and smooth muscle cells. Mutations in *DES* on chromosome 2q35 cause autosomal-dominant, autosomal-recessive, and sporadic skeletal myopathy, cardiomyopathy, or both with marked phenotypic variability—including myofibrillar myopathy (aka, desmin-related myopathy, desminopathy), limb girdle muscular dystrophy, and dilated and hypertrophic cardiomyopathy.[34] Since the first description of desmin-related myopathy by Goldfarb in 1998, 131 mutations in the *DES* gene have been identified including the case of a 30-year-old patient with leg weakness who also harbored the R415 W (c.1243 C > T) mutation.[35–37]

CASE 5

Case Presentation

A 34-year-old man presented with nonprogressive generalized weakness since early childhood. Motor milestones were delayed and he began to walk at age 2 years. As a teen, he underwent lower extremity tendon transfers to correct severe bilateral foot drop. He was previously diagnosed with a congenital myopathy or dystrophy based on clinical and muscle biopsy findings. He denied problems with speech, swallowing, breathing, or sensory symptoms. Past medical history was otherwise unremarkable and there was no history of neuromuscular disease in his deceased parents, 2 brothers, or extended family. Examination was remarkable for thin body habitus with height of 76 inches, weight of 100 pounds, and a body mass index of 12.2. General examination revealed a long thin face, high-arched palate, axial rigidity, finger clinodactyly, genu valgum, and pes cavus and hammertoe deformities (**Fig. 7**). Gait was mildly unsteady with steppage features. He used bilateral ankle-foot orthoses. He was unable to perform a deep knee bend, or stand on heels or tiptoes. He needed to push-off with both hands to arise from a chair. Limb muscles were diffusely thin with the exception of bilateral extensor digitorum brevis muscles, which were prominent. Cranial nerve examination showed mild upper eyelid ptosis and mild facial weakness. Strength testing showed generalized weakness with more severe involvement of finger extensors, intrinsic hand muscles, and foot dorsiflexors (MRC grade 3). There was no percussion or action myotonia. Myotatic reflexes were diffusely hypoactive. Sensory examination was normal.

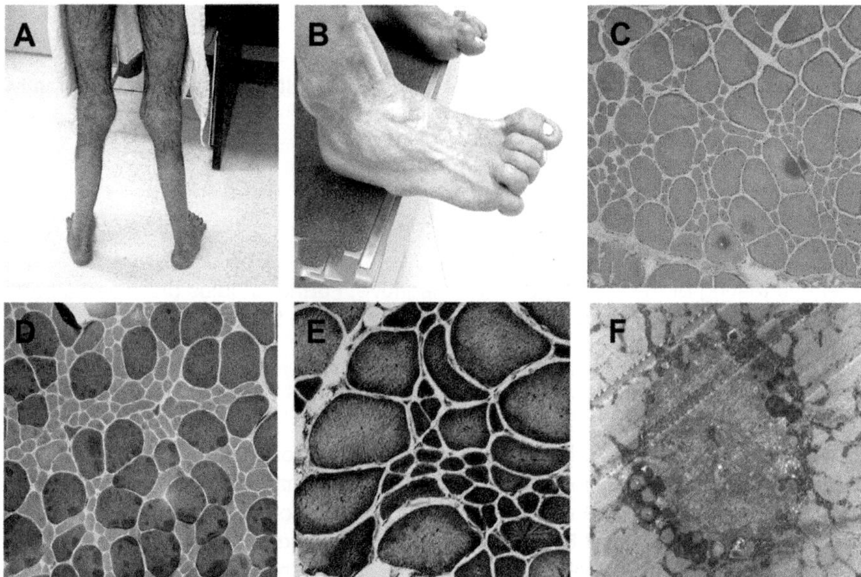

Fig. 7. Photographs and muscle histopathology in case 6 showing genu valgum and foreleg muscle atrophy (*A*), hammertoes and preserved extensor digitorum brevis (*B*), marked variation in myofiber size with bimodal distribution (H&E, x100) (*C*), type 1 myofiber atrophy (ATPase pH 9.4, x100) (*D*), increased central staining on type 1 myofibers (NADH-TR, x200) (*E*), and perinuclear mitochondrial aggregation (electron microscopy, x20000) (*F*).

Diagnostic Studies

Creatine kinase was 67 U/L (reference value, <269 U/L). Comprehensive laboratory testing was normal. Forced vital capacity was 1.67 L (26% of predicted). Electrocardiogram was normal. Echocardiogram disclosed mild mitral regurgitation and prolapse. Left ventricular size and function were normal. Ejection fraction was 50%. Sensory and motor nerve conduction studies were normal. Concentric needle electromyography showed increased (early) recruitment of small polyphasic motor unit action potentials in a diffuse pattern. There were no fibrillation potentials, positive sharp waves, or myotonic discharges. Genetic testing for myotonic dystrophy type 1 was negative. Right vastus lateralis muscle biopsy showed marked variation in myofiber size with a bimodal distribution, including small hypotrophic and large hypertrophic fibers (see **Fig. 7**). Enzyme histochemistry demonstrated fiber type disproportion with the smaller fibers being type 1 and the larger type 2. Most fibers showed internalized nuclei with prominent centralized nuclei in type 1 fibers. NADH-TR sections showed prominently increased central staining with occasional oxidative radial strands. Electron microscopy showed centralized nuclei surrounded by mitochondria. Muscle biopsy findings were consistent with centronuclear myopathy.

Clinical Questions

Myopathies associated with type 1 myofiber atrophy include all of the following except?

1. MYH7 myopathy
2. Centronuclear myopathy

3. *Miyoshi myopathy*
4. Myotonic muscular dystrophy type 1

All of the following gene disorders are associated with centronuclear myopathy except?

1. *MTM1*
2. *ANO5*
3. *DNM2*
4. *BIN1*

Genetic testing of the *MTM1* gene was negative. Further studies disclosed a pathogenic heterozygous mutation (R465 W, c.1393 C > T) in the *DNM2* gene, consistent with centronuclear myopathy type 1 (CNM1).

Discussion

This case highlights the distally predominant weakness occasionally encountered in the congenital myopathies. In keeping with other congenital myopathies, this patient experienced early-onset weakness with slow progression. Other features included distal greater than proximal limb weakness, facial weakness, eyelid ptosis without ophthalmoplegia, and respiratory insufficiency. Muscle histopathology was consistent with a centronuclear myopathy and genetic testing confirmed the diagnosis of CNM1.

The congenital myopathies are a heterogeneous group of genetic muscle disorders causing static or slowly progressive weakness, usually beginning in infancy or childhood—but sometimes delayed into adulthood—initially identified by clinical features, patterns of inheritance, and characteristic muscle pathologic features.[38] Recent genetic discoveries have implicated 44 disease-associated genes and, coupled with the histopathologic and ultrastructural findings, have subclassified the congenital myopathies into 5 major groups: nemaline, core, centronuclear, myosin storage, and congenital fiber type disproportion. Distal-onset weakness may be especially prominent in certain congenital myopathies, including *ACTA1*, *MYH7*, *RYR1*, *NEB*, and *DNM2* gene disorders.

To date, 8 genes have been associated with centronuclear myopathy pathology, including *MTM1*, *DNM2*, *BIN1*, *RYR1*, *TTN*, *MTMR14*, *CCDC78*, and *SPEG*.[9,39] Inheritance patterns include autosomal-dominant, autosomal-recessive, and X-linked transmission. Common to all are the histopathologic findings of increased centralized and internalized nuclei, type 1 myofiber hypotrophy and predominance, darkly stained central areas on oxidative stains, and, in some cases, radiating sarcoplasmic strands and necklace fibers.[40] CNM1 is an autosomal-dominant disorder with symptom onset ranging from infancy to early adulthood. Limb weakness is variable—usually distal more than proximal—progression is slow with many affected patients becoming wheelchair dependent in the fifth or sixth decade.[41] Most published cases describe facial weakness with or without eyelid ptosis and ophthalmoplegia. Cardiac involvement, respiratory insufficiency, and cognitive impairment are less commonly reported. Creatine kinase values are normal or mildly increased. Since the discovery of the genetic cause of CNM1 in 11 families, 54 mutations have been reported in the *DNM2* gene.[9,42] In addition to CNM1, *DNM2*-related disorders include Charcot–Marie–Tooth neuropathies type 2M and dominant intermediate B, and lethal congenital contracture syndrome 5. Recent studies have pointed to impairment of actin-dependent trafficking in muscle cells as a pathologic mechanism in DNM2-associated centronuclear myopathy.[43]

CASE 6

Case Presentation

A 61-year-old man presented with bilateral foot drop and gait difficulties, both slowly progressive for the past 9 years. He denied pain, sensory symptoms, or upper extremity weakness. Past medical history was otherwise unremarkable and he took no medications. There was no known family history of neuromuscular disease. Examination revealed a steppage pattern gait. There was marked atrophy of bilateral tibialis anterior muscles with preserved extensor digitorum brevis muscles (**Fig. 8**). Muscle strength testing revealed weakness of bilateral foot extensors, evertors, and invertors (MRC grade 2). Reflexes and sensory examination were normal. Subtle findings included full eye closure with inability to bury eyelashes and mild humeral muscle atrophy. There was no scapular winging.

Diagnostic Studies

Creatine kinase was 444 U/L (reference value, <308 U/L). Comprehensive laboratory testing was normal. Forced vital capacity was 4.18 L (98% of predicted). Nerve conduction studies were normal. Concentric needle electromyography showed increased (early) recruitment of small polyphasic motor unit action potentials in a diffuse pattern—the abnormalities were particularly prominent in clinically weak muscles. Fibrillation potentials and positive sharp waves were prominent—particularly in the tibialis anterior. Myotonic discharges were absent.

Clinical Questions

Based on the history and clinical findings, the next best diagnostic test is?

1. Muscle biopsy
2. *Next-generation DNA panel for hereditary myopathies*
3. Myotonic dystrophy DNA test
4. *MYH7 DNA* test

All of the following muscular dystrophies may present with prominent distal weakness except?

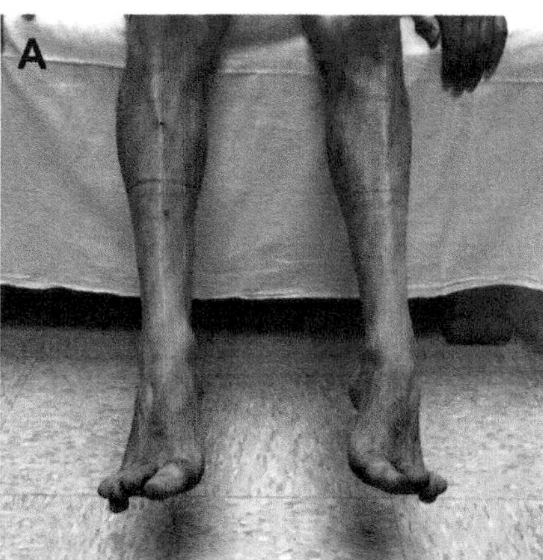

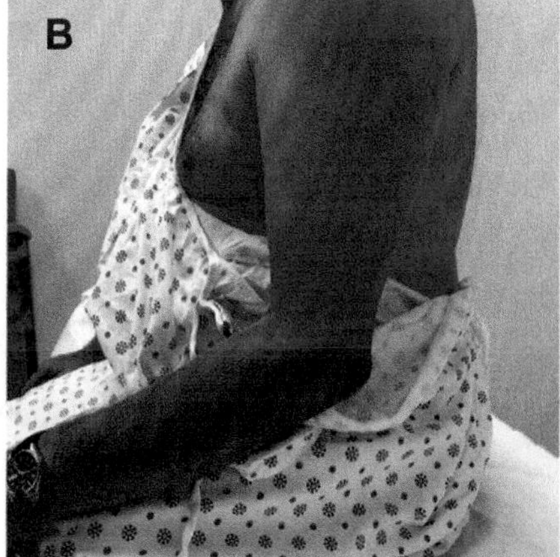

Fig. 8. Photographs in case 7 show marked weakness and atrophy of bilateral tibialis muscles with relatively preserved toe extension (*A*) and humeral muscle atrophy (*B*).

1. FSHD
2. Myotonic muscular dystrophy type 1
3. *Myotonic muscular dystrophy type 2*
4. Emery-Dreifuss muscular dystrophy

Next-generation DNA panel for 105 hereditary myopathy genes disclosed 2 variants of uncertain significance—one in the *COL6A2* gene and the other in the *TTN* gene. FSHD1 DNA test was positive, showing a contraction in D4Z4 repeats on 1 allele of 25 kb in size.

Discussion

This patient developed late-onset bilateral foot drop and gait difficulties. EMG confirmed a primary myopathy, and the fibrillations and positive sharp waves implicated a dystrophic or inflammatory process. Despite the late onset, inclusion body myositis was excluded in the differential diagnosis given the absence of quadriceps and finger flexor weakness. Next-generation DNA panel was nondiagnostic. The mild facial weakness and humeral atrophy—albeit subtle—prompted us to order the FSHD1 DNA test. This test confirmed the diagnosis of FSHD1.

This case highlights 2 points. First, not all patients presenting with a distal myopathy will have one of the classic disorders. Second, other myopathies—including muscular dystrophies, other genetic disorders, and acquired disorders—must be considered when evaluating a new patient with distal myopathic weakness (**Box 1**).[2,3,12,44–51] For the muscular dystrophies, proximal muscle weakness is the typical presenting sign; whereas distal muscle involvement, if present—for example, wrist/finger extensors in FSHD and finger flexors in Becker muscular dystrophy—usually develops concurrently with the proximal weakness or in the later stages of the disease.[3,44] Distal-onset or distal-predominant weakness is less common in these disorders. However, this case and others demonstrate the marked phenotypic variability occasionally encountered in neuromuscular clinical practice, especially in regard to FSHD.

FSHD1 and, the less common, FSHD2 are genetically distinct muscular dystrophies—one owing to contraction of repetitive D4Z4 repeats at 4q35 and the other to mutations in the *SMCHD1* gene.[52] Ultimately, both genetic abnormalities cause a common downstream effect—derepression of the *DUX4* gene leading to the expression of toxic DUX4 protein. Interestingly, some affected patients have both contracted D4Z4 repeats at 4q35 and mutations in the *SMCHD1* gene, implicating FSHD1 and FSHD2 as a disease continuum.[53] The typical clinical features of FSHD include symptom onset in first to second decade; characteristic weakness of facial, shoulder girdle, and humeral muscles; and slow progression.[46,52] Patients with FSHD can also develop weakness of finger, wrist, and foot extensors, usually in association with facial and scapulohumeral involvement. Following the genetic elucidation of FSHD, the clinical spectrum of these disorders expanded to include mild, partial, and atypical phenotypes.[54] These include infantile onset, facial-sparing, limb girdle muscular dystrophy pattern, distal myopathy, chronic external ophthalmoplegia, early joint contractures, and rigid spine, axial-predominant muscle weakness.[3,55–59] A distal myopathy phenotype with prominent foot drop has been previously reported.[3] For a more in-depth discussion of FSHD1 and FSHD2, the reader is referred to the article elsewhere in the issue of *Neurology Clinics*.

CARE AND TREATMENT

Thus far, there are no effective disease-modifying treatments for the distal myopathies. As with all genetic disorder, the hope is that some or all of the potential therapies

Box 1
Other myopathies associated with distal weakness

Congenital myopathies
  Gene disorders: ACTA1, BIN1, CFL2, MTM1, MYH2, NEB, RYR1, SELENON, TNNT1, TPM2, TPM3, TRIM32

Myofibrillar myopathies
  Gene disorders: *BAG3, CRYAB, DES, KY, LDB3, MYOT, PYROXD1, SELENON, TRIM54,* and *TRIM63*

Muscular dystrophies
  Myotonic dystrophy, type 1: *DMPK*
  Fascioscapulomuscular dystrophy: *DUX4,* and *SMCHD1*
  Limb girdle muscular dystrophy type 2G: *TCAP*
  Emery-Dreifuss muscular dystrophy: *EMD, FHL1,* and *LMNA*
  Becker muscular dystrophy: *DMD*
  Oculopharyngodistal myopathy

Multisystem disorders
  HNRNPA1: myopathy, ALS, FTD, PD
  HNRNPA2/B2: myopathy, ALS, FTD, PD
  HSPB1: myopathy, CMT2F, HMN2B
  HSPB8: myopathy, CMT2L, HMN2A
  SQSTM1/TIA1: myopathy, FTD

Other genetic disorders
  Debranching enzyme deficiency: *DBR1*
  POLG-related myopathy: *POLG*
  Neutral lipid storage myopathy: *PNPLA2*
  Cystinosis-associated myopathy: *CTNS*
  Pompe disease: *GAA*

Acquired myopathies
  Sporadic inclusion body myopathy
  Granulomatous myopathy
  Idiopathic inflammatory myopathies
  Hyperthyroid myopathy

Abbreviations: CMT, Charcot-Marie-Tooth neuropathy; FALS, familial amyotrophic lateral sclerosis; FTD, frontotemporal dementia; HMN, hereditary motor neuropathy.

under development—including oligonucleotide-based therapies, small molecule therapies, genome editing, gene replacement, and stem cell therapy—will provide future benefit to affected patients. Until then, disease monitoring, rehabilitative support, physical therapy and exercise programs, and symptomatic treatments are the mainstay of care for patients with distal myopathy. This author recommends referral of these complex patients to neuromuscular centers with experience in the diagnosis and care of patients with genetic neuromuscular disorders. Periodic assessments by a team of providers, including neuromuscular neurologists, physical medicine specialists, cardiologists, pulmonologists and sleep disorder specialists, neuropsychologists, physical and occupational therapists, speech and language pathologists, dietitians, social workers, and respiratory therapists, allow patients to maximize their functional abilities, monitor for potential cardiopulmonary complications, help to navigate insurance and home care issues, provide psychosocial counseling, and, ultimately, improve the quality of life for patients and care givers.[60] In the United States, Muscular Dystrophy Association Care Centers are particularly suited for such care.

SUMMARY

The distal myopathies are a rare and heterogeneous group of disorders. Affected patients present with weakness of the hands, distal lower extremities, or both. Age of onset varies from early childhood to late adulthood. With few exceptions (ie, sporadic inclusion body myositis), most of the disorders causing distal myopathic weakness are genetically based. The list of genetic disorders associated with distal-onset weakness is the ever expanding and further complicated by pronounced genetic heterogeneity, phenotypic variability, and complex multisystem involvement. In addition to the "classic" distal myopathies, other genetic conditions, including myofibrillar, congenital, and dystrophic disorders, warrant consideration when evaluating a new patient or family. Currently, there are no known effective disease-modifying treatments for the distal myopathies. Evaluation, symptomatic management, and periodic monitoring of patients in a multidisciplinary neuromuscular center are the mainstays of care.

DISCLOSURE

Dr K.J. Felice has no relevant disclosures.

REFERENCES

1. Udd B. Distal myopathies – new genetic entities expand diagnostic challenge. Neuromuscul Disord 2012;22:5–12.
2. Udd B. Distal myopathies. Curr Neurol Neurosci Rep 2014;14:434.
3. Felice KJ, Moore SA. Unusual clinical presentations in patients harboring the facioscapulohumeral dystrophy 4q35 deletion. Muscle Nerve 2001;24:352–6.
4. Kazakov VM, Rudenko DI, Stuchevskaya TR. Vladimir Karlovich Roth (1848-1916): the founder of neuromuscular diseases studies in Russia. Acta Myol 2014;33:34–42.
5. Gowers WR. A lecture on myopathy and a distal form: delivered at the National Hospital for the Paralyzed and Epileptic. Br Med J 1902;2:89–92.
6. Welander L. Myopathia distalis tarda hereditaria: 249 examined cases in 72 pedigrees. Acta Med Scand Suppl 1951;265:1–124.
7. Laing NG, Laing BA, Meredith C, et al. Autosomal dominant distal myopathy: linkage to chromosome 14. Am J Hum Genet 1995;56:422–7.
8. Meredith C, Herrmann R, Parry C, et al. Mutations in the slow skeletal muscle fiber myosin heavy chain gene (MYH7) cause Laing early-onset distal myopathy (MPD1). Am J Hum Genet 2004;75:703–8.
9. Gene table of neuromuscular disorders. 2019. Available at: http://www.musclegenetable.fr/. Accessed October 9, 2019.
10. Milone M, Liewluck T. The unfolding spectrum of inherited distal myopathies. Muscle Nerve 2019;59:283–94.
11. ten Dam L, van der Kooi AJ, Verhamme C, et al. Muscle imaging in inherited and acquired muscle diseases. Eur J Neurol 2016;23:688–703.
12. Dimachkie MM, Barohn RJ. Distal myopathies. Neurol Clin 2014;32:817–42.
13. Aoki M. Dysferlinopathy. 2015. Available at: https://www.ncbi.nlm.nih.gov/books/NBK1303/. Accessed October 9, 2019.
14. Fanin M, Angelini C. Progress and challenges in diagnosis of dysferlinopathy. Muscle Nerve 2016;54:821–35.

15. Liu J, Aoki M, Illa I, et al. Dysferlin, a novel skeletal muscle gene is mutated in Miyoshi myopathy and limb girdle muscular dystrophy. Nat Genet 1998;20:31–6.
16. Human gene mutation database. 2019. Available at: http://www.hgmd.cf.ac.uk/ac/index.php. Accessed October 9, 2019.
17. Nguyen K, Bassez G, Krahn M, et al. Phenotypic study in 40 patients with dysferlin gene mutations. Arch Neurol 2007;64:1176–82.
18. Illa I, Serrano-Munuera C, Gallardo E, et al. Distal anterior compartment myopathy: a dysferlin mutation causing a new muscular dystrophy phenotype. Ann Neurol 2001;49:130–4.
19. Han R. Muscle membrane repair and inflammatory attack in dysferlinopathy. Skelet Muscle 2019;1:10.
20. Richard P, Charron P, Carrier L, et al. Hypertrophic cardiomyopathy: distribution of disease genes, spectrum of mutations, and implications for a molecular diagnosis strategy. Circulation 2003;107:2227–32.
21. Dastgir J, Donkervoot S, Meilleur K, et al. MYH7 gene mutation related myopathies of skeletal and cardiac muscle. Neuromuscul Disord 2012;22:817.
22. Lamont P, Laing NG. Laing distal myopathy. 2015. Available at: https://www.ncbi.nlm.nih.gov/books/NBK1433/. Accessed October 9, 2019.
23. Tajsharghi H, Oldfors A. Myosinopathies: pathology and mechanisms. Acta Neuropathol 2013;125:3–18.
24. Marston S. The molecular mechanisms of mutations in actin and myosin that cause hereditary myopathy. Int J Mol Sci 2018;19:2020.
25. Eisenberg I, Avidan N, Potikha T, et al. The UDP-N-acetylglucosamine 2-epimerase/N-acetylmannosamine kinase gene is mutated in recessive hereditary inclusion body myopathy. Nat Genet 2001;29:83–7.
26. O'Ferrall EK, Sinnreich M. GNE-related myopathy. 2013. Available at: https://www.ncbi.nlm.nih.gov/books/NBK1262/. Accessed October 9, 2019.
27. Argov Z, Eisenberg I, Grabov-Nardini G, et al. Hereditary inclusion body myopathy: the Middle Eastern genetic cluster. Neurology 2003;60:1519–23.
28. Weihl CC, Miller SE, Zaidman CM, et al. Novel GNE mutations in two phenotypically distinct HIBM2 patients. Neuromuscul Disord 2011;21:102–5.
29. Carillo N, Malicdan MC, Huizing M. GNE myopathy: etiology, diagnosis, and therapeutic challenges. Neurotherapeutics 2018;15:900–14.
30. Lochmüller H, Behin A, Caraco Y, et al. A phase 3 randomized study evaluating sialic acid extended-release for GNE myopathy. Neurology 2019;92:e2109–17.
31. Batonnet-Pichon S, Behin A, Cabet E, et al. Myofibrillar myopathies: new perspectives from animal models to potential therapeutic approaches. J Neuromuscul Dis 2017;4:1–15.
32. Kley R, Olive M, Schroder R. New aspects of myofibrillar myopathies. Curr Opin Neurol 2016;29:628–34.
33. Selcen D, Engel A. Myofibrillar myopathy. 2012. Available at: https://www.ncbi.nlm.nih.gov/books/NBK1499/. Accessed October 9, 2019.
34. van Spaendonck KY, van Hessem L, Jongbloed JDH, et al. Desmin-related myopathy. Clin Genet 2011;80:354–66.
35. Goldfarb LG, Park KY, Cervenakova L, et al. Missense mutations in desmin associated myopathy with familial cardiac and skeletal myopathy. Nat Genet 1998;19:402–3.
36. Goldfarb LG, Olive M, Vicart P, et al. Intermediate filament diseases: desminopathy. Adv Exp Med Biol 2008;642:131–64.

37. Goldfarb LG, Dalakas MC. Tragedy in a heartbeat: malfunctioning desmin causes skeletal and cardiac muscle disease. J Clin Invest 2009;119:1806–13.
38. North KN, Wang CH, Clarke N, et al. Approach to the diagnosis of congenital myopathies. Neuromuscul Disord 2014;24:97–116.
39. Pelin K, Wallgren-Pettersson C. Update on the genetics of congenital myopathies. Semin Pediatr Neurol 2019;29:12–22.
40. Phadke R. Myopathology of congenital myopathies: bridging the old and the new. Semin Pediatr Neurol 2019;29:55–70.
41. Verma S, Balasubramanian SB. Clinical, electrophysiology, and pathology features of dynamin centronuclear myopathy: a case report and review of the literature. J Clin Neuromuscul Dis 2016;18:84–8.
42. Bitoun M, Maugenre S, Jeannet PY, et al. Mutations in dynamin 2 cause dominant centronuclear myopathy. Nat Genet 2005;37:1207–9.
43. Gonzalez-Jamett AM, Baez-Matus X, Olivares MJ, et al. Dynamin-2 mutations linked to centronuclear myopathy impair actin-dependent trafficking in muscle cells. Sci Rep 2017;7(4580):1–16.
44. Felice KJ. Distal weakness in dystrophin-deficient muscular dystrophy. Muscle Nerve 1996;19:1608–10.
45. van der Sluijs BM, ter Laak HJ, Sheffer H, et al. Autosomal recessive oculopharyngeal myopathy: a distinct phenotypical, histological, and genetic entity. J Neurol Neurosurg Psychiatry 2004;75:1499–501.
46. Tawil R, McDermott MP, Mendell JR, et al. Facioscapulohumeral muscular dystrophy (FSHMD): design of natural history study and results of baseline testing. Neurology 1994;44:442–6.
47. Rowland LP, Fetell M, Olarte M, et al. Emery-Dreifuss muscular dystrophy. Ann Neurol 1979;5:111–7.
48. Griggs RC, Askanas V, DiMauro S, et al. Inclusion body myositis and myopathies. Ann Neurol 1995;38:705–13.
49. Larue S, Maisonobe T, Benveniste O, et al. Distal muscle involvement in granulomatous myositis can mimic inclusion body myositis. J Neurol Neurosurg Psychiatry 2011;82:674–7.
50. DiMauro S, Hartwig G, Hays A, et al. Debrancher deficiency: neuromuscular disorder in 5 adults. Ann Neurol 1979;5:422–36.
51. Barohn RJ, McVey AL, DiMauro S. Adult acid maltase deficiency. Muscle Nerve 1993;16:672–6.
52. Statland JM, Tawil R. Facioscapulohumeral humeral muscular dystrophy. Continnum (Minneap Minn) 2016;22:1916–31.
53. Sacconi S, Briand-Suleau A, Gros M, et al. FSHD1 and FSHD2 form a disease continuum. Neurology 2019;92:e2273–85.
54. Mathews KD, Mills KA, Bosch EP, et al. Linkage localization of facioscapulohumeral muscular dystrophy (FSHD) in 4q35. Am J Hum Genet 1992;51:428–31.
55. Felice KJ, Jones JM, Conway SR. Facioscapulohumeral dystrophy presenting as infantile facial diplegia and late-onset limb-girdle myopathy in members of the same family. Muscle Nerve 2005;32:368–72.
56. Felice KJ, North WA, Moore SA, et al. FSH dystrophy 4q35 deletion in patients presenting with facial-sparing scapular myopathy. Neurology 2000;54:1927–31.
57. Krasnianski M, Eger K, Neudecker S, et al. Atypical phenotypes in patients with facioscapulohumeral muscular dystrophy 4q35 deletion. Arch Neurol 2003;60:1421–5.

58. Papadopoulos C, Zouvelou V, Papadimas GK. Facio-scapulo-humeral dystrophy with early contractures and rigid spine. Acta Myol 2019;38:25–8.
59. Kottlors M, Kress W, Meng G, et al. Facioscapulohumeral muscular dystrophy presenting with isolated axial myopathy and bent spine syndrome. Muscle Nerve 2010;42:273–5.
60. Paganoni S, Nicholson K, Leigh F, et al. Developing multidisciplinary clinics for neuromuscular care and research. Muscle Nerve 2017;56:848–58.

Inflammatory Myopathies

Utility of Antibody Testing

Suur Biliciler, MD[a,*], Justin Kwan, MD[b]

KEYWORDS

- Inflammatory myopathies • Dermatomyositis • Antisynthetase syndrome
- Overlap myositis • Sporadic inclusion body myositis

KEY POINTS

- Inflammatory myopathies can be classified into dermatomyositis; overlap myositis, including antisynthetase syndrome; immune-mediated necrotizing myopathy; inclusion body myositis; and polymyositis. Among the 5, polymyositis is the rarest.
- Dermatomyositis-associated antibodies include MJ(NXP2), TIF1gamma, SAE, Mi-2, MDA-5. Inclusion body myositis is associated with anti-NT5c1A antibodies.
- Cancer risk is increased in older MJ (NXP2) and TIF1 gamma–positive dermatomyositis patients. MDA-5-positive dermatomyositis patients can present with fulminant interstitial lung disease.
- Anti-Jo1, PL-7, PL-12, EJ, OJ, Zo, Ha antibodies, with anti-Jo1 antibody being the most common, can be seen in antisynthetase syndrome. Immune-mediated necrotizing myopathy usually presents with severe weakness and very increased creatine kinase levels. Patients can have anti-signal recognition particle or anti-hydroxy-3-methylglutaryl-coenzyme A reductase antibodies.

 **Video content accompanies this article at http://www.neurologic.theclinics.com.**

CASE CLINICAL PRESENTATION 1

A 76-year-old woman with a medical history of invasive ductal carcinoma of the right breast 2 years ago that was treated with surgical resection and radiation therapy and was in remission who presented for evaluation of 2-week to 3-week history of gradually progressive lower extremity swelling and shortness of breath. She also had difficulty swallowing. Over the preceding week, she also experienced increasing weakness in her arms and legs, and she noticed an increase in her abdominal girth.

[a] Department of Neurology, UT Health Science Center in Houston, McGovern Medical School, 6341 Fannin Street, MSC #466, Houston, TX 77030, USA; [b] Department of Neurology, Temple University, Lewis Katz School of Medicine, 3401 North Broad Street Street, Suite C525, Philadelphia, PA 19410, USA
* Corresponding author.
E-mail address: suur.biliciler@uth.tmc.edu

Neurol Clin 38 (2020) 661–678
https://doi.org/10.1016/j.ncl.2020.05.001
0733-8619/20/Published by Elsevier Inc.

Her general physical examination showed anasarca, pitting edema up to the proximal legs and forearms, hyperpigmented skin lesions on her upper eyelids and knuckles, and ulcerations on her fingertips on the right second and left fourth digits. Her neurologic examination showed mild guttural dysarthria and neck flexor and symmetric proximal muscle weakness. Sensory examination showed mild decrease to vibration in the toes and normal vibration in her fingers. Deep tendon reflexes were hypoactive in the lower extremities.

DIAGNOSTIC STUDIES

Her laboratory studies showed an increase in serum creatinine level of 2.43 mg/dL from her baseline of 0.62 mg/dL, creatine kinase (CK) 6453 U/L, aldolase 78.0 U/L, sedimentation rate 73 mm/h, C-reactive protein 12.7 mg/dL, and thyroid-stimulating hormone 10.1 IU/L. Her antinuclear antibody (ANA), anti-SSA and SSB antibodies, rheumatoid factor (RF), anti–DS DNA antibody, anti-Jo1 antibody, and anticentromere antibody were normal. Her chest computed tomography (CT) with and without contrast showed interstitial lung disease. Her needle electromyography (EMG) study showed fibrillation potentials and positive sharp waves and short-duration, low-amplitude, and polyphasic voluntary motor unit potential with early recruitment pattern in the deltoid, biceps, and triceps muscles consistent with a primary disorder of the muscle with increased membrane irritability.

Which myositis-specific antibody is expected to be positive in this patient?

1. Mi-2
2. MJ/NXP2
3. Anti–melanoma differentiation-associated gene 5 (MDA-5)
4. SAE
5. TIF1 gamma

Answer: 3. MDA-5 antibody. MDA-5 autoantibody has been shown to be associated with rapidly progressive interstitial lung disease (ILD). It is important to identify this subtype of dermatomyositis (DM) because the increased morbidity and mortality caused by ILD requires aggressive treatment using multiple immunosuppressive medications.

TREATMENT AND DEFINITIVE DIAGNOSIS

This patient's history, examination, and diagnostic studies are compatible with DM. Because of her history of breast cancer, cancer antigen 19-9, alpha fetoprotein tumor marker, carcinoembryonic antigen, and a paraneoplastic antibody panel were obtained and were normal. Her PL-7, PL-12, EJ, OJ, signal recognition particle (SRP), Mi-2, TIF1 gamma, MJ/NXP-2, anti-PM/SCL, U2 snRNP, fibrillarin, anti–U1-RNP, anti–SAE, and Ku antibodies were negative. Her MDA-5 antibody titer was increased. Her muscle biopsy showed perifascicular atrophy with focal inflammation compatible with DM.

Based on these findings, the patient was empirically given a 5-day course of intravenous methylprednisolone and intravenous immunoglobulin (IVIg) because of the severity of her weakness, followed by prednisone and monthly IVIg infusions. She was also started on azathioprine. She was treated with a multidrug regimen because of the concern for rapidly progressive ILD. After 3 months of treatment, her CK level decreased to 41 U/L and her strength gradually improved, although she still required the use of a walker to ambulate. All of her skin lesions resolved. Because of the concern that the diagnosis of DM represented a paraneoplastic syndrome, a CT scan of chest, abdomen, and pelvis was obtained that did not show evidence of breast cancer recurrence. She also had follow-up with her oncologist and there was no clinical evidence to suggest cancer recurrence.

DISCUSSION

DM is a subtype of idiopathic inflammatory myopathy in which proximal muscle weakness and cutaneous abnormalities are the most prominent clinical features.[1] The clinical presentation of DM can be heterogeneous, and amyopathic DM is a recognized and well-defined subgroup of DM.[2] Patients diagnosed with DM can have a variety of skin manifestations, varying degrees of muscle weakness, and other systemic disorders. Although the classic skin findings in DM include purplish periorbital edematous rash (heliotrope rash) and erythema and scaly skin lesions over the extensor finger joints (Gottron papules), other skin manifestations include erythematous/violaceous rash over the extensor joints, upper chest, and forehead; erythematous scaly plaques on the scalp; poikiloderma; skin ulcerations; and facial and periorbital edema.[3] Systemic disorders associated with DM include ILD, joint disease, and cardiac disorders such as myocarditis.[4] Muscle biopsy findings in DM can also be variable. Perifascicular atrophy is highly suggestive of DM; however, in some biopsies, only minimal myopathic changes or nonspecific abnormalities are seen.

Autoantibodies are frequently found in patients with DM and include Mi2, TIF1-gamma, MJ/NXP2, SAE, and MDA-5.[5] MDA-5 antibody was first recognized in the Japanese in 2005 and it targets a cytosolic protein involved in innate antiviral immune response.[6,7] In patients who have MDA-5 antibody–associated DM, the skin involvement is often more prominent than the myositis. The most important feature to recognize and the major cause of morbidity in these patients is rapidly progressive ILD, which can result in a high mortality of up to 50%.[7,8] Because of the high mortality in this group of patients, identifying the presence of the MDA-5 antibody and ILD and implementation of early and aggressive therapy in this subgroup of patients with DM is essential. A recent study suggests that a combination therapy using multiple immunosuppressive medications may be more effective in patients who have rapid progressive ILD.[9]

CASE CLINICAL PRESENTATION 2

A 74-year-old woman presented to clinic for progressive weakness and swallowing difficulty for the last 2.5 months. Her past medical history was pertinent for chronic lymphocytic leukemia diagnosed more than 5 years ago, and she had been in remission for the last couple of years. Her family history was noncontributory.

She had normal cranial nerve examination and nasal speech. She was constantly drooling because of swallowing difficulty. She had weakness in neck flexors and proximal muscles in both upper and lower extremities. Her neck flexors were 4 out of 5; deltoid muscles were 3 out of 5 biceps muscles were 4 out of 5; and iliopsoas, gluteus medius and maximus muscles, and hip adductors were 4 out of 5. She had normal deep tendon reflexes and flexor plantar responses bilaterally. Her sensory and cerebellar examinations were also normal. Skin, respiratory, cardiovascular, and gastrointestinal system examination were normal. Her swallowing worsened over a few weeks, requiring a feeding tube.

DIAGNOSTIC STUDIES

The CK level was increased at 845 U/L (normal, 12–191 U/L). ANA, Sjögren antibodies, RF, paraneoplastic panel, and serum protein electrophoresis (SPEP) and urine protein electrophoresis (UPEP) with immunofixation electrophoresis were normal. Her chest, abdomen, and pelvis CT as well as whole-body PET-CT were unremarkable. Her electrodiagnostic studies showed normal nerve conduction responses and the needle EMG revealed increased insertional activity, abnormal spontaneous activity in the form of fibrillation potentials and positive sharp waves, and early recruitment pattern in proximal extremity muscles. A muscle biopsy of the left biceps muscle was performed.

Question:
Based on the pathology seen in the picture (**Fig. 1**) what is the most likely diagnosis?
1. Nemaline rod myopathy
2. DM
3. Inclusion body myositis (IBM)
4. Myotubular myopathy
5. Immune-mediated necrotizing myopathy

Answer: 2. DM. The picture shows perifascicular atrophy, which is typically seen in DM.

TREATMENT AND DEFINITIVE DIAGNOSIS

Perifascicular atrophy is defined as the presence of small fibers observed in the periphery of a muscle fiber fascicle. Some of these fibers result from fiber atrophy, whereas others are regenerating fibers. Perifascicular atrophy is not typically seen in any of the other choices listed.

In addition to perifascicular atrophy, other features seen in DM are collections of mostly perimysial/perivascular inflammatory cells (**Fig. 2**), cytochrome oxidase (COX)–negative fibers mostly located in the perifascicular region (**Fig. 3**), increased expression of major histocompatibility complex class 1 (MHC-1) within the sarcolemma, membrane attack complex deposits in microcapillaries (**Fig. 4**), and MX1 upregulation within the perifascicular region. This case of DM is another in which the patient's myositis autoantibody panel revealed MJ antibody. The patient later developed periungual erythema, Gottron papules (**Fig. 5**), and a rash on her chest and

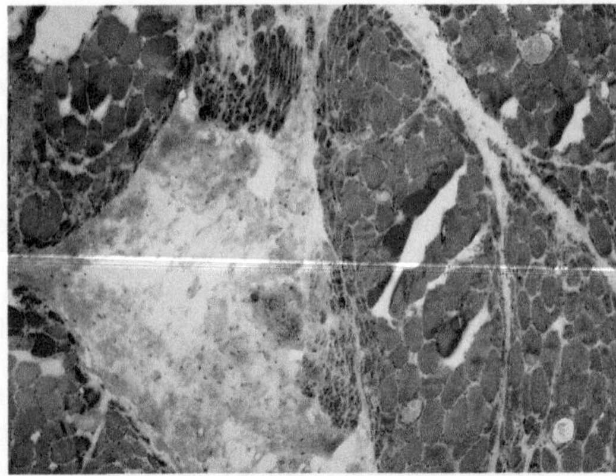

Fig. 1. Perifascicular atrophy/DM (hematoxylin-eosin [H&E, 10x]).

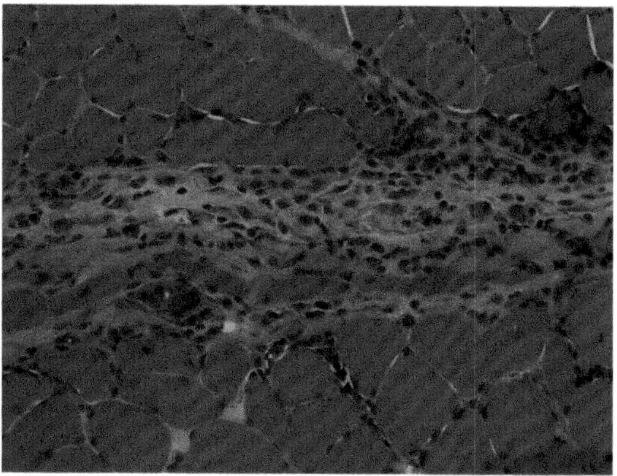

Fig. 2. Perimysial inflammation/DM (H&E, 20x).

knees. She was started on prednisone, to which she responded very well, with improvement of her weakness and dysphagia. The percutaneous endoscopic gastrostomy tube was removed.

DISCUSSION

MJ (NXP2) DM is usually seen in juvenile patients, and calcinosis is observed frequently in MJ (NXP2)-positive patients. The incidence of calcinosis is reported to be higher in juvenile cases.[10–12]

The presence of MJ antibody may portend an increased risk for cancer and may prompt clinicians to search for a malignancy more aggressively. Cancer risk is increased in older patients, especially in individuals older than 39 years of age who harbor TIF1gamma and MJ (NXP2) antibodies.[12,13] In juvenile DM with the same antibodies, an increased risk for malignancies is not observed. The first-line therapy for MJ antibody–associated DM is glucocorticoids. IVIg can also be used.[14] Azathioprine, methotrexate, mycophenolate mofetil, rituximab, cyclophosphamide, cyclosporine, and tacrolimus have all been used as steroid-sparing agents.

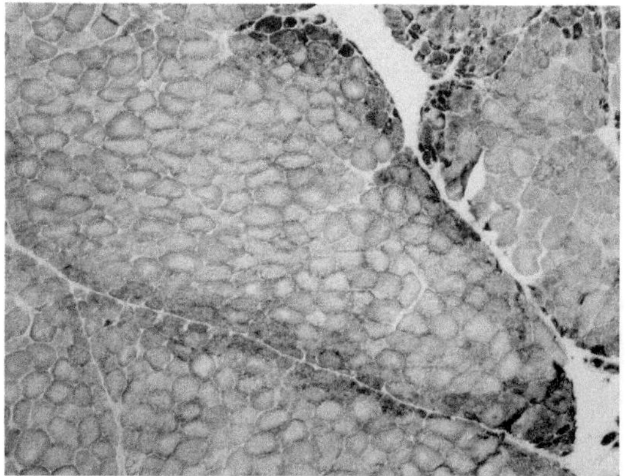

Fig. 3. COX/SDH-COX–negative fibers are densely observed within the perifascicular area/DM. COX/SDH, 10x. SDH, succinyl dehydrogenase.

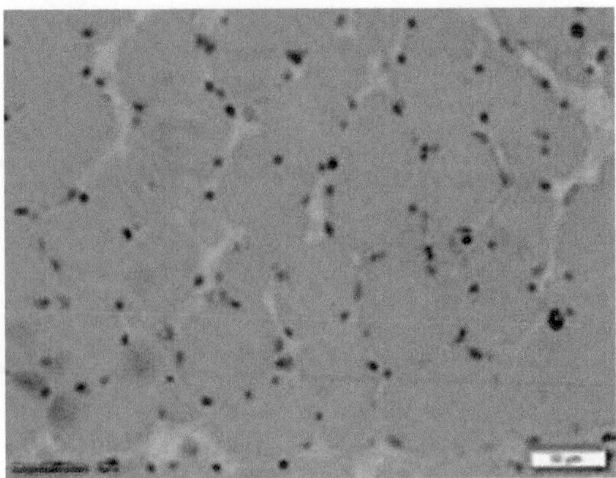

Fig. 4. Presence of MAC deposits within microcapillaries/DM. MAC, 20x. MAC, membrane attack complex.

CASE CLINICAL PRESENTATION 3

A 48-year-old white woman presented to the neuromuscular outpatient clinic complaining of speech problems, swallowing difficulty, and arm and leg weakness for the last 2.5 years. She had slurred speech and could not pronounce the letters as smoothly as she could before the onset of her weakness. She denied having double vision, droopy eyelids, or shortness of breath. Her past medical history was notable

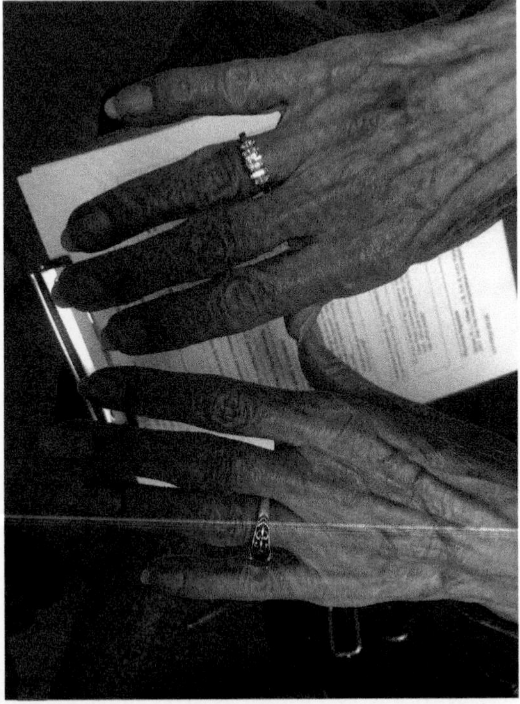

Fig. 5. Gottron papules and periungual erythema/DM.

for hypertension and migraine headaches. There was no family history of muscle disorders or other neurologic or rheumatological disorders. Her neurologic examination showed slurred speech, severe facial weakness, and an inability to close her eyes completely. She had weakness in bilateral deltoid and biceps muscles, left finger flexor muscles, and bilateral iliopsoas and left tibialis anterior muscles. She did not have scapular winging. There were no tongue fibrillations or muscle fasciculations. She had 2+ and symmetric deep tendon reflexes and flexor plantar responses bilaterally. Her sensory examination was normal.

DIAGNOSTIC STUDIES

The CK level was increased at 532 U/L (normal, 12–191 U/L). The rest of her laboratory studies, including complete blood count (CBC), comprehensive metabolic panel (CMP), ANA, RF, erythrocyte sedimentation rate, and C-reactive protein, were normal. Electrodiagnostic studies showed normal nerve conduction studies. Her needle EMG study showed increased insertional activity as well as abnormal spontaneous activity in the form of rare positive waves in quadriceps muscles and early recruitment in biceps, iliopsoas, adductor magnus, and quadriceps muscles.

Question:
What would you do next?

1. Muscle biopsy
2. Genetic testing for hereditary myopathies
3. Treat patient with steroids
4. Check for gelsolin mutation for hereditary amyloidosis
5. Ultrasonography of face, arm, and leg muscles

Answer: 1. Muscle biopsy.

TREATMENT AND DEFINITIVE DIAGNOSIS

This patient is presenting with facial, symmetric proximal, and asymmetric distal muscle weakness in the extremities and mildly increased CK level. There are several hereditary myopathies that can cause facial weakness, such as fascioscapulohumeral dystrophy (FSHD), congenital myopathies (CMs), myotonic dystrophy, and oculopharyngeal muscular dystrophy (OPMD). Facial weakness is not a feature. Even though the possibility of an underlying hereditary myopathy still exists, it is less likely given that the patient lacks several features for the common inherited myopathies mentioned earlier (scapular winging in FSHD, ptosis in myotonic dystrophy and OPMD, and onset at birth or infancy in CM). The progression of her weakness is over 2 years, which is longer than expected in immune-mediated myopathies. There are reports of insidious progression in some immune-mediated necrotizing myopathies (IMNMs), but the CK level is much higher, typically in thousands in IMNMs. Gelsolin mutation is another cause of prominent facial weakness caused by cranial neuropathies. Patients often have sensory symptoms and findings on examination. In individuals who have gelsolin mutation, the kidneys might be affected and lattice cornea is seen on ophthalmologic examination. Our patient did not have any of these clinical findings. Ultrasonography of the muscles can be useful in pattern recognition in some myopathies as well, determining the optimal biopsy site in patients with subtle weakness or inconclusive EMG results. In this patient, the needle EMG findings are consistent with a myopathic disorder (fibrillation potentials are not common in IBM and the pattern is usually that of mixed units of short and long duration) and are helpful enough to choose the muscle to sample.

A biopsy of the left biceps muscle was performed to better understand the underlying muscle disorder. The biopsy showed rimmed vacuoles (**Fig. 6**), several COX-negative fibers (**Fig. 7**), increased expression of MHC-1 on the sarcolemmal membrane, and p62 aggregates (**Fig. 8**) in several fibers, which are all seen in IBM. After the muscle biopsy findings were determined, antibody testing for cytosolic 5′nucleotidase 1A (NT5C1A) was positive. The patient was diagnosed with sIBM. This patient had an uncommon presentation because her main presenting symptom was severe facial weakness. Because of the atypical clinical features, a muscle biopsy was performed first, followed by serologic testing for NT5C1A antibody to confirm the diagnosis. As her disease progressed, the clinical findings became more typical for IBM (current examination, Video 1). She is currently ambulatory and independent in all of her activities of daily living, although she is slowly losing strength. She can no longer play the guitar. She has dysphagia but she can still tolerate an oral diet.

DISCUSSION

sIBM is the most common inflammatory myopathy after the fifth decade of life; it presents with asymmetrical weakness and has a predilection for finger flexor and quadriceps weakness. Dysphagia is one of the common early complaints (reported in one-third of patients), and patients are often referred to see ear, nose, and throat or gastrointestinal specialists before seeking further evaluation by a neurologist. The only antibody associated with sIBM is cytosolic 5′-nucleotidase 1A (NT5c1A) antibody.[15] Studies have showed variable sensitivity and specificity of NT5c1A antibody in diagnosing IBM.[16] Because of this limitation, NT5c1A antibody is currently used in combination with the clinical history and examination (being the most important) and muscle biopsy to confirm the diagnosis of IBM. Facial muscles weakness occurs in one-third of cases. There are no effective treatments for IBM. Standard of care in this patient group is nonpharmacologic. Treatment with immunosuppressive medications such as corticosteroids, azathioprine, and methotrexate was ineffective.[17–19] Even though there are case reports of IVIg being effective in patients with dysphagia, subsequent studies failed to show any long-term efficacy of IVIg treatment to improve strength.[18,20] Clinical trials conducted using anti–T-lymphocyte globulin, alemtuzumab, anakinra, interferon beta-1a, bimagrumab, and simvastatin failed to show any significant clinical benefit.[21–26] Some patients who have upper esophageal relaxation difficulty may benefit from cricopharyngeal myotomy or cricopharyngeal dilatation,

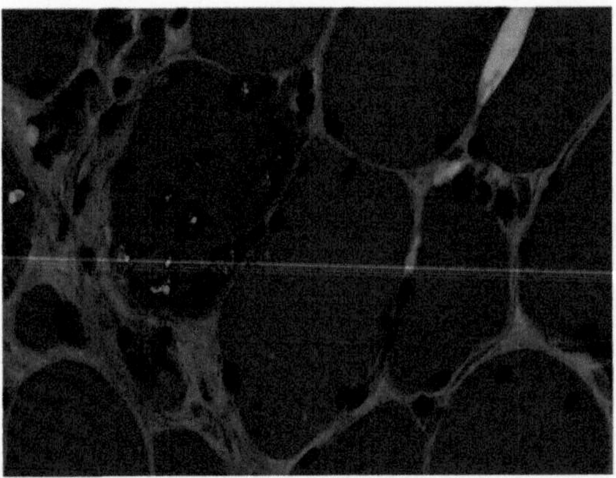

Fig. 6. Rimmed vacuoles/IBM. H&E, 40x.

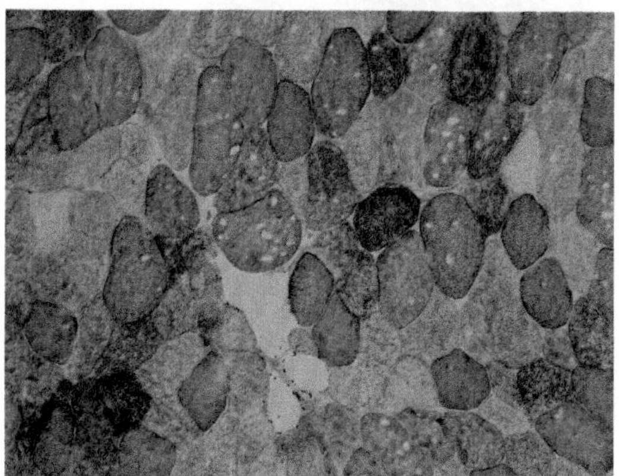

Fig. 7. COX/SDH. Several COX-negative fibers in IBM. COX/SDH stain, 20x.

which can delay the need for a feeding tube placement.[27,28] Focal botulinum toxin injection is also reported to alleviate dysphagia in patients with sIBM and may be useful before myotomy or dilatation.[29] Exercise and physical therapy are recommended.[30] Aerobic exercise was found to improve aerobic capacity in 1 study over a period of 12 weeks.[31]

CASE CLINICAL PRESENTATION 4

A 71-year-old Hispanic woman presented with weakness that has been present for the 1.5 years. The weakness began in her legs then spread to her arms followed by neck involvement over the next 6 months. She denied having speech problems. She had difficulty swallowing when her neck started to bend forward. She was not on statin therapy in the past. Her past medical history was pertinent for breast cancer that was in remission for the last few years. She did not have family members with similar symptoms. Her neurologic examination showed head drop (**Fig. 9**) and proximal muscle weakness in both upper and lower extremities. Her deltoid muscles were 2 out of 5, biceps muscles were 3 out of 5, and hip flexors were 3 out of 5. She had bilateral scapular winging (**Fig. 10**). She had periungual erythema and mechanic's hands. Her

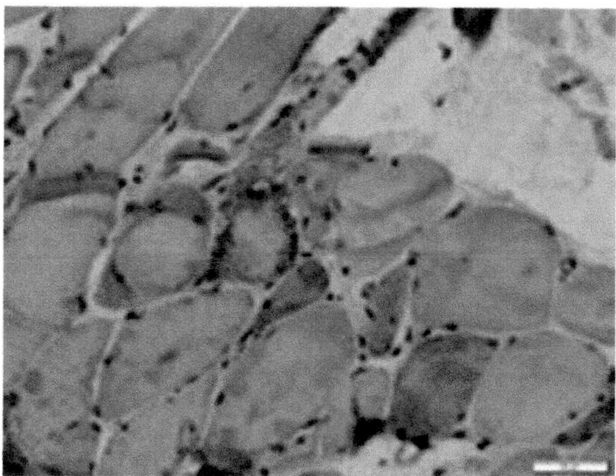

Fig. 8. MHC-1. Upregulation of MHC-1. MHC 1 stain, 40x.

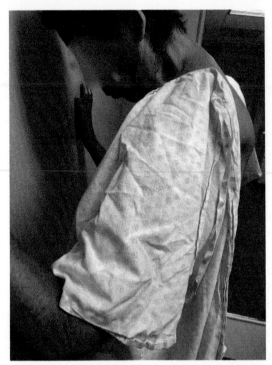

Fig. 9. Head drop in Pm-Scl–positive overlap myositis.

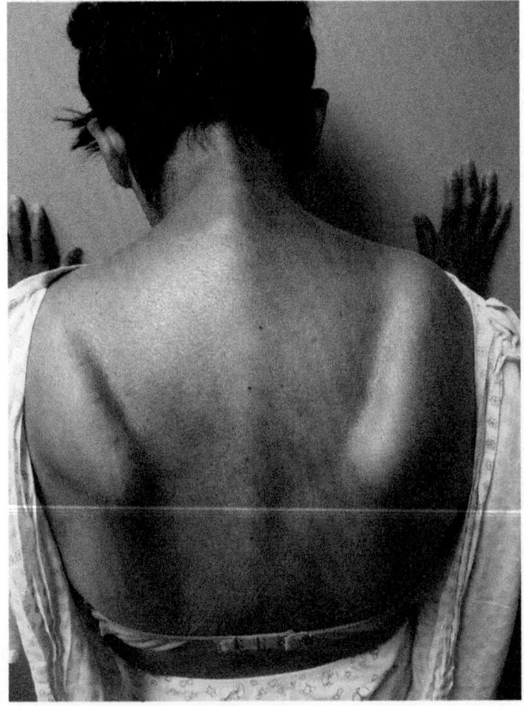

Fig. 10. Scapular winging in Pm-Scl–positive overlap myositis.

cranial nerves, deep tendon reflexes, plantar responses, and sensory examination were normal.

DIAGNOSTIC STUDIES

The CBC; CMP; paraneoplastic panel; FSHD 1 and 2 genetic studies; chest, abdomen, and pelvis CT with contrast; and whole-body PET-CT were normal. The CK level was increased at 1134 U/L (normal, 12–191 U/L).

Electrodiagnostic studies showed mild to moderately increased spontaneous activity in both arms, proximal greater than distal and posterior neck muscles. There was mildly increased spontaneous activity in the proximal leg muscles. Short-duration and polyphasic motor unit potentials were observed in a similar pattern.

Question:
Which antibody is more likely to be positive in this patient?

1. LRP4
2. NT5c1a
3. Contactin
4. Pm-Scl
5. Anti–hydroxy-3-methylglutaryl–coenzyme A reductase (HMGCR)

Answer: 4. Pm-Scl antibody.

TREATMENT AND DEFINITIVE DIAGNOSIS

Contactin antibodies are associated with chronic inflammatory demyelinating polyneuropathies and can be seen in treatment-resistant cases. HMGCR antibodies are present in autoimmune necrotizing myopathy, which does not cause skin rash; however, in some cases, patients can have scapular winging on examination. LRP4 antibodies are found in myasthenia gravis and can present with head drop and acute respiratory failure. These patients do not have cutaneous lesions or scapular winging. NT5c1a is mostly seen in sIBM. PM-Scl is present in overlap myositis, usually in combined myositis and scleroderma. Some patients present with profound cervical brachial involvement, as seen in our patient. This patient's myositis panel showed the presence of Pm-Scl antibody. A muscle biopsy of the left biceps was performed and showed dense collections of inflammatory cells consistent with an inflammatory myopathy (**Fig. 11**). She was treated with IVIg, prednisone, and mycophenolate mofetil. Her leg weakness improved significantly, whereas her upper extremity and neck flexor weakness improved to a lesser degree.

DISCUSSION

Overlap myositis is a subtype of idiopathic inflammatory myopathy and consists of myositis associated with antisynthetase syndrome (ASS) or myositis associated with clinical features of a connective tissue disorder such as systemic lupus erythematosus. This condition is the most common subtype of inflammatory myopathies and accounts for approximately 50% of all the cases.[32] Antibodies associated with overlap myositis excluding the ASS antibodies are anti-Ku, anti-Pm-Scl, anti-Ro/Sjögren syndrome, anti-U1 RNP, and anti-PUF60 antibodies.[33] Anti–Pm-Scl antibodies can be found in patients with overlap of myositis and features of scleroderma. Patients can have mechanic's hands, ILD, arthritis, esophageal dysmotility, and calcinosis.[32] Brachiocervical weakness, head drop, and camptocormia are reported in presence of anti–Pm-Scl or anti-Ku antibodies, with arm abductors being much weaker than hip flexors.[34–36]

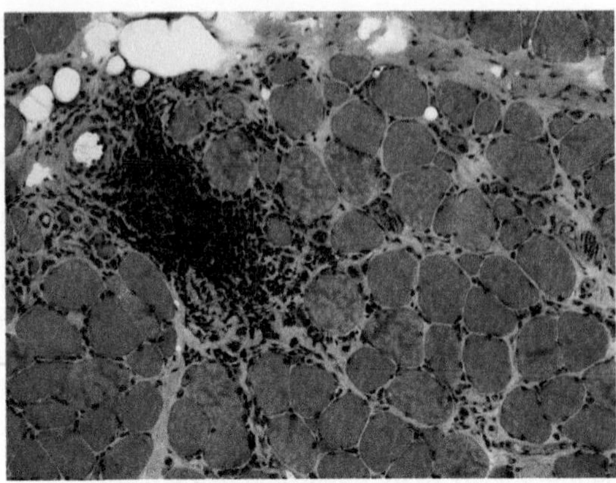

Fig. 11. Collection inflammatory cells (H&E, 20x).

With corticosteroids being the first line of treatment as in other types of myositis, the treatment is also geared toward the underlying systemic disease. Corticosteroid is often used in combination with IVIg, azathioprine, methotrexate, mycophenolate mofetil, or rituximab as steroid-sparing agents.

CASE CLINICAL PRESENTATION 5

An 87-year-old man presented for evaluation of lower extremity weakness progressing over the prior 4 months. He was started on atorvastatin in November 2017 and, by March 2018, he began to have trouble walking. He could not walk as fast as he normally did and had to have help getting out of a vehicle because he was unable to stand up. He also had shortness of breath with exertion, and difficulty climbing the stairs, getting up from the floor, and getting in and out of the bathtub. Because of these symptoms, atorvastatin was discontinued; however, his symptoms did not improve. He did not have muscle pain or cramps and he did not have slurred speech or swallowing difficulty. On physical examination, there was no rash. He had mild facial muscle weakness and symmetric moderate severely proximal muscle weakness. His sensory examination was normal and his deep tendon reflexes were hypoactive in the lower extremities and normoactive in the upper extremities.

DIAGNOSTIC STUDIES

His laboratory studies showed CK level of 6397 U/L, aspartate aminotransferase 229 IU/L, alanine aminotransferase 190 IU/L, and C-reactive protein 7.4 mg/L. His ANA, RF, anti-DS DNA antibody, RNP antibody, anti-SSA and SSB antibodies, anti–Jo-1 antibody, anti–scleroderma-70 antibody, Smith antibody, and anti–centromere B antibodies were normal. His nerve conduction studies showed a median neuropathy across the wrist and his needle electromyography study showed fibrillation potentials and positive waves, and short-duration, low-amplitude, and polyphasic voluntary motor unit potentials with early recruitment in the proximal upper and lower extremity muscles consistent with a primary disorder of the muscle with increased membrane irritability.

Question:

What would you do next?

1. No further testing needed

2. Obtain genetics testing
3. Refer to hand surgery for carpal tunnel syndrome (CTS)
4. Obtain muscle biopsy
5. Obtain anti–cN-1A testing

Answer: 4. Obtain a muscle biopsy. This patient has subacute muscular symptoms after starting statin therapy. A muscle biopsy is helpful to confirm the presence of an autoimmune myopathy.

TREATMENT AND DEFINITIVE DIAGNOSIS

A biceps muscle biopsy was performed that showed rare collections of perimysial perivascular inflammatory cells and many necrotic fibers and upregulation of MHC-1 compatible with a necrotizing myopathy. His Mi-2, Ku, PL-7, PL-2, EJ, and OJ antibodies were negative. His SRP antibody titer was increased. The patient was diagnosed with IMNM with SRP antibodies. His transthoracic echocardiogram showed a normal ejection fraction.

He was treated with a 5-day course of IVIg and 3-day course of intravenous methylprednisolone empirically, followed by oral prednisone and mycophenolate mofetil. Two months after starting treatment, his CK level was 99 U/L and his weakness had markedly improved. He no longer required assistance to get out of a car.

DISCUSSION

IMNM is a subtype of idiopathic inflammatory myopathy defined pathologically by muscle fiber necrosis in the absence or scarcity of inflammatory cell infiltrate on the muscle biopsy.[37] Muscle biopsies from patients who have anti-SRP antibody were the first to be identified as having this pathologic characteristic.[38] Subsequently, muscle biopsies from patients who have HMGCR antibody were also described to have the same pathologic features.[39] Approximately one-third of patients diagnosed with IMNM are seronegative. Patients who have IMNM typically have proximal muscle weakness and high serum CK level, typically in the thousands. Extramuscular manifestation such as myocardial inflammation is more common in patients who have anti-SRP myopathy.[40] Arthritis and mild ILD, which are also most common in anti-SRP myopathy, have also been observed in some patients.[41] Patients who have IMNM may have an increased risk for malignancy, especially in patients who are seronegative, whereas patients who have anti-SRP myopathy have a lower risk.[42] The risk for malignancy in anti-HMGCR is less certain because of conflicting findings in different studies.[42–44]

The diagnosis of IMNM is made by a combination of clinical findings of proximal weakness, highly increased serum CK level, and muscle biopsy that show randomly distributed necrotic muscle fibers.[45] The muscle biopsy typically shows few scattered necrotic fibers, regenerating fibers, inflammatory infiltrates mostly consisting of macrophages, and diffuse sarcolemmal expression of MHC-1. However, a more significant inflammatory cell infiltrate consisting of CD8-positive T cells can be present in up to 25% of the muscle biopsies.[46] Most patients who have IMNM require treatment with a combination of corticosteroids and other immunosuppressive medications. Intravenous gamma globulin, azathioprine, methotrexate, and mycophenolate mofetil are often used in combination with oral or intravenous corticosteroids.[8] Rituximab has been suggested to be more effective in anti-SRP myopathy.[45] The treatment regimen should be tailored to the severity of the disease and other comorbid conditions.

CASE CLINICAL PRESENTATION 6

A 51-year-old woman with a history of Lyme disease confirmed by serologic testing and adequately treated with antibiotics presented for evaluation of a 10-year history of progressive weakness. She first noticed generalized weakness after being diagnosed with Lyme disease. She had trouble with certain activities, such as walking up the stairs, walking up an incline, and getting up from a deep chair. A few years after the onset of her muscular symptoms, her balance became more impaired and she had to be more cautious when walking to prevent falls. Her legs occasionally gave out without warning, causing her to fall. Over the past year, she noticed numbness on her right forearm and mild shortness of breath that was typically associated with physical exertion. On examination, she had mild erythema and edema at the proximal nail folds on all her fingers, hyperkeratotic changes on her fingertips, and fine basilar rales. She had mild proximal arm weakness and moderately severe proximal leg weakness. Her sensory examination was normal and she was areflexic.

DIAGNOSTIC STUDIES

Her laboratory testing showed borderline increased anti-DS DNA antibody level of 5 IU/mL and an increased anti-SSB antibody level. Her antineutrophil cytoplasmic antibodies, CK, C-reactive protein, sedimentation rate, anti–scleroderma-70 antibody, anti-SSA antibody, anti–centromere B antibody, Smith antibody, RNP antibody, anti-ds DNA antibody, and RF were normal. Her thyroid function studies were normal. Her electrophysiologic testing showed an essentially normal nerve conduction study and her needle electromyography showed short-duration and lower-amplitude motor unit potentials with early recruitment in the proximal lower extremity muscles consistent with a primary disorder of the muscle. There was no increased membrane irritability. She had an MRI scan of the right lower thigh, which did not show muscle atrophy or intramuscular edema.

Question:
What would you do next?

1. Repeat Lyme disease testing
2. Start antibiotics therapy
3. Obtain MRI of lumbar spine
4. Obtain myositis-associated antibodies
5. Obtain skin biopsy

Answer: 4. Obtain myositis-associated antibodies or antisynthetase antibodies. This patient presents with a clinical syndrome composed of multisystemic disease involving the skin, lung, and muscle suggesting antisynthetase syndrome. Her cutaneous symptoms do not fit the typical skin changes seen in DM. Myositis-associated antibody testing can be diagnostic in patients who have these clinical features.

TREATMENT AND DEFINITIVE DIAGNOSIS

A biceps muscle biopsy was performed and showed scattered perimysial and perivascular inflammatory infiltrates. Her PL-12 antibody was positive. Her PL-7, Mi-2, Ku, EJ, OJ, SRP, and Jo-1 antibodies were negative. The patient was diagnosed with antisynthetase syndrome based on the findings on her antibody testing. CT chest without contrast was obtained that showed left more than right ground-glass opacification in both lower lobes, and her pulmonary function testing was normal.

She was started on corticosteroids, which were gradually tapered over the next several months. Mycophenolate mofetil was added to her treatment regimen shortly after she began corticosteroid therapy because she had findings of ILD on lung imaging. After being treated with this combination of immunosuppressive therapy for a year, her upper extremity strength was nearly normal; however, she continued to have mild to moderate proximal lower extremity weakness.

DISCUSSION

Antisynthetase syndrome is a heterogeneous group of disorders with main clinical features consisting of myositis, ILD, Raynaud's phenomenon, arthritis, fever, and hyperkeratotic skin changes on the fingers, especially at the tips (known as mechanic's hand).[47] Antisynthetase syndrome is sometimes categorized as a subgroup of overlap myositis because of the association of myositis with other systemic autoimmune disorders. The unifying characteristic of this syndrome is the finding of autoantibodies that target aminacyl–transfer RNA (tRNA) synthetases, which function to attach amino acids to their cognate tRNA as a first step in protein translation. There are currently 10 antisynthetase antibodies identified: Jo-1, PL12, PL7, OJ, EJ, KS, Zo, YRS/Tyr, SC, and JS.[48,49] The most common antibody is anti–Jo-1, followed by PL12 and PL7.

The clinical presentation of myositis antisynthetase syndrome consists of proximal muscle weakness, increased CK level, and changes on needle electromyography compatible with a primary disorder of the muscle. The muscle biopsy can show perifascicular muscle fiber necrosis and an increase in sarcolemmal MHC-1 expression predominantly in the perifascicular region.[50] There are 2 proposed diagnostic criteria for antisynthetase syndrome, and both require the presence of an aminacyl-tRNA synthetase antibody and varying numbers of clinical features.[47,51] In these criteria, the presence of myositis is not required for the diagnosis of antisynthetase syndrome. Treatment of antisynthetase syndrome often requires a combination of immunosuppressive medications and is often dictated by the severity of the ILD. Corticosteroid is given in combination with other agents, including azathioprine, mycophenolate mofetil, and intravenous immunoglobulin because of the high rate of symptom recurrence on tapering of the corticosteroid dose. Other treatment options include rituximab, cyclosporin, and cyclophosphamide, depending on the severity of the ILD.49

DISCLOSURE

The authors have nothing to disclose.

SUPPLEMENTARY DATA

Supplementary data related to this article can be found online at https://doi.org/10.1016/j.ncl.2020.05.001.

REFERENCES

1. Bohan A, Peter JB. Polymyositis and dermatomyositis (first of two parts). N Engl J Med 1975;292(7):344–7.
2. Lundberg IE, Tjarnlund A, Bottai M, et al. 2017 European League Against Rheumatism/American College of Rheumatology Classification Criteria for Adult and Juvenile Idiopathic Inflammatory Myopathies and Their Major Subgroups. Arthritis Rheumatol 2017;69(12):2271–82.

3. Mainetti C, Terziroli Beretta-Piccoli B, Selmi C. Cutaneous manifestations of dermatomyositis: a comprehensive review. Clin Rev Allergy Immunol 2017;53(3):337–56.
4. Marvi U, Chung L, Fiorentino DF. Clinical presentation and evaluation of dermatomyositis. Indian J Dermatol 2012;57(5):375–81.
5. Benveniste O, Goebel HH, Stenzel W. Biomarkers in inflammatory myopathies-an expanded definition. Front Neurol 2019;10:554.
6. Fiorentino D, Chung L, Zwerner J, et al. The mucocutaneous and systemic phenotype of dermatomyositis patients with antibodies to MDA5 (CADM-140): a retrospective study. J Am Acad Dermatol 2011;65(1):25–34.
7. Sato S, Hoshino K, Satoh T, et al. RNA helicase encoded by melanoma differentiation-associated gene 5 is a major autoantigen in patients with clinically amyopathic dermatomyositis: Association with rapidly progressive interstitial lung disease. Arthritis Rheum 2009;60(7):2193–200.
8. Selva-O'Callaghan A, Pinal-Fernandez I, Trallero-Araguas E, et al. Classification and management of adult inflammatory myopathies. Lancet Neurol 2018;17(9):816–28.
9. Tsuji H, Nakashima R, Hosono Y, et al. A multicenter prospective study of the efficacy and safety of combined immunosuppressive therapy with high-dose glucocorticoid, tacrolimus, and cyclophosphamide in interstitial lung diseases accompanied by anti-melanoma differentiation-associated gene 5-positive dermatomyositis. Arthritis Rheumatol 2020;72(3):488–98.
10. Tanboon J, Nishino I. Classification of idiopathic inflammatory myopathies: pathology perspectives. Curr Opin Neurol 2019;32(5):704–14.
11. McHugh NJ, Tansley SL. Autoantibodies in myositis. Nat Rev Rheumatol 2018;14(5):290–302.
12. Fiorentino DF, Chung LS, Christopher-Stine L, et al. Most patients with cancer-associated dermatomyositis have antibodies to nuclear matrix protein NXP-2 or transcription intermediary factor 1gamma. Arthritis Rheum 2013;65(11):2954–62.
13. Hida A, Yamashita T, Hosono Y, et al. Anti-TIF1-gamma antibody and cancer-associated myositis: A clinicohistopathologic study. Neurology 2016;87(3):299–308.
14. Dalakas MC, Illa I, Dambrosia JM, et al. A controlled trial of high-dose intravenous immune globulin infusions as treatment for dermatomyositis. N Engl J Med 1993;329(27):1993–2000.
15. Larman HB, Salajegheh M, Nazareno R, et al. Cytosolic 5'-nucleotidase 1A autoimmunity in sporadic inclusion body myositis. Ann Neurol 2013;73(3):408–18.
16. Felice KJ, Whitaker CH, Wu Q, et al. Sensitivity and clinical utility of the anti-cytosolic 5'-nucleotidase 1A (cN1A) antibody test in sporadic inclusion body myositis: Report of 40 patients from a single neuromuscular center. Neuromuscul Disord 2018;28(8):660–4.
17. Badrising UA, Maat-Schieman ML, Ferrari MD, et al. Comparison of weakness progression in inclusion body myositis during treatment with methotrexate or placebo. Ann Neurol 2002;51(3):369–72.
18. Dalakas MC, Koffman B, Fujii M, et al. A controlled study of intravenous immunoglobulin combined with prednisone in the treatment of IBM. Neurology 2001;56(3):323–7.
19. Leff RL, Miller FW, Hicks J, et al. The treatment of inclusion body myositis: a retrospective review and a randomized, prospective trial of immunosuppressive therapy. Medicine (Baltimore) 1993;72(4):225–35.

20. Takamiya M, Takahashi Y, Morimoto M, et al. Effect of intravenous immunoglobulin therapy on anti-NT5C1A antibody-positive inclusion body myositis after successful treatment of hepatitis C: A case report. eNeurologicalSci 2019;16:100204.
21. Muscle Study G. Randomized pilot trial of betaINF1a (Avonex) in patients with inclusion body myositis. Neurology 2001;57(9):1566–70.
22. Lindberg C, Trysberg E, Tarkowski A, et al. Anti-T-lymphocyte globulin treatment in inclusion body myositis: a randomized pilot study. Neurology 2003;61(2): 260–2.
23. Hanna MG, Badrising UA, Benveniste O, et al. Safety and efficacy of intravenous bimagrumab in inclusion body myositis (RESILIENT): a randomised, double-blind, placebo-controlled phase 2b trial. Lancet Neurol 2019;18(9):834–44.
24. Dalakas MC, Rakocevic G, Schmidt J, et al. Effect of Alemtuzumab (CAMPATH 1-H) in patients with inclusion-body myositis. Brain 2009;132(Pt 6):1536–44.
25. Sancricca C, Mora M, Ricci E, et al. Pilot trial of simvastatin in the treatment of sporadic inclusion-body myositis. Neurol Sci 2011;32(5):841–7.
26. Kosmidis ML, Alexopoulos H, Tzioufas AG, et al. The effect of anakinra, an IL1 receptor antagonist, in patients with sporadic inclusion body myositis (sIBM): a small pilot study. J Neurol Sci 2013;334(1–2):123–5.
27. Murata KY, Kouda K, Tajima F, et al. Balloon dilation in sporadic inclusion body myositis patients with Dysphagia. Clin Med Insights Case Rep 2013;6:1–7.
28. Oh TH, Brumfield KA, Hoskin TL, et al. Dysphagia in inflammatory myopathy: clinical characteristics, treatment strategies, and outcome in 62 patients. Mayo Clin Proc 2007;82(4):441–7.
29. Schrey A, Airas L, Jokela M, et al. Botulinum toxin alleviates dysphagia of patients with inclusion body myositis. J Neurol Sci 2017;380:142–7.
30. Alexanderson H. Exercise in myositis. Curr Treatm Opt Rheumatol 2018;4(4): 289–98.
31. Johnson LG, Collier KE, Edwards DJ, et al. Improvement in aerobic capacity after an exercise program in sporadic inclusion body myositis. J Clin Neuromuscul Dis 2009;10(4):178–84.
32. Fredi M, Cavazzana I, Franceschini F. The clinico-serological spectrum of overlap myositis. Curr Opin Rheumatol 2018;30(6):637–43.
33. Zhang YM, Yang HB, Shi JL, et al. The prevalence and clinical significance of anti-PUF60 antibodies in patients with idiopathic inflammatory myopathy. Clin Rheumatol 2018;37(6):1573–80.
34. Yoshida T, Yoshida M, Mitsuyo K, et al. Dropped head syndrome and the presence of rimmed vacuoles in a muscle biopsy in scleroderma-polymyositis overlap syndrome associated with anti-ku antibody. Intern Med 2018;57(6):887–91.
35. De Lorenzo R, Pinal-Fernandez I, Huang W, et al. Muscular and extramuscular clinical features of patients with anti-PM/Scl autoantibodies. Neurology 2018; 90(23):e2068–76.
36. Chanson JB, Lannes B, Echaniz-Laguna A. Is deltoid muscle biopsy useful in isolated camptocormia? A prospective study. Eur J Neurol 2016;23(6):1086–92.
37. Hoogendijk JE, Amato AA, Lecky BR, et al. 119th ENMC international workshop: trial design in adult idiopathic inflammatory myopathies, with the exception of inclusion body myositis, 10-12 October 2003, Naarden, The Netherlands. Neuromuscul Disord 2004;14:337–45.
38. Miller T, Al-Lozi MT, Lopate G, et al. Myopathy with antibodies to the signal recognition particle: clinical and pathological features. J Neurol Neurosurg Psychiatry 2002;73(4):420–8.

39. Mammen AL, Chung T, Christopher-Stine L, et al. Autoantibodies against 3-hydroxy-3-methylglutaryl-coenzyme A reductase in patients with statin-associated autoimmune myopathy. Arthritis Rheum 2011;63(3):713–21.
40. Kao AH, Lacomis D, Lucas M, et al. Anti-signal recognition particle autoantibody in patients with and patients without idiopathic inflammatory myopathy. Arthritis Rheum 2004;50(1):209–15.
41. Watanabe Y, Uruha A, Suzuki S, et al. Clinical features and prognosis in anti-SRP and anti-HMGCR necrotising myopathy. J Neurol Neurosurg Psychiatry 2016;87(10):1038–44.
42. Allenbach Y, Keraen J, Bouvier AM, et al. High risk of cancer in autoimmune necrotizing myopathies: usefulness of myositis specific antibody. Brain 2016;139(Pt 8):2131–5.
43. Tiniakou E, Pinal-Fernandez I, Lloyd TE, et al. More severe disease and slower recovery in younger patients with anti-3-hydroxy-3-methylglutaryl-coenzyme A reductase-associated autoimmune myopathy. Rheumatology (Oxford) 2017;56(5):787–94.
44. Kadoya M, Hida A, Hashimoto Maeda M, et al. Cancer association as a risk factor for anti-HMGCR antibody-positive myopathy. Neurol Neuroimmunol Neuroinflamm 2016;3(6):e290.
45. Allenbach Y, Mammen AL, Benveniste O, et al. 224th ENMC International Workshop:: Clinico-sero-pathological classification of immune-mediated necrotizing myopathies Zandvoort, The Netherlands, 14-16 October 2016. Neuromuscul Disord 2018;28(1):87–99.
46. Allenbach Y, Arouche-Delaperche L, Preusse C, et al. Necrosis in anti-SRP(+) and anti-HMGCR(+)myopathies: Role of autoantibodies and complement. Neurology 2018;90(6):e507–17.
47. Connors GR, Christopher-Stine L, Oddis CV, et al. Interstitial lung disease associated with the idiopathic inflammatory myopathies: what progress has been made in the past 35 years? Chest 2010;138(6):1464–74.
48. Gallay L, Gayed C, Hervier B. Antisynthetase syndrome pathogenesis: knowledge and uncertainties. Curr Opin Rheumatol 2018;30(6):664–73.
49. Witt LJ, Curran JJ, Strek ME. The diagnosis and treatment of antisynthetase syndrome. Clin Pulm Med 2016;23(5):218–26.
50. Noguchi E, Uruha A, Suzuki S, et al. Skeletal muscle involvement in antisynthetase syndrome. JAMA Neurol 2017;74(8):992–9.
51. Solomon J, Swigris JJ, Brown KK. Myositis-related interstitial lung disease and antisynthetase syndrome. J Bras Pneumol 2011;37(1):100–9.

Case Studies in Management of Muscle Cramps

Hans D. Katzberg, MD, MSc, FRCPC

KEYWORDS

• Muscle cramps • Spasms • Charley horse • Hyperexcitability • Contraction

KEY POINTS

- Muscle cramps are a common symptom that can occur in disease and physiologic states and merits investigations if frequent, severe, and disabling.
- Muscle cramps can occur more commonly in advanced age as well as during pregnancy and during exercise, particularly if associated with dehydration.
- Medical conditions associated with muscle cramps include diabetes, renal dysfunction, and hemodialysis, and neuromuscular conditions associated with cramps include peripheral neuropathy, amyotrophic lateral sclerosis, and metabolic myopathies.
- Peripheral nerve hyperexcitability syndromes include cramp-fasciculation syndrome and immune conditions associated with neuromyotonia and elevated potassium channel antibodies, such as Isaac syndrome and Morvan syndrome.
- There are limited methods of cramp assessment and limited treatment options for muscle cramps, but recent studies have suggested that mexiletine can be effective in patients with muscle cramps.

Video content accompanies this article at http://www.neurologic.theclinics.com.

INTRODUCTION

Muscle cramps are a common symptom encountered by a variety of clinicians, and because cramps can be associated with a variety of neurologic and medical conditions, neurologists often play a major role in the assessment and management of this symptom when it becomes a problem for patients. Muscle cramps are characterized as being acutely painful, have an explosive onset and visible, palpable contraction in a muscle or muscle group, and can have persistent muscle soreness and swelling with a variable rate of improvement, often terminated by stretching.[1] Appropriate management of muscle cramps includes accurate recognition of this phenomenon by the clinician and distinguishing it from other hyperexcitable motor phenomena

Toronto General Hospital / University Health Network, Krembil Brain Institute, University of Toronto, 200 Elizabeth Street, 5ES-306, Toronto, Ontario M6S 4E6, Canada
E-mail address: hans.katzberg@utoronto.ca

Neurol Clin 38 (2020) 679–696
https://doi.org/10.1016/j.ncl.2020.03.011

either through clinical assessment or other methods such as electrophysiologic tests.[2] The clinician should also recognize when cramps warrant simply clinical monitoring and reassurance, screening tests for common medical and neurologic conditions, or more advance investigations for rare and potentially serious syndromes. Similarly, it is important to recognize that not all muscle cramps require treatment and when they do, a rational approach that includes nonpharmacologic in addition to careful prescribing of the limited treatment options available for muscle cramps is required.[3,4] Although muscle cramps can often coexist with neuropathic pain experienced by many patients, treatments are often distinct and need to be treated independently. The following 6 cases aim to illustrate the aforementioned concepts in the management of muscle cramps from the perspective of the clinician.

CASE 1

Clinical Description

A 46-year-old woman has previously experienced occasional muscle cramps throughout her life, but has recently been experiencing calf cramps consistently at the end of long runs, which she is doing every 2 days while training for a half marathon (21 km), during which she sweats profusely. Other cramps are still infrequent, occurring in the calves at bedtime, once every 3 months and brief in duration. General medical and neurologic examination is normal.

Diagnostic Investigations

Screening laboratory work includes complete blood count, creatinine kinase, extended electrolytes, renal function assessed by creatinine, urinalysis, vitamin B12, B6, and D levels, blood sugar tests including 2-h oral glucose tolerance test, hemoglobin A_{1c}, serum protein electrophoresis, and thyroid-stimulating hormone, which are normal. Nerve conduction and electromyography is normal without evidence of neurogenic or myopathic abnormalities.

Treatment and Diagnosis

The patient is reassured that the baseline infrequent muscle cramps are not due to a significant medical or neurologic condition, and this is further confirmed by the normal examination, screening labs and electrophysiology. Counseling is given on B-complex vitamin supplementation and stretching of the calves before bed to minimize occurrence of infrequent cramps. Excessive salt loss through sweating is thought to be the reason for the exercise-induced cramps, and salt tablets and aggressive hydration during races helps to minimize these cramps and allow participation in races without limitation.

Multiple-Choice Question 1

A neurogenic muscle cramp has which characteristic signature on needle electromyography?

a. Spontaneous 3- to 10-Hz discharge potentials
b. Spontaneous 50- to 150-Hz discharge potentials
c. Voluntary 10-Hz discharge potentials
d. Electrical silence on needle electromyography

Discussion

Muscle cramps as a symptom are ubiquitous throughout the lifespan, starting usually after age 8 and increasing in prevalence with advancing age.[5–7] Cramps that occur in otherwise healthy persons are usually brief, infrequent, short in duration, and seldom disabling, as in this case.[8] The pathophysiology of neurogenic muscle cramps has numerous peripheral and central targets implicated[9–15] (**Fig. 1**). In the case that a muscle cramp is captured with needle electromyography, the characteristic spontaneous high-frequency 50- to 150-Hz continuous discharge (**Fig. 2**) can distinguish it from other hyperexcitable muscle phenomena (**Table 1**).[8] These conditions include myotonia, myokymia, and neuromyotonia, which have characteristic electromyography patterns and characterized with delayed relaxation or electrical discharges occurring at various frequencies and intervals. In cases where concerning neurologic symptoms or signs including weakness, reflex changes, and sensory disturbance are present, advanced, directed serology and imaging are required; otherwise, simple screening laboratory tests for common and reversible medical conditions, as performed in this case, are recommended.[16] Although many nonpharmacologic treatments have been attempted to help prevent muscle cramps, there is a paucity of high-level evidence proving that any of these efforts help to reduce muscle cramps.[17] Among these many suggestions, there does seem to be modest evidence that stretching before bed and B-complex vitamins can help reduce the frequency of idiopathic or benign muscle cramps.[17–19]

During certain periods of physiologic stress, muscle cramps can become more frequent and bothersome. One common reason for this is strenuous or prolonged exercise, particularly in a deconditioned muscle, which is particularly worsened in the setting of sweating or excessive heat, as in this case, or situations including dehydration or malnutrition (**Table 2**).[20] Adequate treatment would be a gradual buildup of endurance training to optimize muscle conditioning and ensuring adequate

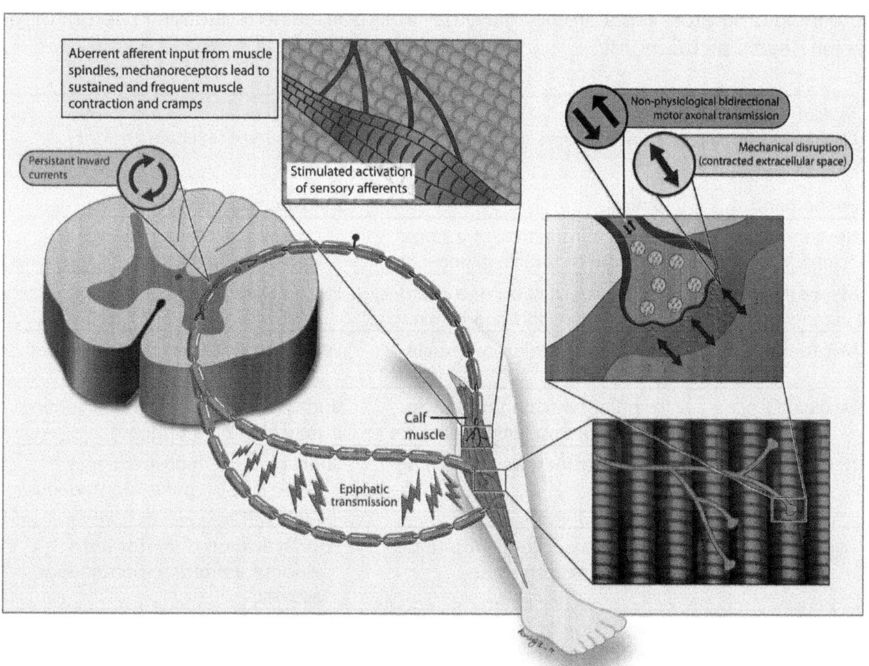

Fig. 1. Pathophysiology underlying neurogenic muscle cramps.

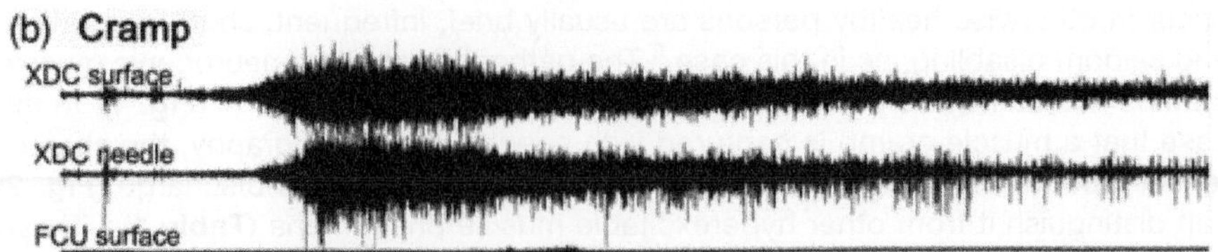

Fig. 2. High-frequency continuous cramp discharge seen on needle and surface electromyography. (*From* Veltkamp R et al. Progressive nonatrophic arm weakness and tonic spasm: isolated manifestation of multifocal motor neuropathy in the brachial plexus. *Muscle Nerve* 2003, 28:242–245; with permission.)

replacement of electrolytes (eg, through salt tablets or other concentrated electrolyte solutions) during prolonged exercise.[21]

CASE 2

Clinical Description

A 32-year-old woman who is 6 months pregnant has noticed that she has developed cramps that have progressively increased in frequency, occurring every day and keeping her up at night, interfering with sleep. She does not want to use any agent that might be harmful in pregnancy, and would like to understand why she has more cramps now and what she might do to prevent them. General neurologic examination is normal.

Diagnostic Investigations

Screening laboratory tests are normal other than borderline reduction in serum magnesium levels at 1.6 mg/dL.

Table 1
Clinical and electrographic features of muscle cramps and other hyperexcitable motor phenomena

Phenomena	Clinical	Electromyography
Neurogenic muscle cramps	Painful contraction of a single muscle or muscle group	Spontaneous, 50- to 150-Hz electrical discharges
Myopathic muscle cramps	Painful contraction of a muscles, usually precipitated by exercise	Electrically silent
Myotonia	Delayed relaxation of muscle	Waxing and waning "dive-bomber" spontaneous discharges
Myokymia	Irregular twitching of muscle giving a rippling appearance	Bursts of electrical activity ("soldiers marching on a bridge")
Neuromyotonia	Muscle stiffness and twitching	Short bursts of high-frequency (>150 Hz), irregular spontaneous discharges
Hypertonia	Stiffness associated with upper motor neuron signs	Poor activation of motor units without abnormal spontaneous activity
Dystonia	Contraction of agonist and antagonist muscles	Continuous firing of motor units in agonist and antagonist muscles
Stiff limb syndrome	Painful, sudden muscle spasms triggered by sudden stimuli	Continuous low-frequency firing in agonist and antagonist muscles

Table 2
Comparison between the development of the electrolyte depletion and dehydration hypothesis, and the neuromuscular hypothesis

Electrolyte Depletion and Dehydration Hypothesis	Neuromuscular Hypothesis
Massive sweating unbalanced by an appropriate reintroduction of liquids	Repetitive exercises in unfavourable environment
↑ osmolarity of the extracellular fluid	Muscle fatigue
Migration of the interstitial fluid toward the extracellular space	↑ afferent excitatory drive; ↓ afferent inhibitory drive
↑ pressure on specific nerve pathways due to a loss of interstitial volume	↑ α motoneuron activity
Altered excitability	↑ muscle cell activity
Muscle cramp	*Muscle cramp*

Adapted from Giuriato G, et al. Muscle cramps: A comparison of the two-leading hypothesis. 2018 Aug; 41:89-95; with permission.

Treatment and Diagnosis

The patient is diagnosed with pregnancy-related muscle cramps, and magnesium citrate 5 mmol in the morning and 10 mmol in the evening is prescribed, which has a significant impact on muscle cramps, nearly resolving them. Cramps completely resolve after the pregnancy and magnesium supplements are discontinued.

Multiple-Choice Question 2

Which of the following statements about magnesium supplementation for muscle cramps is true?

a. Magnesium supplements can help patients with pregnancy-related cramps and idiopathic cramps
b. Magnesium supplements have only been proved to work in pregnancy-related cramps
c. Intramuscular and serum magnesium levels are often equivalent
d. Magnesium citrate, glycinate, and lactate have been tested in trials for muscle cramps

Discussion

Muscle cramps are a common symptom in pregnancy. One theory underlying responsible pathogenesis thought to be low intramuscular magnesium levels not reflected on serum magnesium levels. Magnesium replacement in the setting of pregnancy, even in the setting of normal serum magnesium levels, have thus been tested and have produced modest evidence for benefit in contrast to other supplements including calcium and sodium supplementation. The primary study showing this was performed by Dahle and colleagues,[22] who evaluated 73 patients 22 to 36 weeks pregnant, comparing magnesium citrate or lactate dosed at 5 mmol in the morning and 10 mmol in the evening versus placebo. A significantly higher proportion of patients taking the magnesium supplements at 3 weeks was either cramp free or considerably improved compared with placebo. Although magnesium supplementation has been shown to be helpful in the setting of pregnancy-related cramps, there is no such evidence that this treatment is helpful outside the setting of pregnancy.[23]

CASE 3

Clinical Description

A 19-year-old woman presents with a history of muscle cramps that occur bilaterally in the lower extremities involving the thighs, hamstrings, and calves during periods of high-intensity exercise after 5 minutes of running and other sports. Symptoms have been occurring consistently over the past 10 years since she was a child, and she now feels weakness of the proximal lower extremities and has had multiple episodes of dark-colored urine. Physical examination reveals fixed hip and shoulder girdle weakness graded at 4+/5, without changes in reflexes and normal sensory examination. There is no family history of neuromuscular disorder.

Diagnostic Investigations

Nerve conduction studies are normal but needle electromyography shows occasional short-duration, low-amplitude polyphasic motor unit action potentials (MUAP) with early (myopathic) recruitment from the deltoid, tensor fascia latae, vastus lateralis, and paraspinal muscles. Creatinine kinase (CK) is elevated at 980 U/L. Forearm exercise testing shows low (<2-fold) lactate peak (lactate is expected to be elevated after ischemia or repetitive exercise) as well as exaggerated 10-fold increase (>2.5 fold is considered abnormal) ammonia peak, with elevated ammonia-to-lactate ratio. Muscle biopsy is performed and shows absence of myophosphorylase activity, and increased glycogen in vacuoles one hematoxylin-eosin and periodic acid-Schiff staining as well as electron microscopy, which shows non-membrane-bound glycogen in subsarcolemmal and intermyofibrillar regions. Genetic testing reveals homozygous p.R50X mutations in the PYGM gene.

Diagnosis and Treatment

Needle electromyography and elevated CK indicates a myopathic process, and the abnormal forearm exercise test and muscle biopsy are suggestive of a glycogen storage disorder (GSD), specifically GSD type V or McArdle disease. The patient is informed of the diagnosis and counseled on the signs of rhabdomyolysis, advised to avoid prolonged isometric contractions or strenuous exercise, and instead encouraged to work with a trainer to gradually build exercise capacity and fitness to raise the threshold for triggering myalgia and cramps, as well as to use adequate hydration during exercise with ample rest (>48 hours) between periods of exercise.

Multiple-Choice Question 3

Which of the following metabolic myopathies is less often associated with myogenic muscle cramps?

a. McArdle disease
b. Carnitine palmitoyl transferase 2 (CPT2) deficiency
c. Myoclonic epilepsy with ragged red fibers
d. Phosphofructokinase deficiency

Discussion

In contrast to more random and paroxysmal presentations characteristic of neurogenic muscle cramps discussed throughout most of this review, this case reflects myogenic muscle cramps. Myogenic muscle cramps are mostly present in cases of metabolic muscle disease, whereby disrupted energy production in myocytes occur in McArdle disease and other disorders of glycogen metabolism such as phosphorylase kinase B deficiency, phosphofructokinase deficiency, and phosphoglycerate kinase and mutase deficiency (**Fig. 3**). In addition, fatty acid oxidation disorders including carnitine deficiency and CPT2 deficiency are also associated with muscle cramps but with symptoms arising after more prolonged exercise.[24] Muscle relaxation is an active process that requires ATP, such that in the state of ATP deficiency muscle fibers remain in the contracted state and actin and myosin chains cannot disengage, which in turn results in electrically silent muscle cramp (ie, contracture). The underlying enzymatic defect may result in accumulation of metabolites, which can further aggravate the ATP-deficient state. Over time fixed weakness can occur, and diagnosis relies on measurement of elevated CK levels, myopathic pattern on electromyography, abnormal forearm exercise tests, findings consistent with metabolic myopathy on muscle biopsy, and abnormal genetic testing. This case is an example of GSD type V or McArdle disease, an autosomal recessive condition caused by mutations in the PYGM gene that lead to myophosphorylase enzyme deficiency and abnormal accumulation of glycogen in myocytes (**Fig. 4**).[25] This condition manifests most commonly during sustained isometric contraction or repetitive high-intensity activity with occasional occurrence of a "second-wind" phenomenon whereby exercise intolerance is temporarily alleviated if intensity is lowered after initiation of the exercise. Symptoms include exercise intolerance, episodes of rhabdomyolysis, and elevated CK and myogenic hyperuricemia as well as weakness later in the disease course, as in this case.[26] Treatment is supportive, encouraging avoidance of strenuous or unconditioned activity and ensuring adequate hydration to avoid discomfort from muscle cramps and complications from muscle breakdown and myoglobulinuria.

CASE 4

Clinical Description

A 51-year-old obese patient with type 2 diabetes and chronic renal failure on hemodialysis and treated with metformin, atorvastatin, and hydrochlorothiazide has experienced burning, numbness, and tingling in the feet for 5 years. Over the past year the patient has also been experiencing cramps in the feet and calves, and most recently hands and biceps, and has noticed that cramps are particularly prominent during hemodialysis. Examination shows glove-and-stocking pattern reduction in light touch, pinprick, and vibration in the extremities, 4/5 weakness in the foot intrinsic and distal leg muscles, hyporeflexia at the knees, and unobtainable ankle jerks.

Diagnostic Investigations

Nerve conduction studies show an axonal sensorimotor polyneuropathy, and needle electromyography detects occasional fibrillations and neurogenic recruitment in a length-dependent pattern in the intrinsic foot muscles and distal legs. Screening laboratory tests reveal increased hemoglobin A_{1c} at 12% and elevated creatinine consistent with end-stage renal disease.

Diagnosis and Treatment

The patient is diagnosed with multifactorial causes contributing to muscle cramps, including diabetes, neuropathy, end-stage renal dysfunction, and hemodialysis-associated cramps as well as medication-related cramps from statins and diuretics. To manage the cramps, the nephrology team adjusts the dialysate used during hemodialysis while the medical team switches the statin to an alternative cholesterol-lowering agent (atorvastatin to ezetimibe) and antihypertensive (hydrochlorothiazide to ramipril), leading to a significant improvement in muscle cramps.

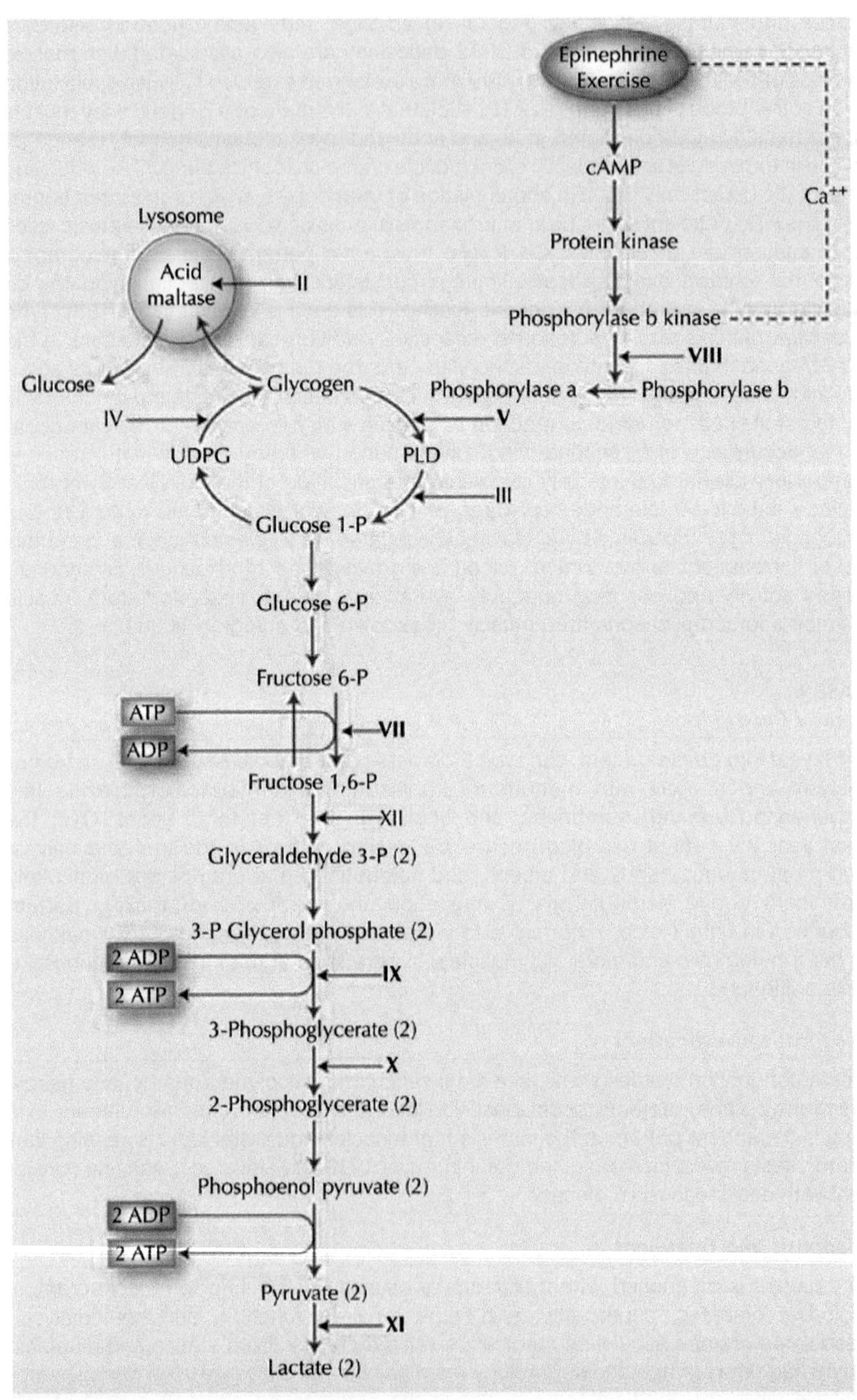
Epinephrine
Exercise
cAMP
Ca++
Protein kinase
Phosphorylase b kinase
VIII
Phosphorylase a
Phosphorylase b
Lysosome
Acid maltase
II
Glucose
Glycogen
IV
V
UDPG
PLD
III
Glucose 1-P
Glucose 6-P
Fructose 6-P
ATP
ADP
VII
Fructose 1,6-P
XII
Glyceraldehyde 3-P (2)
3-P Glycerol phosphate (2)
2 ADP
2 ATP
IX
3-Phosphoglycerate (2)
X
2-Phosphoglycerate (2)
Phosphoenol pyruvate (2)
2 ADP
2 ATP
Pyruvate (2)
XI
Lactate (2)

Fig. 3. Glycogen metabolism and glycolysis. Roman numerals denote muscle glycogenoses caused by defects in the following enzymes: II, acid maltase; III, debrancher; IV, brancher; V, myophosphorylase; VII, phosphofructokinase; VIII, phosphorylase b kinase; IX, phosphoglycerate kinase; X, phosphoglycerate mutase; XI, lactate dehydrogenase; XII, aldolase. Bold numerals designate glycogenoses associated with exercise intolerance, cramps, and myoglobinuria. Nonbold numerals correspond to glycogenoses causing weakness. ADP, adenosine diphosphate; ATP, adenosine triphosphate; cAMP, cyclic adenosine monophosphate; PLD, phospholipase D; UDPG, uridine diphosphoglucose. (*Adapted from* Hirano, M. Metabolic myopathies. In: Gilman, S., editor. Neurobiology of Disease. San Diego, CA. Elsevier Academic Press; 2007. p. 947-956; with permission.)

Multiple-Choice Question 4

Which of the following is the most relevant independent risk factor for development of muscle cramps in patients with diabetes?

a. Nephropathy
b. Hemoglobin A_{1c} level

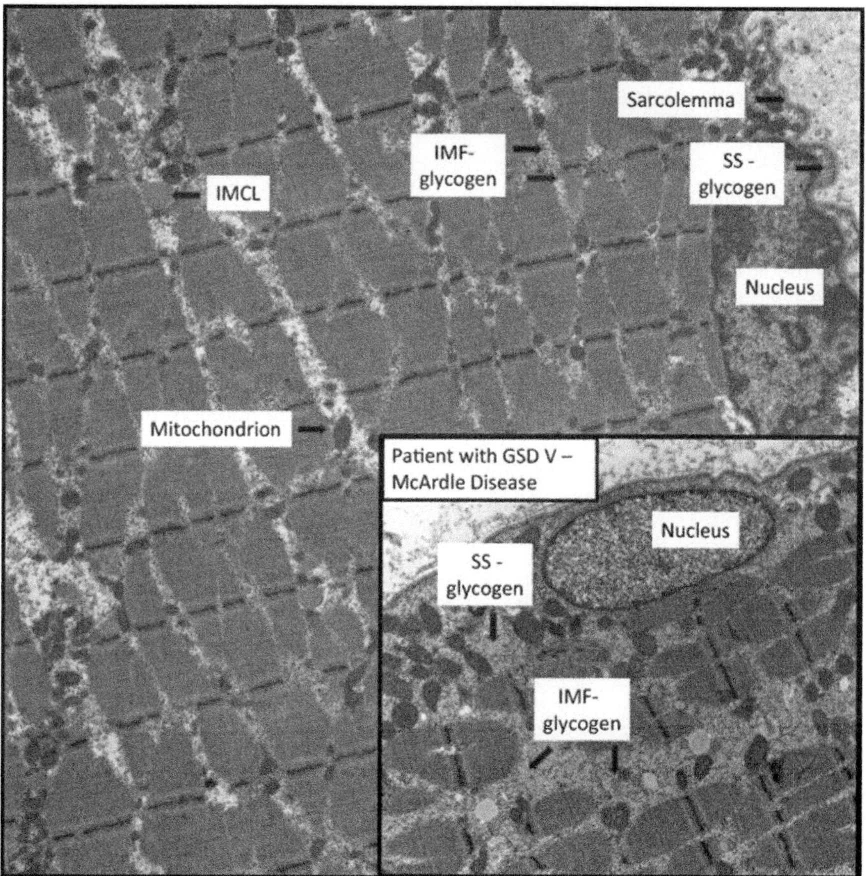

Fig. 4. Electron microscopy of human skeletal muscle. IMCL, intramyocellular lipid; IMG, intermyofibrillar; SS, subsarcolemmal. (*Adapted from* Tarnopolsky MA. Myopathies Related to Glycogen Metabolism Disorders. Neurotherapeutics (2018) 15:915–927; with permission.)

c. Neuropathy
d. Vascular insufficiency

Discussion

In this case, several medical and neurologic conditions could be contributing to muscle cramps.[26,27] **Table 3** includes a list of common physiologic, medical, and neurologic causes of muscle cramps. Patients with diabetes not only have a higher prevalence of muscle cramps than healthy volunteers but suffer more frequent, prolonged, severe, and disabling cramps, which are most common in distal lower extremities but can also present in a non-length-dependent pattern including involvement of the upper extremities.[28] In the setting of diabetes, muscle cramps can occur without the presence of concurrent medical conditions, presumably because of metabolic derangement and nephropathy; however, the most relevant independent risk factor for development of cramps is neuropathy. Patients with advanced renal failure who are on hemodialysis are particularly prone to muscle cramps as part of the dialysis disequilibrium syndrome, whereby changes in dialysate parameters and flow rates can mitigate development of cramps and other symptoms including hypotension, dizziness, and light-headedness.[29] The most common medications associated with muscle cramps include thiazide diuretics and statin medications as in this case, with cramps also reported in patients taking β-agonists, acetylcholinesterase inhibitors (often used for treatment of myasthenia gravis), certain immunosuppressants, and psychotropic medications.[30–32]

CASE 5

Clinical Description

A 49-year-old man, previously healthy other than remote right knee injury and surgery, on no medications and with normal screening laboratory tests, has had worsening diffuse twitching and muscle cramps in the back, torso, arms, and legs as well as cramps in the gluteal muscles, calves, shoulders, and back (bilateral calf twitching is demonstrated in Video 1). No clinical weakness is identified throughout the serial evaluations over 1 year; however, there is progression in muscle stiffness and cramps, which have started to impede mobility and functioning. In addition, the patient has

Table 3
Causes of muscle cramps

Physiologic	Neuromuscular disorders
• Idiopathic	• Amyotrophic lateral sclerosis
• Exercise-induced	• Charcot-Marie-Tooth
• Pregnancy	• Radiculopathy
• Nocturnal leg cramps of the elderly	• Acquired neuropathy
• Dehydration	• Cramp-fasciculation syndrome
Metabolic	• Isaac syndrome (neuromyotonia)
• Cirrhosis	• Metabolic myopathies (McArdle)
• Uremia/hemodialysis	Other neurologic conditions
• Hypothyroidism	• Parkinson disease
• Malnutrition (vitamin B, vitamin D, magnesium deficiency)	• Dystonia
Medications	• Multiple sclerosis
• Diuretics	• Stroke
• Statins	
• β-Agonists	

started to complain of constipation, postural dizziness, erectile dysfunction, and hyperhidrosis.

Diagnostic Investigations

Repeat clinical assessments and electromyography over a period of 24 months show fasciculations but no fibrillations, changes in recruitment, or MUAP morphologic changes. Given the normal screening laboratory tests, additional laboratory tests are ordered including antinuclear antibody, rheumatoid factor, erythrocyte sedimentation rate, C-reactive protein, serum anti-SSA (Sjögren syndrome–related antigen A), anti-SSB, antinuclear cytoplasmic antibodies, glutamic acid decarboxylase antibodies, and anti-GM1 antibodies, which are all normal. On most recent assessment, electromyography has shown myokymia, and slow repetitive nerve stimulation at 1 Hz in the ulnar hand muscles shows prominent cramp afterdischarges (**Fig. 5**) and neuromyotonia (**Fig. 6**). Serum and cerebrospinal fluid is sent for analysis and shows markedly elevated contactin-associated protein (CASPR) potassium channel antibodies.

Diagnosis and Treatment

Elevated potassium channel antibodies in the context of peripheral nerve hyperexcitability seen on electromyography along with coexisting autonomic dysfunction is suggestive of Isaac syndrome. Symptomatic treatment with carbamazepine, 200 mg 3 times daily, is prescribed and helps reduce the muscle cramps but not completely, while the autonomic dysfunction persists. Plasmapheresis and additional chronic immunotherapy including prednisone and steroid-sparing medication with azathioprine is started and helps to further control all the symptoms.

Multiple-Choice Question 5

Which of the following features are more commonly associated with Morvan syndrome versus Isaac syndrome?

a. Hyperhidrosis
b. Autonomic dysfunction

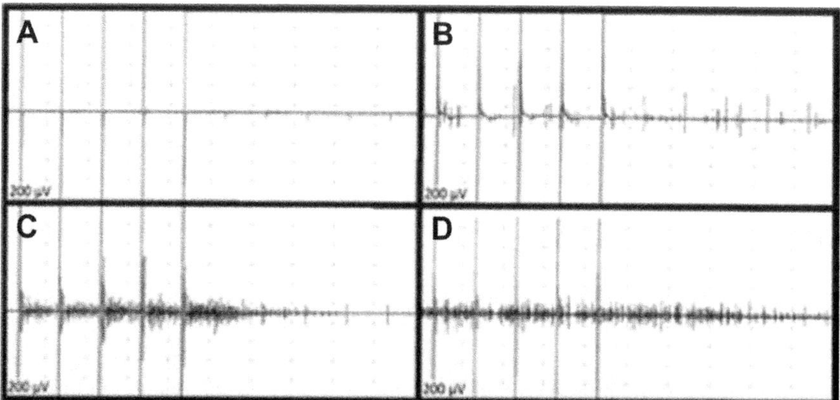

Fig. 5. Cramp potentials and afterdischarges in response to slow repetitive nerve stimulation. (*A–C*) Increasing levels of after-cramp discharges. (*D*) Continuous cramp potential in response to 1-Hz repetitive nerve stimulation of the tibial nerve and recording from the abductor hallicus.

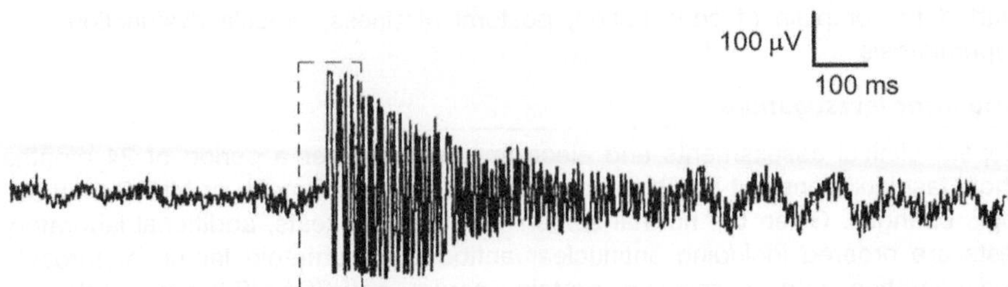

Fig. 6. Neuromyotonic discharge. Note the decrementing response. The top is recorded with a long sweep speed of 100 ms/division while the inset is at a regular sweep speed of 10 ms/division. Note the very high-frequency (150–250 Hz) repetitive discharge of a single motor unit. (*From* Preston DC, Shapiro BE. (2013). Electromyography and neuro- muscular disorders, third edn. London: Elsevier/Saunders, with permission.)

c. Neuromyotonia
d. Encephalopathy

Discussion

Nerve conduction studies and electromyography tests are critical here to confirm peripheral nerve hyperexcitability as evidenced by myokymia, neuromyotonia, fasciculations, and afterdischarges on slow repetitive nerve stimulation and absence of weakness or additional denervating changes.[33,34] Another syndrome to consider in this case early in the process and on the benign end of the peripheral nerve hyperexcitability spectrum is cramp-fasciculation syndrome.[35] In this more common condition, cramp potentials and fasciculations can be observed but electromyographic changes such as myokymia and neuromyotonia are not usually seen. When neuromyotonia, a >150-Hz high-frequency, irregular abnormal discharge, is seen on electromyography and is accompanied by hyperhidrosis and other signs of autonomic dysfunction as in this case, Isaac syndrome, an immune condition associated with with elevations in CASPR2 and LGI1 potassium channel antibodies in the serum and cerebrospinal fluid, should be considered.[36] Peripheral nerve hyperexcitability syndromes, whether benign or associated with active immune dysfunction, are often responsive to antiepileptic medications including carbamazepine, which have sodium channel–blocking properties. If this syndrome is additionally accompanied by central neurologic dysfunction such as agitation, memory loss, encephalopathy, and sleep disturbance, the term Morvan syndrome is used. **Table 4** delineates the characteristic clinical findings in cramp-fasciculation syndrome, Isaac syndrome, and Morvan syndrome. In Morvan and Isaac syndromes, immunotherapy including intravenous immunoglobulin, plasmapheresis, steroids, and steroid-sparing agents are often used with the goal of immunosuppression or immunomodulation, which can lead to an improvement in symptoms.

CASE 6

Clinical Description

A 63-year-old man presents with right leg muscle cramps in the calf, hamstring, and gluteal muscles along with progressive, painless weakness of these muscles leading to buckling of the right leg and falls over the past 4 months. Examination shows multimyotomal weakness and fasciculations in the right leg and right arm and leg hyperreflexia, upgoing toes, and normal sensory examination.

Table 4
Clinical characteristics distinguishing cramp-fasciculation syndrome, Isaac syndrome, Morvan syndrome

Characteristic Clinical Findings in Patients with Acquired Peripheral Nerve Hyperexcitability Syndromes			
	Cramp-Fasciculation Syndrome	**Isaacs Syndrome**	**Morvan Syndrome**
Muscle stiffness	+	++	++
Muscle twitching	++	++	++
Muscle cramps	++	++	++
Fasciculation potentials	++	+	+
Myokymic discharges	-	++	++
Neuromyotonic discharges	-	++	+++
Autonomic features	-	++	++
Agitation	-	-	++
Memory loss	-	-	+
Insomnia	-	-	+
VGKC-complex antibodies	+/–	+	+

Adapted from Katirji B. Peripheral nerve hyperexcitability. Handbook Clin Neurol 2019;161:281-290; with permission.

Diagnostic Investigations

Screening laboratory tests are normal and MRI of the brain and whole spine does not show significant intra-axial or compressive disorder to explain the clinical findings. Nerve conduction studies are normal without evidence of amplitude reduction, conduction slowing, or block on motor nerve testing, and sensory responses are normal. Needle electromyography shows prominent fibrillations, positive sharp waves, and complex fasciculations along with reduced recruitment and polyphasia from all right leg muscles tested in the proximal and distal L2-S1 myotomes, most prominently from the L5 and S1 innervated muscles. The left leg shows similar active denervation and reinnervation from the L5 and S1 myotomes, the right arm shows active and chronic C8/T1 denervation in the right arm, and the lumbar and thoracic paraspinals also show fibrillations and fasciculations.

Diagnosis and Treatment

Normal imaging, serology, and nerve conduction studies in the context of lower motor neuron changes at the cervical, thoracic, and bilateral lumbar levels along with upper motor neuron changes at the cervical and bilateral lumbar levels is suggestive of amyotrophic lateral sclerosis/motor neuron disease (ALS/MND). As part of the symptomatic management, mexiletine, 100 mg 3 times daily, for 2 weeks causes a reduction in muscle cramps by 25% with improvement in the pain and discomfort associated with muscle cramps. An increase to 200 mg thrice daily after 4 weeks leads to a 75% reduction in frequency of muscle cramps and further improvement in severity of these symptoms.

Multiple-Choice Question 6

Which of the following is true about muscle cramps in ALS?

a. Muscle cramps are present more often early in the course of the disease and lessen as weakness progresses
b. Muscle cramps are present more commonly later in the course of the disease after weakness is prominent
c. Pharmacologic agents including gabapentin and calcium-channel blockers have good evidence for efficacy in patients with ALS
d. Quinine has an excellent safety profile when used in the treatment of muscle cramps

Discussion

In contrast to case 5, this case is characterized by weakness and signs of denervation in addition to the cramps and fasciculations seen clinically and on needle electromyography in a pattern and course characteristic of ALS/MND. In ALS/MND, cramps can be a prominent early symptom that can cause significant disability, and although these cramps can persist throughout the entire course of the disease they can become less frequent and severe as the disease progresses, particularly in muscles that have undergone complete denervation.[37]

There are limited options for the the treatment of muscle cramps associated with aggressive and relentless damage to motor neurons. In addition to the nonpharmacologic options mentioned earlier, medications that have been tried but have shown either limited or lack of success include calcium-channel blockers and gabapentin.[38,39] Other treatment options that do show some evidence for efficacy in patients with muscle cramps are outlined in **Table 5**.[8] Quinine sulfate has been used since the 1920s for the treatment of muscle cramps because of its effects on stabilizing sodium-channel conduction, as demonstrated by 2 class I studies showing efficacy in improving muscle cramps, albeit with significant safety concerns.[40–42] In addition to more common symptoms of problems hearing

Table 5
Prescription medications for muscle cramps

Medication	Dose	Adverse Events
Quinine sulfate[a]	300 mg qhs	Cinchonism, thrombocytopenia, TTP, palpitations, nausea, blurry vision, bitter taste
Mexiletine[b]	Up to 300 mg tid	Nausea, vomiting, dizziness, tremor, palpitation, arrhythmia
Diltiazem	30 mg daily	Edema, headache, nausea, dizziness, rash, asthenia, arrhythmia
Leveteracitam[b]	Up to 1500 mg bid	Fatigue, headache, insomnia, arthralgia, edema
Carbamazepine[c]	Up to 1600 mg daily	Confusion, dizziness, nausea, rash, SIADH, hyponatremia
Phenytoin	300 mg daily	Confusion, dizziness, nausea, rash
Baclofen	Up to 50 mg daily	Confusion, dizziness, nausea, flaccid weakness, ataxia, withdrawal

Abbreviations: bid, twice per day; qhs, every bedtime; SIADH, syndrome of inappropriate antidiuretic hormone secretion; tid, three times per day; TTP, thrombotic thrombocytopenia purpura.

[a] Food and Drug Administration warning against use for treatment of muscle cramps in the United States.

[b] Studied in amyotrophic lateral sclerosis.

[c] Studied in cramp-fasciculation syndrome.

(cinchonism), bitter taste, and abnormal visual disturbances, more serious adverse effects including thrombocytopenia, thrombotic thrombocytopenia purpura, and arrhythmia have been reported with quinine, particularly at doses over and above the usual 300 mg every bedtime, which is the most commonly studied.[43] Given this safety concern, a Food and Drug Administration advisory was posted against use of quinine sulfate for the treatment of muscle cramps in 2006.[44] Since then other medications with a similar mechanism of action but better safety profiles have been studied, including 2 recent studies evaluating mexiletine for the treatment of muscle cramps in patients with ALS. Although there was no disease-modifying effect, mexiletine at doses of 300 to 900 mg per day was shown in these studies to be effective in reducing the frequency and severity of muscle cramps, with favorable safety profiles. The most common adverse events with mexiletine were dizziness and nausea, most prominent at the higher doses (highest with doses of 900 mg/day).

As newer agents are tried for the treatment of muscle cramps, it is imperative to have reliable and validated tools to evaluate the severity of the symptoms. In trials to date this has most commonly been cramp frequency, and a recent scale in ALS has been proposed, which also incorporates cramp location, severity, and cramp precipitants in addition to cramp frequency.[45] A recent patient-reported, qualitative study analyzing cramp impact in patients with cramps of multiple causes confirms these cramp characteristics in addition to effects of cramps on daytime functioning and sleep. Mental health may be another important component in measuring and capturing the entire cramp experience.[46]

SUMMARY

Adequate recognition of muscle cramps as a common and potentially disabling symptom in patients across the spectrum of healthy and disease states is vital for all clinicians and especially important for neurologists who have the expertise to evaluate and treat the various medical and neurologic conditions encountered. Much of this assessment can be done through a thorough history, general medical and neurologic examination, and screening laboratory tests; however, on occasion imaging, electrophysiology including nerve conductions and electromyography, and additional advanced testing is required to identify the cause of the muscle cramps. Although many circumstances in which cramps occur are benign and do not need treatment, there are general nonpharmacologic recommendations that can be provided to help abort cramps when they occur and prevent the development of cramps. When these approaches are not helpful, prescription-level medications, which may include antispasmodic medications, antiepileptics, and sodium-channel blockers, are used, with careful attention paid to potentially bothersome and serious side effects. There is currently a need for the development of novel, targeted, and safe treatment options for muscle cramps as well as a need for validated clinical and paraclinical scales and biomarkers, which could further aid clinicians and patients in the follow-up assessment of muscle cramps as well as in clinical trials studying this common and important symptom.

DISCLOSURE

The author disclose that some of this work was supported by a New Initiatives grant from the Division of Neurology at the University of Toronto.

SUPPLEMENTARY DATA

Supplementary data to this article can be found online at https://doi.org/10.1016/j.ncl.2020.03.011.

REFERENCES

1. Layzer RB. The origin of muscle fasciculations and cramps. Muscle Nerve 1994;17:1243–9.
2. Jansen PH, Gabreëls FJ, van Engelen BG. Diagnosis and differential diagnosis of muscle cramps: a clinical approach. J Clin Neuromuscul Dis 2002;4(2):89–94.
3. Jansen PH, Joosten EM, Vingerhoets HM. Muscle cramp: main theories as to etiology. Eur Arch Psychiatry Neurol Sci 1990;239(5):337–42.
4. Miller TM, Layzer RB. Muscle cramps. Muscle Nerve 2005;32:431–42.
5. Leung AK, Wong BE, Chan PY, et al. Nocturnal leg cramps in children: incidence and clinical characteristics. JAMA 1999;91(6):329–32.
6. Abdulla AJ, Jones PW, Pearce VR. Leg cramps in the elderly: prevalence, drug and disease associations. Int J Clin Pract 1999;53:494–6.
7. Butler JV, Mulkerrin EC, O'Keeffe ST. Nocturnal leg cramps in older people. Postgrad Med J 2002;78:596–8.
8. Katzberg HD. Neurogenic muscle cramps. J Neurol 2015;262(8):1814–21.
9. Matzner O, Devor M. Hyperexcitability at sites of nerve injury depends on voltage-sensitive Na channels. J Neurophysiol 1994;72:349–59.
10. Mense S. Group III and IV receptors in skeletal muscle: are they specific or polymodal? Prog Brain Res 1996;110:125–35.
11. Baldissera F, Cavallari P, Dworzak F. Motor neuron 'bistability'. A pathogenetic mechanism for cramps and myokymia. Brain 1994;117(5):929–39.
12. Graven-Nielsen T, Mense S. The peripheral apparatus of muscle pain: evidence from animal and human studies. Clin J Pain 2001;17:2–10.
13. Obi T, Mizoguchi K, Matsuoka H, et al. Muscle cramp as the result of impaired GABA function—an electrophysiological and pharmacological observation. Muscle Nerve 1993;16(11):1228–31.
14. Jentsch TJ, Stein V, Weinreich F, et al. Molecular structure and physiological function of chloride channels. Physiol Rev 2002;82:503–68.
15. Conte Camerino D, Tricarico D, Pierno S, et al. Taurine and skeletal muscle disorders. Neurochem Res 2004;29:135–42.
16. Sawlani K, Katirji B. Peripheral nerve hyperexcitability syndromes. Continuum (Minneap Minn) 2017;23(5):1437–50.
17. Katzberg HD, Khan AH, So YT. Assessment: symptomatic treatment for muscle cramps (an evidence-based review): Report of the therapeutics and technology assessment subcommittee of the American Academy of Neurology. Neurology 2010;74(8):691–6.
18. Chan P, Huang TY, Chen YJ, et al. Randomized, double-blind, placebo-controlled study of the safety and efficacy of vitamin B complex in the treatment of nocturnal leg cramps in elderly patients with hypertension. J Clin Pharmacol 1998;38:1151–4.
19. Coppin RJ, Wicke DM, Little PS. Managing nocturnal leg cramps: calf-stretching exercises and cessation of quinine treatment: a factorial randomised controlled trial. Br J Gen Pract 2005;55:186–91.
20. Eichner ER. Muscle cramping in the heat. Curr Sports Med Rep 2018;17(11):356–7.

21. Getzin AR, Milner C, Harkins M. Fueling the triathlete: evidence-based practical advice for athletes of all levels. Nutr Ergogenic Aids 2018;16(4):240–6.
22. Dahle LO, Berg G, Hammar M, et al. The effect of oral magnesium substitution on pregnancy induced leg cramps. Am J Obstet Gynecol 1995;173:175–80.
23. Maor NR, Alperin M, Shturman E, et al. Effect of magnesium oxide supplementation on nocturnal leg cramps a randomized clinical trial. JAMA Intern Med 2017;177(5):617–23.
24. Kishnani PS, Chen YT. V glycogen storage disease. In: Kliegman RM, Stanton BF, St Geme J, et al, editors. Nelson textbook of pediatrics. 19th edition. Philadelphia: Elsevier; 2011. p. 492–501.
25. Tarnopolsky MA. Myopathies related to glycogen metabolism disorders. Neurotherapeutics 2018;15:915–27.
26. Amato A, Russell JA. Neuromuscular disorders. New York: McGraw Hill; 2008.
27. Weiner IH, Weiner HL. Nocturnal leg muscle cramps. JAMA 1990;150:511–8.
28. Katzberg H, Kokokyi S, Halpern E, et al. Prevalence of muscle cramps in patients with diabetes. Diabetes Care 2014;37(1):17–8.
29. Arieff AI. Dialysis disequilibrium syndrome: current concepts on pathogenesis and prevention. Kidney Int 1994;45:629–35.
30. Kanaan N, Sawaya R. Nocturnal leg cramps. Clinically mysterious and painful-but manageable. Geriatrics 2001;56(6):39–42.
31. Naylor JR, Young JB. A general population survey of rest cramps. Age Ageing 1994;23:418–20.
32. Garrison SR, Dormuth CR, Morrow RL, et al. Nocturnal leg cramps and prescription use that precedes them: a sequence symmetry analysis. Arch Intern Med 2012;172:120–6.
33. Harrison TB, Benatar M. Accuracy of repetitive nerve stimulation for diagnosis of the cramp-fasciculation syndrome. Muscle Nerve 2007;35:776–80.
34. Minetto MA, Holobar A, Botter A, et al. Discharge properties of motor units of the abductor hallucis muscle during cramp contractions. J Neurophysiol 2009;102:1890–901.
35. Tahmoush AJ, Alonso RJ, Tahmoush GP, et al. Cramp-fasciculation syndrome: a treatable, hyperexcitable peripheral nerve disorder. Neurology 1991;41:1021–4.
36. Shillito P, Molenaar PC, Vincent A, et al. Acquired neuromyotonia: evidence for autoantibodies directed against K? channels of peripheral nerves. Ann Neurol 1995;38:714–22.
37. Ganzini L, Johnston W, Hoffman W. Correlates of suffering in amyotrophic lateral sclerosis. Neurology 1999;52(7):1434–40.
38. Voon WC, Sheu SH. Diltiazem for nocturnal leg cramps. Age Ageing 2001;30:91–2.
39. Miller RG, Moore DH, Gelinas DF, et al. Phase III randomized trial of gabapentin in patients with amyotrophic lateral sclerosis. Neurology 2001;56:843–8.
40. Connolly PS, Shirley EA, Wasson JH, et al. Treatment of nocturnal leg cramps: a crossover trial of quinine vs vitamin E. Arch Intern Med 1992;152:1877–80.
41. Jansen PH, Veenhuizen KC, Wesseling AI, et al. Randomised controlled trial of hydroquinine in muscle cramps. Lancet 1997;349:528–32.
42. Diener HC, Dethlefsen U, Dethlefsen-Gruber S, et al. Efficacy of quinine in treating muscle cramps: a double- blind, placebo-controlled, parallel-group, multicentre trial. Int J Clin Pract 2002;56:243–6.
43. Bateman DN, Dyson EH. Quinine toxicity. Adverse Drug React Acute Poisoning Rev 1986;4:215–33.

44. Food and Drug Administration, Department of Health and Human Services. Drug products containing quinine; enforcement action dates. Fed Reg 2006;71: 75557–60.
45. Mitsumoto H, Chiuzan C, Gilmore M, et al. A novel muscle cramp scale (MCS) in amyotrophic lateral sclerosis. Amyotroph Lateral Scler Frontotemporal Degener 2019;20:328–35.
46. Katzberg HD, Bril V, Riaz S, et al. Qualitative, patient-centered assessment of muscle cramp impact and severity. Can J Neurol Sci 2019;46(6):735–41.

Differential Diagnoses of Inclusion Body Myositis

Vinojini Vivekanandam, MBBS, FRACP[a], Enrico Bugiardini, MD[a], Ashirwad Merve, FRCPath[b], Matthew Parton, MD[c], Jasper M. Morrow, FRACP[a], Michael G. Hanna, FRCP, FMedSci[c], Pedro M. Machado, MD, PhD[a,d,*]

KEYWORDS

• Inclusion body myositis • Muscular dystrophy • Muscle biopsy
• Magnetic resonance imaging • Inflammatory myopathy • Diagnosis

KEY POINTS

- Inclusion body myositis (IBM) is a slowly progressive myopathy with characteristic early involvement of quadriceps and long finger flexors. Less common presentations (eg, dysphagia), however, are important to recognize.
- Clinical assessment complemented by neuromuscular magnetic resonance imaging (MRI) is useful in choosing the optimal muscle to biopsy.
- Clinicopathologic correlation is imperative in interpretation of the muscle biopsy and guiding further staining.
- MRI also can be useful in delineating patterns of muscle involvement to differentiate IBM from other primary muscle conditions, namely inherited myopathies.
- Inflammatory features on muscle biopsy can be seen in the idiopathic inflammatory myopathies (polymyositis, dermatomyositis, IBM, and immune-mediated necrotizing myopathies) and in some inherited muscle conditions, such as facioscapulohumeral muscular dystrophy, and other genetic muscular dystrophies, in particular dysferlinopathies.

[a] Department of Neuromuscular Diseases, Queen Square Centre for Neuromuscular Diseases, University College London, 1st Floor, Russell Square House, 10-12 Russell Square, London WC1B 5EH, UK; [b] Department of Neuropathology, UCL Institute of Neurology, 1st Floor, Queen Square House, 22 Queen Square, London WC1N 3BG, UK; [c] Department of Neuromuscular Diseases, Queen Square Centre for Neuromuscular Diseases, University College London, Ground Floor, 8-11 Queen Square, London WC1N3BG, UK; [d] Division of Medicine, Centre for Rheumatology, University College London, 1st Floor, Russell Square House, 10-12 Russell Square, London WC1B 5EH, UK

* Corresponding author. Department of Neuromuscular Diseases, Queen Square Centre for Neuromuscular Diseases, University College London, 1st Floor, Russell Square House 10-12 Russell Square, London WC1B 5EH, UK.
E-mail address: p.machado@ucl.ac.uk

Neurol Clin 38 (2020) 697–710
https://doi.org/10.1016/j.ncl.2020.03.014

neurologic.theclinics.com

INTRODUCTION

The term, *inclusion body myositis* (*IBM*), was first coined in 1971. A subsequent case series 8 years later described the characteristic early pattern of weakness involving the quadriceps and long finger flexors.[1] Understanding of the condition has since improved substantially.

IBM has an estimated prevalence of 139 per million in the population above the age of 50 and an overall estimated prevalence of 46 per million.[2] Although it typically is thought of as affecting those over age 50, approximately 20% develop symptoms in their 40s.[3] There is a male predominance. Whites are more affected, although the exact racial differences are not clear, because studies tend to cluster in the same geographic areas.

Although IBM is slowly progressive, there currently is no effective treatment and the resultant disability can be significant. Estimated health care costs are significant and several comorbidities, including hypertension, hyperlipidemia, and ischemic heart disease, have been associated with IBM.[4] Using a bayesian survival model for IBM, an increased risk of premature death compared with the general population of the same age and gender recently has been suggested for IBM.[5]

Together with increased use of MRI, muscle biopsies, and natural history studies, understanding of pathogenesis has improved, leading to instigation of treatment trials. Treatment approaches that recently have been tested in IBM include the inhibition of the myostatin pathway with follistatin gene therapy[6] and bimagrumab,[7] and targeting protein dyshomeostasis with arimoclomol[8] and rapamycin.[9] A large randomized, double-blind, placebo-controlled phase 2 clinical trial of arimoclomol for the treatment of IBM currently is under way (NCT02753530).

Prevalence figures are probably underestimates because of the high rate of misdiagnosis. Moreover, there is a 4-year to 6-year delay in diagnosis.[1] Accurate diagnosis is pivotal in providing prognostic information and support in the home as well as accessing clinical trials. Five cases are described that illustrate key diagnostic challenges and important differential diagnoses to consider.

CASE A: A LUMP IN THE THROAT

A 69-year-old gentleman presented with an 8-year history of swallowing difficulty. He previously had had a hemithyroidectomy for follicular adenoma and took amlodipine for hypertension. He lived with his wife on a farm. He was active and maintained his farm.

He first noticed difficulty with dry foods but went on to have difficulty with liquids, needing to gulp them down and swallow several times. He initially was assessed by an ear, nose, and throat surgeon with no cause found and was referred to speech and language therapy. He was able to manage cut-up solid foods but liquidized vegetables, including beans and leeks.

Over time, he had increasing difficulty with solids, taking 2 hours to eat a meal. He unintentionally lost approximately 8 kg over 8 years. He coughed a lot when eating and had 1 chest infection over this period. He remained active on his farm but more recently had noticed some difficulty climbing stairs.

He went on to have investigations, including barium swallow, magnetic resonance imaging (MRI) of the brain and cervical spine, electromyography (EMG), anticholinesterase, and anti-MUSK antibodies, all of which were nondiagnostic. An elevated creatinine kinase (CK) level of 746 IU/L led to referral to a muscle specialist.

Examination at this stage demonstrated normal facial strength with normal eye movements. There was no fatigable ptosis and no tongue wasting or fasciculations. In the upper limb, bulk was normal; however, there was subtle weakness of distal finger flexors. In the lower limbs, quadriceps muscle wasting was noted. Lower limb strength Medical Research Council (MRC) strength testing was normal (5) in all groups. He was unable, however, to stand from a squat. Reflexes, sensory examination, and coordination all were normal.

He went on to have lower limb MRI, which demonstrated fatty infiltration of the anterior thigh compartment typical of IBM. Subsequent left vastus lateralis biopsy demonstrated features supportive of a diagnosis of IBM, including prominent vacuoles, several cytochrome C oxidase (COX)-negative fibers, and major histocompatibility complex (MHC) class I up-regulated protein 62 (p62)-positive fibers.

He went on to have a percutaneous endogastric tube inserted to supplement diet and boost nutrition.

Clinical Questions

What percentage of patients with IBM present with dysphagia?

1. 25% to 50%
2. 11% to 25%
3. 4% to 10%
4. Less than 4%

Answer: 3

What other neuromuscular conditions can present with dysphagia?

1. Myasthenia gravis
2. Motor neuron disease
3. Chronic inflammatory demyelinating polyneuropathy
4. All of the above

Answer: 4

Discussion

Dysphagia is an important feature to recognize as part of IBM. The prevalence of dysphagia varies between cohorts, ranging from 46% to 86%; however, it tends to present later in the disease course.[10–13] A review of patients with IBM seen at the MRC Centre for Neuromuscular Diseases in 2013 found 4 of 51 patients (7.8%) reported symptom onset was with dysphagia.[12] Similarly, 4.4% of patients first presented with swallowing difficulty in a cohort of 140 patients from 2 centers in Paris and Oxford[11] and 9% of 64 patients in a Dutch cohort.[13] Disease onset with dysphagia is rare but important to recognize in order to guide management and prevent aspiration and excessive weight loss.

Patients initially report dysphagia to solid foods followed by increasing difficulty with liquids and secretions.[14] The oropharyngeal weakness responsible for dysphagia also may cause obstructive sleep apnea.[10]

Considering muscle diseases in the differential diagnosis for dysphagia is important. The diagnosis of IBM in particular is important to look for. Identifying symptoms pertaining to characteristic muscle groups affected in IBM may be helpful:

- Difficulty climbing stairs or rising from a low chair or the floor, which may suggest subtle proximal lower limb weakness
- Difficulty with writing and fine motor tasks, in particular, gripping a pen

These features may suggest early weakness in characteristic muscle groups affected in IBM. Clinical examination of these muscles in a patient presenting with dysphagia also is important:

- Long finger flexors (flexor digitorium profundus)
- Knee extension (quadriceps femoris)
- Hip flexion (iliopsoas, rectus femoris, and proximal leg muscles)
    - Knee extension is characteristically weaker than hip flexion.

As in case A, muscle MRI additionally may demonstrate characteristic patterns of involvement, which may be subtle and not clinically obvious.

Differential diagnoses for neuromuscular causes of dysphagia are important to appreciate and are illustrated in **Box 1**.

Management of dysphagia is important for patients with IBM. Assessment and recommendations from a speech and language therapist include swallowing methods, such as the Mendelsohn maneuver, and dietary adjustment. Symptomatic improvement with cricopharyneal myotomy and pharyngoesophageal dilation is reported.[15] In more advanced disease, percutaneous endogastric tube insertion may be required.

CASE B: THIRD TIME LUCKY

A 64-year-old gentleman presented with a 3-year history of difficulty climbing stairs. His medical history is significant for spondylosis and varicose veins. He was retired but continued work as a Scouts Commissioner.

He first noticed difficulty after slipping while walking upstairs. Managing stairs became more difficult, progressing to needing to use a handrail at all times. Getting out of low chairs also became difficult.

Most recently he noticed that he could no longer give the Scout salute at parades. He found that fingers on his right hands seemed to curl in. There were no other cranial nerve or sensory symptoms.

Box 1
Neuromuscular differential diagnosis for dysphagia

Primary muscle disease
- Idiopathic inflammatory myopathies
    - IBM
    - Polymyositis
    - Dermatomyositis
    - Immune-mediated necrotizing myopathies
- Dystrophies
    - Oculopharyngeal muscular dystrophy
    - Myotonic dystrophy
    - Advanced Duchenne muscular dystrophy
    - Advanced FSHD
- Myotonia congenita (rare cause)

Neuromuscular junction disorders
- Myasthenia gravis
- Lambert-Eaton syndrome (rare cause)
- Botulism (rare cause)

Neuropathy
- Guillain-Barré syndrome
- Chronic inflammatory demyelinating polyradiculopathy
- Infectious (eg, diphtheria) (rare cause)

Neuronopathy
- Bulbospinal muscular atrophy (Kennedy disease) (rare cause)
- Motor neuron disease
- Spinal muscular atrophy (adult onset) (rare cause)

EMG was consistent with a myopathy and CK level was 444 IU/L. Investigations for inflammatory or immune causes of a myopathy, however, were not diagnostic. He went on to have a muscle biopsy of the quadriceps, which demonstrated only fibrous tissue. A second biopsy of the left deltoid was performed but did not demonstrate any significant changes. Subsequent referral to a muscle specialist to investigate for other adult-onset myopathies was made.

On examination, cranial nerves were normal. Upper limb examination demonstrated mild weakness of the distal finger flexors. In the legs, there was marked quadriceps wasting and severe knee extension weakness. Reflexes, sensation, and coordination were normal.

Further review of the clinical history did not reveal any additional features, developmental delay, or family history.

Proximal lower limb muscles were severely involved and provided a low yield biopsy. Proximal upper limb muscles were unaffected and also low yield on biopsy. As such, a distal forearm muscle which was mild to moderately affected, was chosen to perform a repeat muscle biopsy.

Histopathology demonstrated features of IBM (**Fig. 1**). The features include myopathic changes, rimmed vacuoles, up-regulation of MHC class I, p62-positive inclusions, several COX-deficient fibers, up-regulation of MHC class I (HLA-ABC), chronic inflammatory cell infiltrate in the endomysium, and several fibers with COX deficiency.

Clinical Questions

What is a differential diagnosis for an adult-onset myopathy?

1. Duchenne muscular dystrophy
2. Spinal muscular atrophy type 1
3. Pompe disease
4. Myotonia congenita

Answer: 3

Which factor is ideal for the choice of muscle to biopsy?

1. An atrophic muscle
2. A clinically weak muscle
3. A clinically strong muscle
4. A muscle normal on MRI

Answer: 2

Do all IBM biopsies have rimmed vacuoles? Which statement is true?

1. 50% of biopsies have rimmed vacuoles.
2. 15% to 20% of biopsies have rimmed vacuoles.
3. 15% to 20% of biopsies do not have rimmed vacuoles.
4. All muscle biopsies in IBM have rimmed vacuoles.

Answer: 3

Discussion

Other causes of myositis, such as dermatomyositis, polymyositis, and immune-mediated necrotizing myopathies, often are associated with a more acute onset and more rapid progression. IBM, however, has a more insidious course. In this case, subtle proximal weakness was present for 3 years. Over the subsequent 3 years to 5 years, a more characteristic pattern became apparent. At initial presentation, however, an

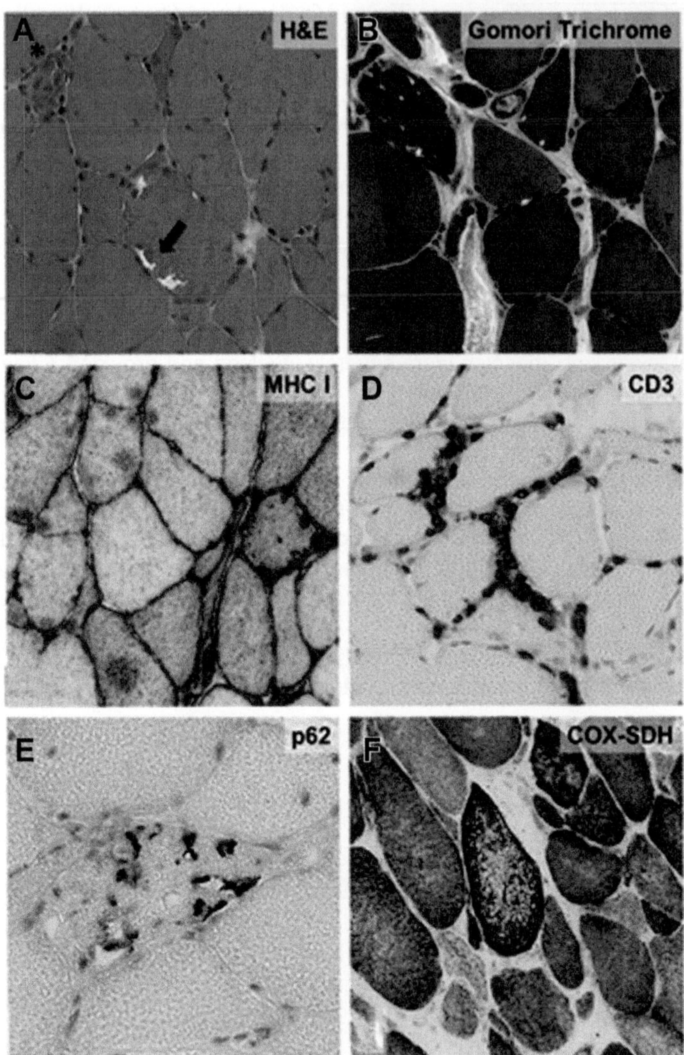

Fig. 1. Histopathologic changes in IBM. (*A*) H&E staining showing myopathic changes, including variation in fiber size, neurogenic atrophy (angular shaped fibers), increase in internal nuclei, and regenerating and necrotic (*asterisk*) fibers, along with fibers with rimmed vacuoles (*arrow*), which are typical for IBM. (*B*) Gomori trichrome stain showing a ragged red fiber (*asterisk*), with same fiber containing rimmed vacuoles. (*C*) MHC class I (HLA-ABC) showing diffuse sarcolemmal up-regulation with internal expression in some fibers, suggestive of an immune inflammatory process. (*D*) Cluster of differentiation 3 (CD3) stain showing T-lymphocyte infiltrate within the endomysium with focal infiltrate in intact fibers (not shown). (*E*) The vacuolated fibers contained globular inclusions typical for IBM highlighted with p62 antibody. (*F*) Mitochondrial abnormality often is seen in IBM, which is represented as COX and succinate dehydrogenase (SDH)-deficient fiber (*blue* [*center*]) on COX-SDH stain (magnifications: [*A*]–[*D*] ×20; [*E*] ×40; and [*F*] ×20).

Table 1
Key differential diagnoses for an adult-onset myopathy

Myopathy	Features
IBM	Classically long finger flexor and quadriceps weakness CK level moderately elevated
FSHD	Classically asymmetric shoulder girdle weakness with relative sparing of the deltoid; prominent scapular winging CK level mildly elevated
Limb girdle muscular dystrophy	Typically, proximal weakness and elevated CK level
Late-onset congenital myopathies	Central core disease Centronuclear myopathy Nemaline myopathy
Myofibrillar myopathy	Proximal weakness; CK level normal or elevated May have cardiac or respiratory involvement
Myotonic dystrophy type 2	Myotonia clinically and on EMG
Pompe disease	Autosomal recessive Acid maltase deficiency Limb girdle weakness; may have diaphragmatic weakness CK level mildly elevated
McArdle disease	Autosomal recessive Shoulder girdle weakness in a subset Exercise-provoked cramp, fatigue, myoglobulinuria, second-wind CK level markedly elevated >1000 at times
Mitochondrial myopathy	Proximal weakness Extraocular weakness, fatigue CK level normal to mildly elevated Can be accompanied by multisystem involvement
Endocrine myopathy	Thyroid myopathy Hyperadrenocorticism in Cushing syndrome. Hyperparathyroidism

adult-onset slowly progressive proximal lower limb weakness has a broad differential (**Table 1**). Adult-onset myopathies may mimic IBM and vice versa.

In addition to clinical characteristics, muscle biopsy has an important role in differentiating between these diagnoses. In this case, the first biopsy of quadriceps was nondiagnostic and showed only fibrous replacement of muscle fibers. A second biopsy of the deltoid was near normal, and only the third biopsy yielded diagnostic features. Carefully selecting an appropriate muscle to biopsy is important in increasing diagnostic yield and preventing repeated procedures. A clinically weak muscle, which is not too severely wasted, is the ideal choice. MRI can be useful in muscle choice. Severely fat infiltrated or atrophic muscle is likely to consist mostly of fibrous or fatty tissue, whereas an unaffected muscle on MRI is likely to be near normal. Anticytosolic 5′-nucleotidase 1A (encoded by NT5C1A) has been identified in IBM but testing still is not universally available, and diagnostic performance (ie, sensitivity and specificity) varies widely in the literature.

The classic histologic features on a muscle biopsy in IBM are shown in **Fig. 1**. On hematoxylin-eosin (H&E) stain, myopathic features, endomysial inflammation, and eosinophilic inclusions can be seen. MHC class I up-regulation and increased number of COX-negative fibers also can be seen. Microscopy may demonstrate tubulofilamets.[16] Characteristic rimmed vacuoles may be seen; however, 15% to 20% of cases may not have rimmed vacuoles.[17] Additional immunohistochemical staining, for example, for dystrophin, calpain-3, or myophosphorylase, is useful in excluding alternative diagnoses. Congophilic material adjacent to the vacuoles is useful and is part of the diagnostic criteria. Clinicopathologic correlation is imperative in guiding this additional staining and interpretation of histology.

CASE C: AN UPHILL BATTLE

A 62-year-old man presented with difficulty climbing stairs. He has a past medical history significant for restrictive lung disease, cataracts, eczema, and rheumatoid arthritis, managed primarily on sulfasalazine. He also has ischemic heart disease and, prior to symptom onset, had been commenced on atorvastatin, 40 mg daily.

He presented with a 3-year history of progressive difficulty in climbing stairs. Most recently, he had to use the handrail and at times took each step at a time. He also noted difficulty raising his arms above his head. He developed difficulty opening jars, doing buttons, and taking his socks off.

At review, it was felt that his rheumatoid arthritis was active. He then was commenced on methotrexate.

On examination, he had normal cranial nerves. Periscapular wasting and bilateral winging was noted as well as more distal upper limb wasting. There was severe proximal weakness, shoulder abduction strength MRC grade 2. Distal weakness was worst at the distal interphalangeal joint, with MRC grade 3. There was marked quadriceps wasting in the lower limbs with knee extension strength reduced to MRC grade 4. Upper limb reflexes and the knee jerks were reduced or absent. Sensation and coordination were normal. The CK level was 700 IU/L.

The clinical picture was thought to be atypical for a statin-related myopathy; however, given the proximity of symptom onset to commencing atorvastatin, it was stopped. Despite this, symptoms continued to worsen.

Given the autoimmune history, myositis was suspected. Myositis-specific antibodies, including anti-hydroxymethylglutaryl coenzyme A reductase antibodies, were negative. A left deltoid muscle biopsy, however, was performed. This muscle was chosen clinically at the time because it was definitely affected by the disease process. The biopsy demonstrated severe atrophy and chronic inflammation.

A subsequent treatment trial with steroids reduced the CK level from a range of 600 IU/L to 900 IU/L to 200 IU/L to 400 IU/L; however, there was no corresponding clinically significant improvement. He went on to have 3 courses of intravenous immunoglobulin (IVIG), again with no objective clinical improvement.

MRI of lower limb muscles demonstrated severe selective quadriceps involvement. Given the lack of treatment response that would be expected in an (inflammatory) myositis, a repeat muscle biopsy was performed of left vastus lateralis, which demonstrated mild inflammation, rimmed vacuoles, COX-negative fibers, eosinophilic inclusions, and p62-positive fibers, supportive of a diagnosis of IBM.

Clinical Questions

Which condition is a differential diagnosis for severe preferential quadriceps wasting?

1. Facioscapulohumeral muscular dystrophy (FSHD)
2. Dystrophinopathy
3. Myotonic dystrophy (MD)

4. Becker muscular dystrophy

Answer: 1

What is the role for IVIG or other immunomodulators in IBM?

1. There is good level I evidence for the use of IVIG and immunosuppressive treatment.
2. There is no evidence for the use of IVIG and immunosuppressive treatment.
3. There is evidence that IVIG is helpful for severe phenotypes.
4. There is evidence that methotrexate is helpful for severe phenotypes.

Answer: 2

Discussion

In this case, the presenting feature was quadriceps involvement, with difficult climbing stairs. The patient went on to develop quadriceps wasting. Quadriceps involvement is seen characteristically in IBM but also can be seen in other muscle conditions, including dystrophinopathies, sarcoglycanopathies, and laminopathies.[18] A femoral neuropathy, lumbosacral plexopathy, or L3-4 radiculopathy should not be forgotten, although these often are unilateral and associated with sensory involvement.

In this case, the coexistence of active autoimmune comorbidities favored the diagnosis of an immune-mediated myositis. There are reports of association of IBM with autoimmune diseases (13%–24%), most commonly Sjögren syndrome (13%–24%).[1] An association with large granular lymphocytic leukemia also has been reported. There are several aspects, however, that reduced the likelihood of an immune-mediated myositis. The onset and progression in this case were more insidious than often are seen in an immune-mediated process. The CK level is not as high as often is seen in immune-mediated myositis, particularly in necrotizing myositis.

Importantly, there was no objective clinical response to treatment with steroids, methotrexate, or IVIG. The evidence to date establishes that IBM is resistant to immunosuppressive treatment.[16] A small retrospective trial demonstrated transient improvement with IVIG only.[19] Clearly defining measures to demonstrate failure to respond to treatment is important. The IBM functional rating scale, 6-minute walk distance test, and timed up and go test alongside manual muscle testing are validated assessments that may be helpful.

CASE D: NOT WHAT IT SEEMS

A 69-year-old gentleman presented with a 5-year history of progressive lower limb weakness. His CK level was 385 IU/L. At initial presentation, lower limb weakness with a subsequent muscle biopsy demonstrating inflammation led to a probable diagnosis of IBM.

The patient was monitored annually. On review in the muscle clinic 10 years later, very slow progression was noted. He noted some additional upper limb involvement.

On examination at this stage, shoulder girdle wasting with weak shoulder abduction and external rotation was seen. There was no scapula winging. Distal upper limb strength, including finger flexors, was strong. There was mild weakness in all lower limb muscle groups, with marked dorsiflexion weakness with foot drop.

This progression and distribution of weakness were thought atypical for IBM, prompting reinvestigation. The initial muscle biopsy was re-reviewed with additional immune stains. These stains demonstrated cytoplasmic immunoreactivity in several fibers with p62 and myotilin and less so for desmin. This pattern of staining suggested a myofibrillary myopathy.

Subsequent genetic testing by direct sequencing of exons 2 to 10 of the myotilin (MYOT) gene revealed a pathogenic heterozygous c.179 C > G (p.Ser60Cys) variant consistent with a diagnosis of myotilin-associated myofibrillar myopathy. Desmin (DES) and FSHD genetic testing were negative.

A diagnosis of myofibrillar myopathy was made, prompting appropriate screening. Cardiac screening revealed a previous silent myocardial infarction.

Clinical Questions

Which of the following features is seen in the typical MRI pattern seen in IBM?

1. Relative sparing of rectus femoris
2. Marked fatty infiltration of rectus femoris
3. Marked fatty infiltration of tibialis anterior
4. Relative sparing of quadratus femoris

Answer: 1

Which muscular dystrophy(ies) can have cardiac or respiratory involvement and should not be missed?

1. Oculopharyngeal muscular dystrophy
2. Duchenne muscular dystrophy
3. Lamin A/C deficiency
4. 2 and 3

Answer: 4

Discussion

This case is particularly important in illustrating the need for clinicopathologic correlation, which prompted additional staining on the muscle biopsy leading to the ultimate diagnosis.

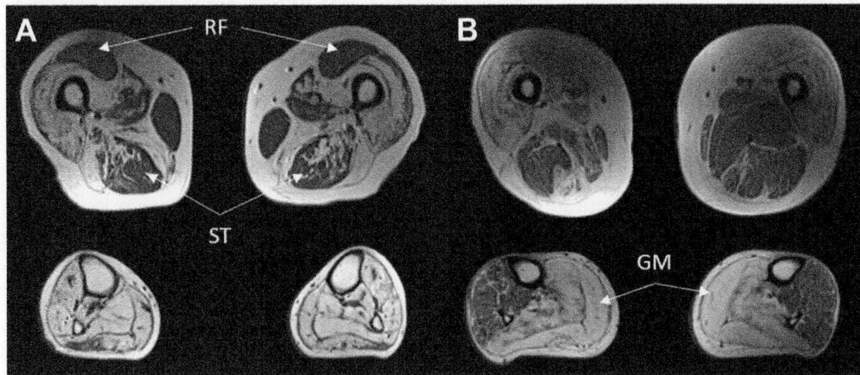

Fig. 2. MRI changes in case D of MYOT p.Ser60Cys mutation (*A*) versus MRI changes found in a case of IBM (*B*). In MYOT-related myopathy, there is a pattern of muscle involvement characterized by posterior compartment involvement (semimembranosus and biceps femoris) in the thigh, with relative sparing of semitendinosus [ST]). In the anterior compartment, vastus intermedius typically is affected, followed by vastus lateralis. Rectus femoris (RF) usually is spared. In IBM, in the thigh, quadriceps typically is affected (sometimes with relative sparing of the rectus femoris, not observed in this figure) whereas the posterior compartment is less frequently involved. In the calf, gastrocnemius medialis (GM) typically is the most severely affected muscle.

Muscle MRI is now more readily available and is a useful tool in diagnosis. Characteristic patterns can be seen in muscle conditions, which then can direct more targeted genetic testing and biopsy staining. The pattern seen in myotilin-associated myofibrillar myopathy is distinct from IBM[20] (**Fig. 2**). In IBM, the typical pattern is fatty replacement, preferentially in the quadriceps femoris, with relative sparing of the rectus femoris and preferential fat accumulation within the medial head of gastrocnemius (in comparison with soleus and lateral gastrocnemius).

Making an accurate diagnosis has important implications in screening for respiratory and cardiac involvement. Myofibrillar myopathies may present with proximal weakness, and some muscle biopsy features can cross over with IBM. Considering this differential and performing appropriate genetic diagnostics are important for accurate diagnosis and subsequent cardiac and respiratory monitoring, as is needed in myofibrillar myopathy. Cardiomyopathy also is seen in Duchenne muscular dystrophy, Emery-Dreifuss muscular dystrophy, lamin A/C deficiency, Becker muscular dystrophy, sarcoglycanopathy, and dystroglycanopathy. Respiratory impairment is seen in lamin AC deficiency, sarcoglycanopathy, and dystroglycanopathy.

CASE E: PURSUING A DIAGNOSIS

A 52-year-old gentleman presented with right knee clicking and giving way. He subsequently underwent right knee arthroscopy. Over the next 2 years, however, skiing became more difficult. He felt the right leg, in particular, was weak.

This progressed slowly and he found that he could no longer run and he had difficulty with tasks, such as climbing stairs, carrying a heavy load, and going downstairs. Getting off the floor from lying was increasingly difficult. The slow progression and distribution of weakness made the diagnosis of IBM likely.

EMG was nondiagnostic and muscle biopsy was arranged. Biopsy of right vastus lateralis demonstrated myopathic features with some inflammatory components, including MHC class I up-regulation, all seen in IBM. No vacuolation or eosinophilic inclusions, however, were seen. Additionally, prominent lobulated and ring fibers, although nonspecific, suggested genetic myopathies, including myotonic dystrophy type 2 (DM2).

Additional tests, including a CK level of 356 IU/L, and slow progression continued to remain consistent with probable IBM. Given some atypical muscle biopsy changes, however, genetic testing was pursued. Testing for the CNBP expansion mutation seen in DM2 was negative.

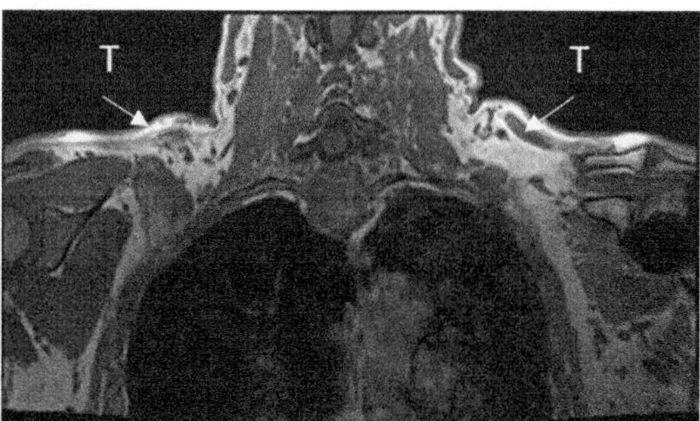

Fig. 3. Upper limb MRI in FSHD. Upper limb girdle MRI showed asymmetric muscle atrophy and fatty infiltration of right trapezius (T) and left serratus anterior.

An MRI of the limbs was performed, which demonstrated asymmetric thigh involvement with fat replacement. Clinically, the upper limbs were normal with no evidence of wasting; however, upper limb MRI demonstrated reduced bulk and fatty signal in the right trapezius and left serratus anterior (**Fig. 3**). This pattern of muscle involvement on MRI and marked asymmetry prompted investigation for FSHD.

FSHD genetic testing returned positive, with a partial deletion of the D4Z4 4q35 repeat region with a 31-kb fragment demonstrated (pathogenic <39 kb). Given the patient's mild/atypical clinical phenotype, second-line FSHD testing was requested, namely permissive haplotype analysis. Further genetic testing using the 4qA probe revealed that the 31-kb fragment was associated with the 4qA haplotype in this patient.

Clinical Questions

Which diagnosis also can demonstrate inflammatory features on muscle biopsy?

1. FSHD
2. Myotonia congenita
3. Spinal muscular atrophy
4. Motor neuron disease

Answer: 1

Discussion

Myopathic muscle biopsies with inflammatory features can be seen in several conditions beyond classic myositis (idiopathic inflammatory myopathies). It is important to consider other myopathies when faced with a biopsy with inflammatory cells. Up to a third of muscle biopsies in FSHD can have an inflammatory infiltrate.[17] The infiltrate is composed of $CD4^+$ and $CD8^+$ lymphocytes; however, invasion of intact muscle fibers rarely is seen. In dysferlinopathies, up to a third can have an inflammatory infiltrate, predominantly of T cells and macrophages. A small number of calpainopathies can have an eosinophilic infiltrate.

In this case, the clinical picture was informative, and reviewing the phenotype over the disease course was helpful. The upper limb involvement demonstrated on MRI and marked lower limb asymmetry prompted investigation for conditions that more classically demonstrate this pattern of muscle involvement. In this case, again neuromuscular MRI was useful in detecting patterns of involvement.

SUMMARY

This article describes 3 cases with atypical or challenging aspects in diagnosing IBM as well as 2 cases of inherited myopathies that may mimic IBM. Atypical presentations, such as dysphagia, may prompt investigation for alternative etiologies; however, IBM also should be considered in the differential diagnosis. Specifically examining and imaging other characteristically affected muscle groups may aid diagnosis.

The presence of inflammation on muscle biopsy is an important aspect to discuss. Inflammatory features are seen in conditions beyond dermatomyositis, polymyositis, and immune-mediated necrotizing myopathy. Similar inflammatory features can be seen in IBM and also FSHD, which should be considered in the differential diagnosis. Clinicopathologic correlation in multidisciplinary meetings are helpful in interpreting biopsy changes in clinical context and guiding further biopsy staining. Treatment resistance to immunosuppression should additionally prompt investigation for IBM.

MRI can be an extremely helpful tool in accurate diagnosis. As illustrated, specific patterns can be seen in IBM compared with other inherited myopathies. MRI also is useful in selection of muscle to biopsy.

Clinical characteristics, appropriate muscle biopsy with clinically guided staining, and neuromuscular MRI patterns in combination are likely to improve diagnostic rates in IBM and its mimics.

ACKNOWLEDGMENTS

P.M. Machado is supported by the National Institute for Health Research (NIHR), University College London Hospitals (UCLH), and Biomedical Research Centre (BRC). The views expressed are those of the authors and not necessarily those of the UK National Health Service, the NIHR, or the UK Department of Health.

DISCLOSURE

P.M. Machado has received consulting/speaker's fees from Abbvie, BMS, Celgene, Eli Lilly, Janssen, MSD, Novartis, Pfizer, Roche, and UCB.

REFERENCES

1. Greenberg SA. Inclusion body myositis: clinical features and pathogenesis. Nat Rev Rheumatol 2019;15(5):257–72.
2. Callan A, Capkun G, Vasanthaprasad V, et al. A systematic review and meta-analysis of prevalence studies of sporadic inclusion body myositis. J Neuromuscul Dis 2017;4(2):127–37.
3. Badrising UA, Maat-Schieman MLC, Van Houwelingen JC, et al. Inclusion body myositis: clinical features and clinical course of the disease in 64 patients. J Neurol 2005;252(12):1448–54.
4. Keshishian A, Greenberg SA, Agashivala N, et al. Health care costs and comorbidities for patients with inclusion body myositis. Curr Med Res Opin 2018;34(9): 1679–85.
5. Capkun G, Schmidt J, Ghosh S, et al. Development and validation of a Bayesian survival model for inclusion body myositis. Theor Biol Med Model 2019; 16(1):1–10.
6. Mendell JR, Sahenk Z, Al-Zaidy S, et al. Follistatin gene therapy for sporadic inclusion body myositis improves functional outcomes. Mol Ther 2017;25(4):870–9.
7. Hanna MG, Badrising UA, Benveniste O, et al. Safety and efficacy of intravenous bimagrumab in inclusion body myositis (RESILIENT): a randomised, double-blind, placebo-controlled phase 2b trial. Lancet Neurol 2019;18(9):834–44.
8. Ahmed M, MacHado PM, Miller A, et al. Targeting protein homeostasis in sporadic inclusion body myositis. Sci Transl Med 2016;8(331):28–31.
9. Benveniste O, Hogrel J-Y, Annoussamy M, et al. Rapamycin Vs. Placebo for the treatment of inclusion body myositis: improvement of the 6 min walking distance, a functional scale, the FVC and muscle quantitative MRI [abstract]. ACR/ARHP Annu Meet. 2017:11–2. Available at: http://www.myositis.org/storage/documents/IBM_Published_Research/Rapamycin_Vs_Placebo_for_the_Treatment_of_Inclusion_Body_Myositis_ACR_abstract_2017.pdf. Accessed February 10, 2020.

10. Langdon PC, Mulcahy K, Shepherd KL, et al. Pharyngeal dysphagia in inflammatory muscle diseases resulting from impaired suprahyoid musculature. Dysphagia 2012;27(3):408–17.
11. Benveniste O, Guiguet M, Freebody J, et al. Long-term observational study of sporadic inclusion body myositis. Brain 2011;134(11):3176–84.
12. Cortese A, Machado P, Morrow J, et al. Longitudinal observational study of sporadic inclusion body myositis: Implications for clinical trials. Neuromuscul Disord 2013;23(5):404–12.
13. Cox FM, Titulaer MJ, Sont JK, et al. A 12-year follow-up in sporadic inclusion body myositis: An end stage with major disabilities. Brain 2011;134(11):3167–75.
14. Mulcahy KP, Langdon PC, Mastaglia F. Dysphagia in inflammatory myopathy: self-report, incidence, and prevalence. Dysphagia 2012;27(1):64–9.
15. Oh TH, Brumfield KA, Hoskin TL, et al. Dysphagia in inclusion body myositis. Am J Phys Med Rehabil 2008;87(11):883–9.
16. Machado P, Brady S, Hanna MG. Update in inclusion body myositis. Curr Opin Rheumatol 2013;25(6):763–71.
17. Michelle EH, Mammen AL. Myositis mimics. Curr Rheumatol Rep 2015; 17(10):1–8.
18. Mercuri E, Muntoni F. Muscular dystrophies. Lancet 2013;381(9869):845–60.
19. Dobloug C, Walle-Hansen R, Gran JT, et al. Long-term follow-up of sporadic inclusion body myositis treated with intravenous immunoglobulin: a retrospective study of 16 patients. Clin Exp Rheumatol 2012;30(6):838–42.
20. Bugiardini E, Morrow JM, Shah S, et al. The diagnostic value of MRI pattern recognition in distal myopathies. Front Neurol 2018;9(JUN):1–11.

Immune-Mediated Neuropathies

Kelly G. Gwathmey, MD*, A. Gordon Smith, MD

KEYWORDS

- Guillain-Barré syndrome • CIDP • Miller-Fisher syndrome
- Multifocal motor neuropathy • Vasculitic neuropathy • Sensory neuronopathy
- Nodo-paranodopathy • Autoimmune neuropathy

KEY POINTS

- The differential diagnosis of immune-mediated neuropathies is broad. Recognition of specific clinical patterns focuses the differential diagnosis.
- Electrodiagnostic testing plays a pivotal and sometimes confirmatory diagnostic role.
- Our understanding of the autoimmune demyelinating neuropathies is rapidly evolving with the identification of nodal and paranodal antibodies in some cases.
- Many immune-mediated neuropathies overlap with systemic autoimmune disorders and connective tissue diseases.
- Prompt recognition of immune-mediated neuropathies is mandatory. Delays in identification and treatment may result in permanent disability.

Video content accompanies this article at http://www.neurologic.theclinics.com.

CASE 1. A NEW YEAR'S EVE TO REMEMBER

A 65-year-old librarian with a past medical history of hypertension developed conjunctivitis with ocular erythema and discharge 1 week before New Year's eve. These symptoms resolved with antibiotic eye drops. On New Year's eve, she developed bilateral hand clumsiness resulting in difficulty typing. Within 1 day, her gait deteriorated significantly. She was admitted to a community hospital where she developed progressive dyspnea requiring intubation. Cerebrospinal fluid (CSF) protein, glucose, leukocyte counts, Gram stain, and culture were normal. She was given 1.5 g/kg of intravenous immune globulins (IVIg) divided over 3 days for presumed Guillain-Barré syndrome (GBS) before transfer to a tertiary care hospital. After transfer, an MRI of the spine with and without gadolinium demonstrated nerve root enhancement and enlargement (**Fig. 1**).

Department of Neurology, Virginia Commonwealth University, 1101 East Marshall Street, PO Box 980599, Richmond, VA 23298-0599, USA
* Corresponding author.
E-mail address: Kelly.Gwathmey@vcuhealth.org

Neurol Clin 38 (2020) 711–735
https://doi.org/10.1016/j.ncl.2020.03.008

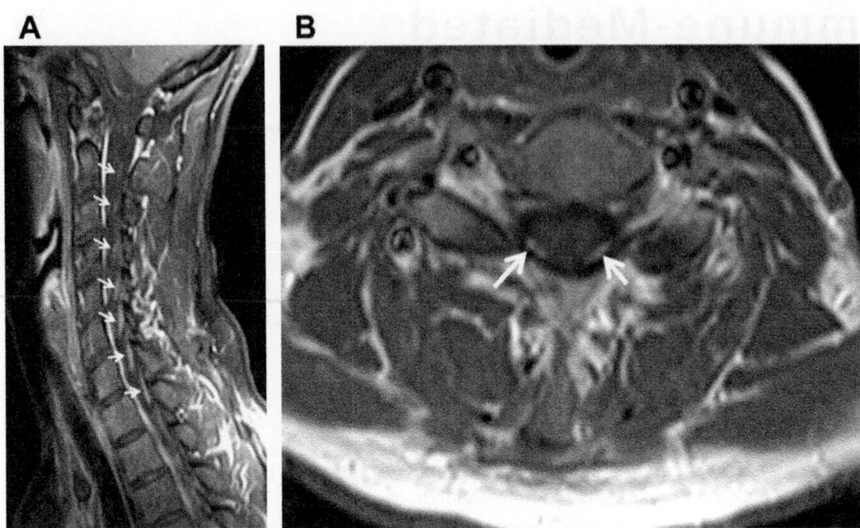

Fig. 1. (*A*) Postcontrast T1 sagittal MRI and (*B*) postcontrast T1 axial MRI demonstrating contrast enhancement and enlargement of the nerve roots (*arrows*).

Nerve conduction studies revealed absent F responses. Although this can be an isolated finding in early GBS, it could also be explained by the sedation given in the intensive care unit and the patient's asleep state.[1]

Clinical Questions

Most aspects of this patient's history and presentation are consistent with GBS. What feature is *atypical* for GBS?

1. Upper respiratory and gastrointestinal infections typically precede GBS rather than conjunctivitis.
2. The normal CSF protein level (ie, lack of cytoalbuminologic dissociation).
3. Her rapid decline resulting in respiratory failure.

In general, which of the following diagnostic studies argues *against* a diagnosis of GBS?

1. Cytoalbuminologic dissociation on CSF analysis
2. Enlarged, enhancing nerve roots on MRI studies of the spine
3. Positive CSF cytology
4. Prolonged or absent F waves and H reflexes on electrodiagnostic studies

All the following are appropriate next steps in management *except*:

1. Admission to the intensive care unit for monitoring and respiratory support
2. Close monitoring for development of dysautonomia
3. Administration of an additional 0.5 g/kg of IVIg
4. Initiation of plasma exchange

Discussion

- GBS is an autoimmune, acute-onset demyelinating polyradiculoneuropathy.
- GBS typically follows either a gastrointestinal or respiratory infection by 10 to 14 days.

- The most commonly associated preceding infection is *Campylobacter jejuni*. Other common pathogens include *Mycoplasma pneumoniae*, Epstein-Barr virus, hepatitis E virus, cytomegalovirus, enterovirus, and influenza A.[2–5]
- In recent years Zika virus, a flavivirus with large outbreaks in Asia, South America, and Central America, has been associated with an increased incidence of GBS.[6]
- In 1976, there was a greater incidence of GBS associated with the swine flu vaccine. Additionally, there was a slightly increased risk after the 2009 H1N1 influenza vaccine. Given that influenza infection portends a higher risk of GBS than the vaccination, vaccination continues to be recommended.[7]

Clinical Presentation

- GBS presents with rapidly progressive proximal and distal weakness with areflexia or hyporeflexia, which reaches nadir within 4 weeks. Most patients report neuropathic pain in their lower back and legs.
- Other common examination findings include:
  - Cranial nerve involvement occurs in one-half of patients (usually facial weakness).[8]
  - Respiratory impairment necessitating intubation and ventilation occurs in one-third of patients.[8]
  - Autonomic involvement, including tachycardia, bradycardia, fluctuating blood pressure, urinary retention, and gastric dysmotility, is common, particularly in patients with severe weakness.

Diagnostic Approach

- A clinical diagnosis of GBS is supported by CSF cytoalbuminologic dissociation (elevated protein and with a normal cell count). The CSF protein is normal, such as in our patient, in one-half in the first week and elevated in up to 88% at 2 weeks after symptom onset.[9,10] Pleocytosis (elevated white blood cell count) raises the question of a malignant or infectious process (human immunodeficiency virus, Lyme, cytomegalovirus) or sarcoidosis.
- The electrodiagnostic hallmarks of an acquired demyelinating neuropathy may take days or even weeks to develop. Prolonged and absent H reflexes and F waves are often the earliest feature, along with the pattern of a normal sural sensory amplitude with reduced median sensory amplitude ("sural sparing"). With time, other electrodiagnostic features of primary demyelination become apparent including partial motor conduction block, temporal dispersion, and nonuniform slowing of motor conduction velocities.
- MRI of the spine may demonstrate hypertrophic, contrast-enhancing nerve roots. When anterior spinal roots are solely involved, GBS should strongly be considered.[11] Ultrasound examination may demonstrate enlargement of nerve roots and peripheral nerves.[12]

Treatment

- Respiratory function must be monitored closely with frequent measurement of forced vital capacity and maximal expiratory and inspiratory pressures.
- Autonomic function should also be closely monitored with particular vigilance for cardiac arrhythmias, urinary retention, and constipation.
- The 2 first-line treatments for GBS, IVIg and plasma exchange are equally efficacious.[13–15] Either should be started immediately in patients with clinically defined GBS, even in the setting of normal electrodiagnostic studies and CSF analysis.
  - The standard dosing for IVIg is 2 g/kg divided over 2 to 5 days.

- Alternatively, 4 to 6 plasma exchanges on alternate days may be used. Caution must be used with plasma exchange owing to the risk of hypotension in someone with autonomic dysfunction. The usefulness of either is not proven after 2 months of onset if there is a lack of improvement.
- Physical therapy, occupational therapy, and neurorehabilitation are imperative.
- Patients should be queried regarding neuropathic pain, and appropriate therapy instituted.

> Treatment-related fluctuations occur in about 10% of patients within the first 2 months.[16] It is recommended to treat the patient with IVIg or plasma exchange, whichever treatment they responded to initially. Clinical deterioration beyond the first 2 months should raise the possibility of acute-onset chronic inflammatory demyelinating polyradiculoneuropathy (CIDP).

CASE 2. A MAN WITH DOUBLE VISION AND GAIT IMBALANCE

A 47-year-old man with a history of juvenile rheumatoid arthritis presented to the emergency department with a 1-week of blurry vision, intermittent diplopia, and gait instability. He had a sinus infection treated with antibiotics 1 week before the onset of neurologic symptoms. He denied any dysarthria, dysphagia, dyspnea, or generalized weakness. He reported patchy sensory changes that were resolving. On examination, he had complete ophthalmoplegia (Video 1), areflexia, and impaired tandem gait.

Brain MRI and CSF analysis were normal. Electrodiagnostic studies were normal apart from reduced recruitment of the right frontalis muscle.

Clinical Questions

Which of the following would be in your differential diagnosis?

1. Wernicke's encephalopathy
2. Miller-Fisher syndrome
3. Parinaud's syndrome
4. Myasthenia gravis

Which of the following laboratory studies would support a diagnosis of Miller-Fisher syndrome?

1. Anti-GM1 antibodies
2. Anti-MAG antibodies
3. Anti-GQ1b antibodies
4. Antineurofascin antibodies

This patient's anti-GQ1b titer was positive at a titer of 1:1600 (normal <1:100).

Discussion

- Miller-Fisher syndrome, a GBS variant, is characterized by the classic clinical triad of ophthalmoplegia, ataxia, and areflexia.[17] Other cranial neuropathies, dysesthesia, and micturition problems may also occur.
- Miller-Fisher syndrome comprises 5% to 10% of GBS cases in Western countries and a higher proportion in Asia. It often follows *C jejuni* or *Haemophilus influenzae* infection.[18] For description of other GBS variants please refer to (**Table 1**).
- The characteristic anti-GQ1b ganglioside antibodies react with *C jejuni* surface epitopes supporting molecular mimicry between nerve and bacteria.
- Electrodiagnostic studies may demonstrate sensory predominant axonopathy.[20]

- The prognosis is generally good, regardless of whether IVIg or plasma exchange is given. For this reason, many experts do not treat patients with classic Miller-Fisher syndrome, although patients with progressive weakness and ophthalmoplegia ("ophthalmoplegic GBS") should be treated.

Table 1
GBS variants

GBS Variant	Clinical Features	Associated Antibodies	Specific Comments
MFS	Ataxia Areflexia, Ophthalmoplegia	GQ1b, GT1a, GD1b	5%–10% of GBS cases. Higher incidence in Asia. Prognosis is good regardless of treatment.
Bickerstaff's brainstem encephalitis	Impaired consciousness Hyperreflexia Ophthalmoplegia Ataxia	GQ1b	Considered a variant of MFS (10%).
Pharyngeal-brachial variant	Facial and pharyngeal weakness May spread to arms Normal reflexes	GT1a, GD1a, GQ1b	3% of GBS.
Sensory GBS	Acute onset Symmetric sensory deficits No clinical motor involvement	None	Demyelinating features on motor nerve conduction studies.
Acute sensory ataxic neuropathy	Acute onset sensory ataxia Areflexia No ophthalmoplegia Positive Romberg sign Follows antecedent infection	GD1b	Considered an incomplete MFS subtype, Excellent recovery,
Ataxic GBS	Acute onset cerebellar-like ataxia No ophthalmoplegia Negative Romberg sign Follows antecedent infection	GQ1b	Considered an incomplete MFS subtype. Excellent recovery.
Acute autonomic sensory neuropathy	Acute onset sensory and autonomic deficits Reach clinical nadir within 1 mo Motor system spared	None	Sensory axonopathy on NCS. Likely responds to IVIg, PLEX, or steroids, but insufficient data to support use[19]
Acute motor axonal neuropathy	Rapid onset pure motor deficits. Minimal dysautonomia DTRs present/increased.	GM1, GD1a	Major subtype in Asia, Central and South America May be classified as a nodal or paranodal neuropathy owing to rapid reversal of conduction block.
Acute motor and sensory axonal neuropathy	Rapid onset, severe motor and sensory deficits Minimal dysautonomia	GM1, GD1a	—

Abbreviations: GBS, Guillain-Barré syndrome; MFS, Miller-Fisher syndrome.

CASE 3. THE 61-YEAR-OLD BANKER WITH DIABETES WITH PROGRESSIVE WEAKNESS

A 61-year-old man with type 2 diabetes presented with 4 months of progressive muscle weakness. It affected his arms and legs symmetrically, both proximally and distally. He went from walking independently, to using a cane, then a walker, and ultimately became wheelchair bound. The progressive finger and hand weakness resulted in trouble with activities of daily living. He reported mild numbness in the feet, but no paresthesia or neuropathic pain. He denied bowel, bladder, or bulbar dysfunction.

On examination the patient had symmetric weakness of his proximal and distal lower extremities (Medical Research Council grade 4/5 throughout, except dorsiflexion was a 3/5). Pinprick sensation was decreased to the level of the knees and hands. Vibratory sensation was absent to the level of the ankles and normal in the fingers. He was areflexic.

Clinical Questions

Which of the following clinical features would support a diagnosis of CIDP?

1. Autonomic dysfunction
2. Symmetric proximal and distal weakness
3. Respiratory impairment
4. Dysphagia

What would be the highest yield diagnostic study at this point?

1. CSF analysis
2. Nerve conduction studies and electromyography
3. Voltage-gated calcium channel antibodies
4. MRI of the brain

On nerve conduction studies, there were no elicitable sensory responses. The motor nerve conduction studies illustrated in **Table 2**.

In multiple motor nerves, there are prolonged distal latencies, slowed conduction velocities, and partial motor conduction block as represented in the left median–abductor pollicis brevis compound muscle action potential waveforms (**Fig. 2**):

Unlike GBS, CIDP is often managed with which treatment?

1. Plasma exchange
2. IVIg
3. Prednisone or other corticosteroid
4. Rituximab

Discussion

- CIDP is the most common, chronic autoimmune polyneuropathy.
- The estimated incidence is 0.33 per 100,000 and prevalence 2.81 per 100,000.[21]
- Both cellular and humoral mechanisms are involved.[22]

Clinical Presentation

- CIDP is an acquired demyelinating polyradiculoneuropathy that primarily involves large diameter myelinated nerve fibers resulting in weakness, loss of sensation, and sensory ataxia.

Table 2
Case 3 Motor Nerve Conduction Studies

Nerve/Sites	Muscle	Latency, ms	Ref., ms	Amplitude, mV	Ref., mV	Segments	Distance, mm	Lat Diff, ms	Velocity, m/s	Ref., m/s
R median - APB										
Wrist	APB	**6.6**	≤4.5	**4.0**	≥3.0	Wrist - APB	70			
Elbow	APB	15.1		**1.3**		Elbow-Wrist	252	8.5	**30**	≥48
L median-APB										
Wrist	APB	**8.4**	≤4.5	**3.1**	≥3.0	Wrist - APB	70			
Elbow	APB	17.2		**1.3**		Elbow-Wrist	258	8.8	**29**	≥48
R ulnar-ADM										
Wrist	ADM	**4.9**	≤3.6	**0.7**	≥5.0	Wrist - ADM	70			
B. Elbow	ADM	16.7		**0.3**		Wrist - B. Elbow	260	−11.7	**22**	≥48
A. Elbow	ADM	19.6		**0.3**		B. Elbow - A. elbow	90	−2.9	**31**	≥48
						A. Elbow-wrist		14.6		
L Radial - EIP										
Forearm	EIP	3.4		**0.7**	≥2.0	Forearm - EIP	60			
Elbow	EIP	11.1		**0.1**	≥2.0	Elbow - forearm	190	7.7	**25**	≥48
R peroneal - EDB										
Ankle	EDB	**NR**	≤6.6	**NR**	≥2.0	Ankle - EDB	80			
Fibula head	EDB	**NR**		**NR**		Ankle - fibula head		**NR**		≥42
R tibial - AH										
Ankle	AH	**NR**	≤6.6	**NR**	≥2.0	Ankle - AH	80			
Popliteal fossa	AH	**NR**		**NR**		Popliteal fossa - ankle		**NR**		≥42

In multiple motor nerves, there are prolonged distal latencies, slowed conduction velocities, and conduction block Abnormalities are bolded.

Abbreviations: ADM, abductor digiti minimi; AH, abductor hallucis; APB, abductor pollicis brevis; diff, difference; EDB, extensor digitorum brevis; EIP, extensor indicis proprius; L, left; lat, latency; NR, no response; R, right; ref, reference.

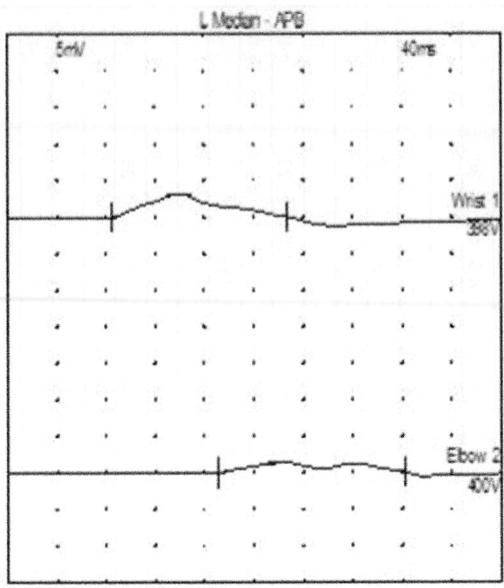

Fig. 2. Conduction block is represented in the left median–abductor pollicis brevis compound muscle action potential waveforms.

- One-half of patients have typical CIDP, which is characterized by symmetric, proximal, and distal generalized weakness; distal large fiber sensory impairment; and areflexia.
- A postural tremor may accompany the typical features of CIDP and is often treatment refractory.
- In contrast with GBS, CIDP usually spares the cranial nerves, respiratory muscles, and autonomic function.
- Patients reach clinical nadir more than 2 months after symptom onset.
- The disease course may be monophasic, relapsing remitting, or progressive.

Diagnostic Approach

- Electrodiagnostic testing is mandatory in patient with suspected CIDP. Classic features include:
  - Prolonged distal motor and peak sensory latencies
  - Slowing of motor conduction velocity that varies between nerves (nonuniform slowing)
  - Prolonged minimal F-wave latencies
  - Partial motor conduction block and abnormal temporal dispersion
  - A sural-sparing pattern (similar to GBS)
- Certain laboratory studies are necessary, including:
  - Serum electrophoresis, immunofixation, and free light chains to screen for a monoclonal gammopathy. Monoclonal gammopathies can be associated with CIDP. Other demyelinating neuropathies associated with hematologic malignancies are Waldenstrom's macroglobulinemia and osteosclerotic myeloma in polyneuropathy, organomegaly, endocrinopathy, M-protein, and skin changes, both of which portend a poorer prognosis and require a different treatment approach.

- Laboratory testing to exclude alternative causes of neuropathy such as glycosylated hemoglobin, liver, renal, thyroid function studies, vitamin B_{12} level.
- CSF analysis is not required for all cases of CIDP, but when collected also classically demonstrates cytoalbuminologic dissociation.
- MRI may demonstrate contrast enhancing, hypertrophied nerve roots, plexuses, and proximal peripheral nerves.[23,24]
- There are more than 15 electrodiagnostic criteria published for CIDP.[25] The European Federation of Neurologic Societies/Peripheral Nerve Society criteria are recommended, given their well-balanced sensitivity and specificity and high diagnostic accuracy.[26,27]

Treatment Approach

- There are 3 first-line treatments for CIDP including IVIg, subcutaneous immune globulins, and corticosteroids. Plasma exchange is considered second line given the logistical challenges of administering it chronically in the outpatient setting.
  - IVIg is typically administered at a 2 g/kg dose divided over 2 to 5 days, followed by every 3 to 4 week doses of approximately 1 g/kg. The dose and frequency should constantly be assessed and adjusted depending on treatment response.
  - Subcutaneous immune globulins is administered at a dose of 0.4 g/kg/wk for 5 weeks followed by maintenance dose of either 0.2 or 0.4 g/kg weekly. The PATH study led to its approval by the US Food and Drug Administration in 2018.[28]
  - Corticosteroids (prednisone at a daily dose of 1–1.5 g/kg, high-dose dexamethasone 40 mg/d for 4 days every 4 weeks, or IV methylprednisolone weekly) are options for induction therapy. Three months may be necessary for corticosteroids to be efficacious. Once there is clinical improvement, corticosteroids should be tapered.
- Plasma exchange is considered in refractory disease with 5 to 10 exchanges over 2 to 4 weeks followed by 1 to 2 sessions every 3 to 4 weeks.
- Steroid-sparing agents such as mycophenolate mofetil and azathioprine are often used to facilitate tapering of corticosteroids.[29,30]
- In patients refractory to these approaches, pulse intravenous cyclophosphamide 1 g/m^2 monthly for 6 months may be effective. The dose should be assessed and appropriately modified based on nadir white blood cell counts.[31]

> The overall likelihood of improvement on one of these first-line CIDP treatments is approximately 70%. This likelihood increases to approximately 80% when patients are included who switch to a different first-line therapy.[32]

CASE 4. A 68-YEAR-OLD WITH LEFT HAND WEAKNESS

The patient presented with left hand weakness upon waking up in the morning. Months later, she realized she has difficulty pressing the gas pedal or the brakes completely with her right foot. On examination, she had a left finger and wrist drop as well as right foot drop (**Fig. 3**). Electrodiagnostic studies confirmed conduction blocks of multiple motor nerves at noncompressive sites suggesting a diagnosis of multifocal motor neuropathy (MMN).

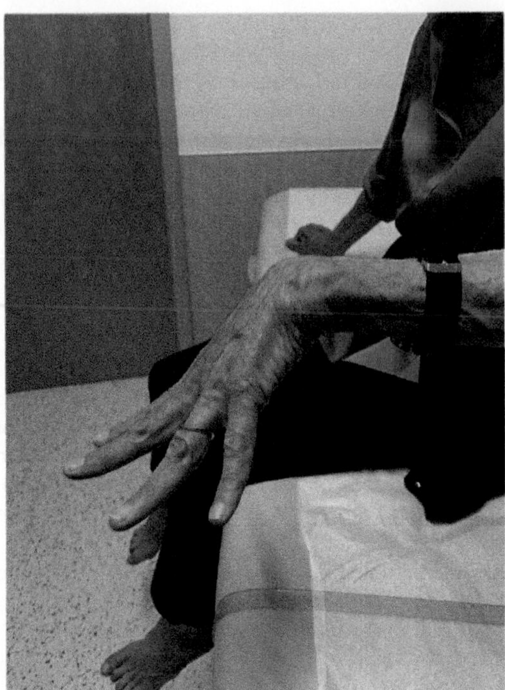

Fig. 3. Left wrist and finger drop.

Clinical Questions

Which of the following autoantibodies is present in approximately 50% of MMN patients?

1. Anti-GQ1b antibodies
2. Anti-GD1a antibodies
3. Anti-MAG antibodies
4. Anti-GM-1 antibodies

Which of the following treatments, which is effective for CIDP, may worsen MMN?

1. Corticosteroids
2. Plasma exchange
3. IVIg
4. Rituximab

Discussion

- MMN is an acquired neuropathy that affects individual motor nerves.
- Nerve conduction studies demonstrate multiple areas of partial motor conduction block in 60% of patients. Evolving evidence suggests GM1 antibodies impair function at the node of Ranvier, calling into question whether MMN is truly a demyelinating neuropathy or a nodopathy.[33]
- Males are affected more than females at a ratio of 2.7:1.[34]

Clinical Presentation

- The initial site of onset is the distal upper extremity in the majority of patients, with one-third first experiencing foot drop.[34]

- Cramps and fasciculations may occur.
- Cold often exacerbates symptoms.
- Sensory signs and symptoms should not exist.

MMN is considered in the differential diagnosis for motor neuron diseases owing to its painless, progressive weakness.

- MMN has weakness affecting individual peripheral nerves, whereas amyotrophic lateral sclerosis has weakness in a myotomal pattern.
- Amyotrophic lateral sclerosis is associated with upper motor neuron signs, whereas MMN is a pure lower motor neuron syndrome.

Diagnostic Approach

- Electrophysiologic studies, which confirm the clinical diagnosis, demonstrate conduction block at nonentrapment sites.
  - The ulnar and median nerves are most commonly affected.
- Anti-GM1 antibodies are present in approximately 50%, and may be monoclonal.[35]
- MRI may demonstrate enlargement and enhancement of the roots, plexuses, and peripheral nerves. Ultrasound examination similarly may demonstrate multifocal nerve enlargement.

Treatment

- IVIg is clearly the first choice treatment for MMN.[36] Subcutaneous immune globulins is also likely beneficial.[37,38]
- Cyclophosphamide and rituximab are considered only in the setting of treatment-refractory disease.[34]
- Corticosteroids are ineffective and have been reported to worsen disease.[36]

CASE 5. THE 40-YEAR-OLD WITH RELENTLESSLY PROGRESSIVE WEAKNESS

A 40-year-old man presented as a second opinion for CIDP. He developed numbness of the soles of his feet acutely approximately 6 months before presentation. Over the following 2 months, the numbness ascended his legs and into his hands, followed by progressive weakness, resulting in a steppage gait. His initial electrodiagnostic studies demonstrated a demyelinating neuropathy and he was started on IVIg. Despite repeated doses, his weakness progressed, resulting in needing a rolling walker and then a wheelchair. He was treated with several doses of intravenous methylprednisolone followed by 60 mg of prednisone daily without improvement. He lacked bulbar or autonomic dysfunction. His CSF protein was 733 mg/dL with 3 white blood cells per high power field.

Upon presentation to our institution, his motor examination was remarkable for Medical Research Council grade 2 to 3/5 strength proximally and 0/5 strength distally in the upper and lower extremities. He had profound loss of small and large fiber-mediated sensation in a length-dependent pattern. Deep tendon reflexes were unobtainable. He was nonambulatory. His electrodiagnostic studies were repeated (**Table 3**).

The study was interpreted as consistent with a severe length-dependent sensorimotor demyelinating neuropathy with secondary axonal degeneration.

Clinical Questions

Which of the following are distinctive features of this patient's presentation, which raise the possibility of a nodo-paranodopathy?

Table 3
Repeat electrodiagnostic studies

Nerve/Sites	Rec. Site	Peak Lat, ms	Ref., ms	B-P Amp, μV	Ref., μV	Segments	Distance, mm	Velocity, m/s
Sensory nerve conduction studies								
R Median - Ulnar Digit II and V								
Wrist (median)	Dig II	**NR**	≤3.7	**NR**	≥15	Wrist (median) - Dig II	130	**NR**
Wrist (ulnar)	Dig v	**NR**	≤3.1	**NR**	≥5	Wrist (ulnar) - Dig V	110	**NR**
R Radial - Anatomic snuff box (forearm)								
Forearm	Wrist	**NR**	≤2.5	**NR**	≥14	Forearm - wrist	100	**NR**
						Forearm - wrist	100	**NR**
L Radial - Anatomic snuff box (forearm)								
Forearm	Wrist	**NR**	≤2.5	**NR**	≥14	Forearm - wrist	100	**NR**
						Forearm - wrist	100	**NR**
R Sural – ankle (calf)								
Calf	Ankle	**NR**	≤4.8	**NR**	≥5	Calf - ankle	140	**NR**
						Calf - ankle	140	**NR**

Nerve/Sites	Muscle	Latency, ms	Ref., ms	Amplitude, mV	Ref., mV	Segments	Distance, mm	Lat Diff, ms	Velocity, m/s	Ref., m/s
Motor nerve conduction studies										
R Median - APB										
Wrist	APB	**12.8**	≤4.5	**0.2**	≥3.0	Wrist - APB	70			
Elbow	APB	26.4		0.2		Elbow - wrist	263	13.6	**19**	≥48
L Median - APB										
Wrist	APB	**12.3**	≤4.5	**0.3**	≥3.0	Wrist - APB	70			
Elbow	APB	21.9		0.1		Elbow - wrist	240	9.5	**25**	≥48
R Ulnar - ADM										
Wrist	ADM	**8.4**	≤3.6	**1.3**	≥5.0	Wrist - ADM	70			
B. Elbow	ADM	16.8		1.2		Wrist - B. elbow	235	−8.4	**28**	≥48

L Ulnar - ADM										
Wrist	ADM	**7.4**	≤3.6	**2.0**	≥5.0	Wrist - ADM	70			
B. Elbow	ADM	15.2		1.7		Wrist - B. elbow	217	–7.7	**28**	≥48
R Peroneal - EDB										
Ankle	EDB	**NR**	≤6.6	**NR**	≥2.0	Ankle - EDB	80			
R Tibial - AH										
Ankle	AH	**NR**	≤6.6	**NR**	≥4.0	Ankle - AH				

Abbreviations: ADM, abductor digiti minimi; AH, abductor hallucis; APB, abductor pollicis brevis; B-P Amp, baseline-peak amplitude; EDB, extensor digitorum brevis; EIP, extensor indicis proprius; lat, latency; NR, no response; Rec, recording; Ref, reference.

Abnormalities are bolded.

(*From* Collins MP, Dyck PJB, Gronseth GS, et al. Peripheral Nerve Society Guideline on the classification, diagnosis, investigation, and immunosuppressive therapy of non-systemic vasculitic neuropathy: executive summary. J Peripher Nerv Syst. 2010;15(3):176–184; with permission.)

1. Refractoriness to IVIg
2. Severely prolonged distal latencies
3. Lack of tremor
4. Lack of dysautonomia
5. Distal predominant weakness

How would you manage this patient?

1. Admission to start plasma exchange
2. Continue the current treatment plan (IVIg and prednisone)
3. Rituximab
4. Initiate azathioprine

Given the patient's presentation, a demyelinating neuropathy panel including antibodies to neurofascin-155, neurofascin-140, and contactin-1 was sent. Neurofascin-155 antibodies returned positive. The patient was admitted to the hospital for a series of 5 plasma exchanges. He ultimately was discharged with twice weekly exchanges that have been spaced to every 2 weeks. He has experienced a dramatic clinical improvement (**Fig. 4**, Video 2). Rituximab was chosen as the next treatment to allow hopefully for discontinuation of the plasma exchange.

Discussion

- Ten percent of patients with CIDP will have antibodies directed to paranodal or nodal cell adhesion proteins.[39]
- These antibodies are associated treatment refractoriness and distinctive clinical presentations (**Table 4**).
- Antibodies may be directed toward contactin-1 in the axons and neurofascin-155 in the myelin at the paranodal region. Together these proteins, with contactin-associated protein 1, form a complex that allows for gathering of voltage-gated sodium channels at the nodes and voltage-gated potassium channels at the juxtaparanodes.[40]
- Autoantibodies may also attack the nodal form of neurofascin isoforms 186 and 140.
- These antibodies are of the IgG4 subtype.
- CSF protein is remarkably elevated even more than typical CIDP cases.

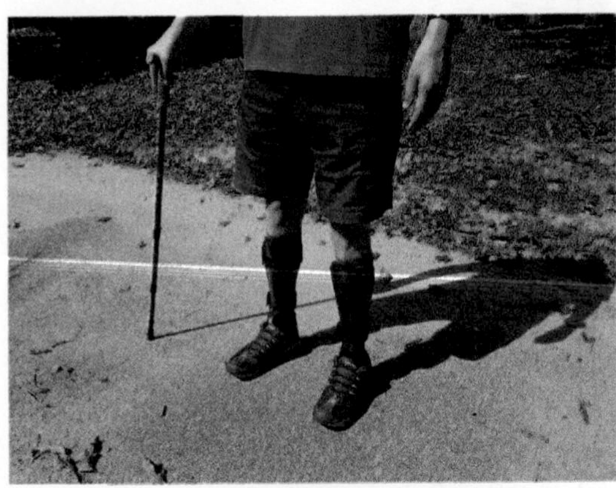

Fig. 4. Patient standing with ankle foot orthotics and a cane.

Table 4
Neuropathies associated with nodal and paranodal proteins

Autoantibody	Location	Presentation	Treatment Response
Anti-CNTN1	Axons in paranodal region	Motor predominant neuropathy or Sensory ataxic neuropathy May mimic GBS	Refractory to IVIg Steroid responsive May respond to B-cell depletion (rituximab)
Anti-NF155	Myelin in paranodal region	Young patients Distal weakness Ataxia (with cerebellar component) 3–5 Hz tremor High association with HLA-DRB 15	Refractory to IVIg May respond to B-cell depletion (rituximab)
Anti-NF186/140	Nodal region	Subacute sensory ataxia No tremor Associated nephrotic syndrome and retroperitoneal fibrosis reported	Better response to IVIg May respond to B-cell depletion (rituximab)

Abbreviations: CNTN1, contactin-1; NF-155, neurofascin-155; NF186/140, neurofascin isoforms 186 and 140.

CASE 6. THE 55-YEAR-OLD WITH PAINFUL FOOT DROP

A 55-year-old woman developed right wrist and forearm pain without any weakness. This pain was followed by numbness and tingling in her right foot, which then spread to her left foot. While out at dinner, she noted she was dragging her left foot. She consulted with her internist who sent the following laboratory studies: erythrocyte sedimentation rate of 82 (reference value, <20), cytoplasmic antineutrophil cytoplasmic antibody titer of 1:40 (reference value, <1:20), and perinuclear antineutrophil cytoplasmic antibody of less than 1:20. The internist noted the patient had raised, red-purple spots on her extremities (**Fig. 5**). Given the concern that the rash was palpable purpura (leukocytoclastic vasculitis) and the pattern of her neurologic presentation, the patient was then referred for electrodiagnostic studies (**Fig. 6**, **Table 5**).

Clinical Questions

This patient's clinical presentation and electrodiagnostic studies are highly suggestive of which diagnosis?

1. Wartenburg's migratory sensory neuritis
2. Neurolymphomatosis
3. Scleroderma-associated polyneuropathy
4. Antineutrophil cytoplasmic antibody–associated vasculitic neuropathy

What is the definitive test for vasculitic neuropathies?

1. Histopathologic evidence of a necrotizing vasculitis.
2. Demonstration of positive antineutrophil cytoplasmic antibodies in the peripheral blood.
3. Electrophysiologic evidence of multiple partial motor conduction blocks.
4. Elevated serum neurofilament light chains.

Ultimately, the patient was referred for a right superficial peroneal biopsy (**Fig. 7**).

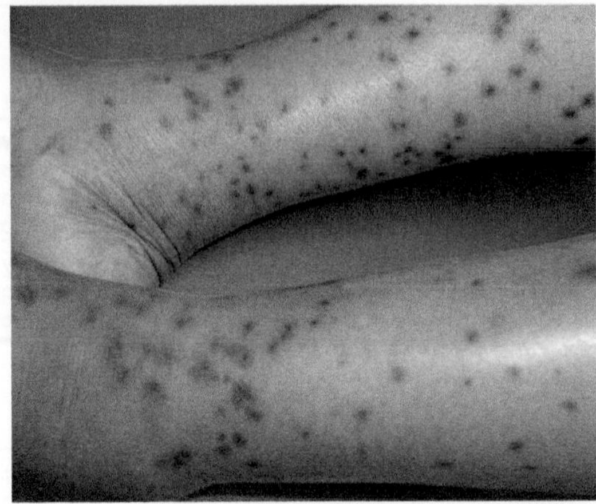

Fig. 5. Leukocytoclastic vasculitis (ie, palpable purpura).

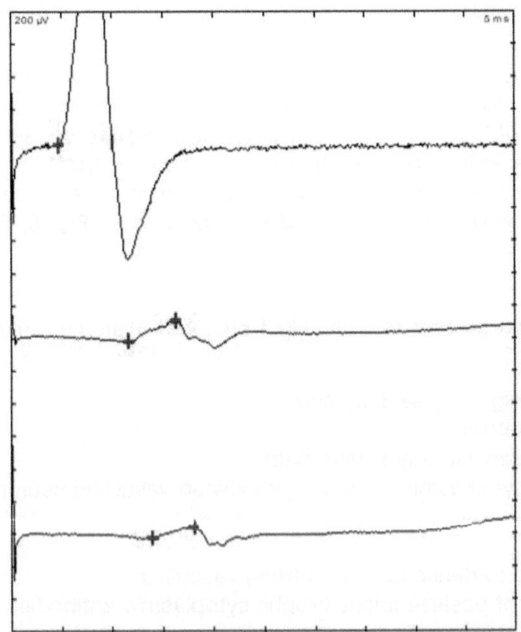

Fig. 6. Nerve conduction studies were performed and were interpreted as an asymmetric, motor-predominant polyneuropathy. There were several nerves that demonstrated partial motor conduction block. The right peroneal nerve compound muscle action potential wave-forms and data are included to the left and below for illustrative purposes.

Table 5
Right peroneal-EDB compound muscle action potentials

Nerve/ Sites	Muscle	Latency, ms	Ref., ms	Amplitude, mV	Ref., mV	Segments	Distance, mm	Lat Diff, ms	Velocity, m/s	Ref., m/s
R Peroneal - EDB										
Ankle	EDB	4.8	≤6. 6	**1.3**	≥2.0	EDB - ankle	80	4.8		
Fibula (head)	EDB	11.7		**0.1**		Ankle - fibula (head)	295	6.9	43	≥42
Popliteal fossa	EDB	14.0		**0.1**		Ankle - popliteal fossa	413	9.2	45	

Abbreviations: Diff, difference; Dist, distance; mNl, normal; R, right.

Given the histopathologic findings on nerve biopsy demonstrating a necrotizing vasculitic neuropathy, the patient was started on 60 mg/d of prednisone. Despite this she experienced spread of weakness to her hands and worsening neuropathic pain.

Which of the following would be the *most appropriate* next management step?

1. Rituximab
2. Mycophenolate mofetil
3. Azathioprine
4. IVIg
5. Plasma exchange

She was then treated with rituximab 1 g twice separated by 2 weeks. Her corticosteroids were gradually tapered with some improvement in strength and neuropathic pain.

Discussion

- Vasculitic neuropathies result from inflammatory cell infiltration of the vasa nervorum and resultant ischemia of the peripheral nerves.
- These neuropathies may occur in the context of systemic vasculitis.

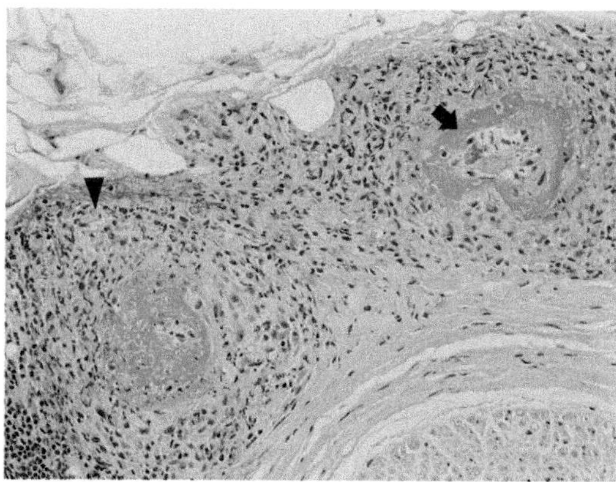

Fig. 7. Hematoxylin and eosin stain of the right superficial peroneal nerve demonstrated transmural inflammation in epineurial blood vessels (*arrowhead*), with focal fibrinoid necrosis of the vessel walls (*arrow*) and a partially occluded lumen.

  - Primary systemic vasculitis includes systemic disorders resulting in multiorgan dysfunction such as eosinophilic granulomatosis with polyangiitis and polyarteritis nodosa.
  - Secondary systemic vasculitis is associated with specific triggers, such as viral infection, connective tissue disease, and paraneoplastic disease (**Box 1**).

Box 1
Classification of vasculitides associated with neuropathy according to the Peripheral Nerve Society Guideline of 2010

I. Primary systemic vasculitides
   a. Predominantly small vessel vasculitis
      i. Microscopic polyangiitis
      ii. Churg-Strauss syndrome (eosinophilic granulomatosis with polyangiitis)
      iii. Wegener granulomatosis (granulomatosis with polyangiitis)
      iv. Essential mixed cryoglobulinemia (non–hepatitis C related)
      v. Henoch-Schölein purpura
   b. Predominantly medium vessel vasculitis
      i. Polyarteritis nodosa
   c. Predominantly large vessel vasculitis
      i. Giant cell vasculitis

II. Secondary systemic vasculitides association with 1 of the following:
   a. Connective tissue diseases
      i. Rheumatoid arthritis
      ii. Systemic lupus erythematosus
      iii. Sjögren syndrome
      iv. Systemic sclerosis
      v. Dermatomyositis
      vi. Mixed connective tissue disease
   b. Sarcoidosis
   c. Behcet disease
   d. Infection (hepatitis B, hepatitis C, human immunodeficiency virus, cytomegalovirus, leprosy, Lyme disease, HTLV-1)
   e. Drugs
   f. Malignancy
   g. Inflammatory bowel disease
   h. Hypocomplementemic urticarial vasculitis syndrome

III. Nonsystemic/localized vasculitis
   a. NSVN (includes nondiabetic radiculoplexus neuropathy and some cases of Wartenberg migrant sensory neuritis)
   b. Diabetic radiculoplexus neuropathy
   c. Localized cutaneous/neuropathic vasculitis
      i. Cutaneous polyarteritis nodosa
      ii. Others

Abbreviation: HTLV-1, human T-cell leukemia virus type 1.

From Collins MP, Dyck PJB, Gronseth GS, et al. Peripheral Nerve Society Guideline on the classification, diagnosis, investigation, and immunosuppressive therapy of non-systemic vasculitic neuropathy: executive summary. *J Peripher Nerv Syst*. 2010;15(3):176–184.

- Vasculitis may also be isolated to the peripheral nervous system (ie, nonsystemic vasculitic neuropathy [NSVN]) or may focally affect the roots, plexus, and nerves such as in the radiculoplexus neuropathies (eg, diabetic lumbosacral radiculoplexus neuropathy [DLRPN]).

Clinical Presentation

- Classically, patients develop sequential involvement of individual peripheral nerves, the so-called mononeuritis multiplex or multiple mononeuropathy pattern. This painful, progressive neuropathy starts acutely or subacutely. Initially, numbness and weakness are asymmetric, but over time may become symmetric ("confluent").
- In those with systemic vasculitis, other organ involvement is commonplace, resulting in respiratory impairment, gastrointestinal symptoms, hematuria, and rash. Constitutional symptoms such as weight loss, fevers, chills, and night sweats often coexist. In contrast, NSVN is not associated with any extraneural manifestations.

Diagnostic Evaluation

- Laboratory studies
  - The following laboratory studies are necessary in all suspected vasculitic neuropathy patients: erythrocyte sedimentation rate, C-reactive protein, antineutrophil cytoplasmic antibodies, rheumatoid factor, complete blood count, comprehensive metabolic panel, hepatitis B and C and cryoglobulins.
  - Antineutrophil cytoplasmic antibodies are antibodies directed against polymorphonuclear cell antigens. Most often, cytoplasmic antineutrophil cytoplasmic antibodies are associated with antibodies directed against proteinase 3 and perinuclear antineutrophil cytoplasmic antibodies are associated with myeloperoxidase antibodies. Microscopic polyangiitis and eosinophilic granulomatosis with polyangiitis are associated with perinuclear antineutrophil cytoplasmic antibody, whereas cytoplasmic antineutrophil cytoplasmic antibody is associated with granulomatosis with polyangiitis.
- Electrodiagnostic studies
  - Multiple nerves with side-to-side comparisons should be studied to assess for multifocality and asymmetry.
  - Nerve conduction studies can also identify an affected nerve for biopsy.
  - A characteristic finding, which is occasionally identified, is pseudoconduction block, as was observed in this patient. This finding occurs in the setting of acute nerve infarct, resulting in failure of conduction and apparent conduction block when the nerve is stimulated proximal to the infarct site. Within days Wallerian degeneration results in the expected axonal changes.
- Nerve biopsy
  - Sensory nerve biopsy, usually with a neighboring muscle, is imperative in cases of suspected NSVN and in systemic vasculitic neuropathy if another organ has not demonstrated histopathologic evidence of vasculitis. Biopsy of a nearby muscle increases diagnostic yield by 25%.[41]
  - Vasculitic neuropathies can be classified based on size of the affected blood vessels into nerve large arteriole (affecting blood vessels that range from 75 to 300 μm in diameter) and microvasculitis (affecting blood vessels <40 μm in diameter).
  - Common histopathologic features, regardless of the size of involved blood vessels, include perivascular inflammation, axonal degeneration, macrophages laden with hemosiderin, immune complex deposition, and neovascularization and fibrinogen in the epineurial vessel walls. Fascicle-to-fascicle

variation in axon loss may also be observed. Diagnostic criteria for pathologic diagnosis of vasculitic neuropathies exist.[42]
  - Fibrinoid necrosis of the tunica media and intima is a finding in nerve large arteriole vasculitis.

Treatment

- Treatment can be considered in 2 categories: induction and maintenance.
  - Induction therapy
    - Induction therapy is conventionally high dose corticosteroids (prednisone 1.0 mg/kg/d).
    - In antineutrophil cytoplasmic antibody-associated vasculitis, corticosteroids are often combined with cyclophosphamide or rituximab.[43,44]
    - In NSVN, combination therapy (corticosteroids with cyclophosphamide or methotrexate) is recommended over corticosteroid monotherapy.[45] Additionally rituximab is likely a first-line alternative to cyclophosphamide in induction therapy for severe NSVN.
    - Plasma exchange and IVIg can be considered for refractory vasculitis.
    - In localized forms of vasculitic neuropathy, if the diagnosis is made quickly (eg, DLRPN), short-term treatment with IVIg or intravenous corticosteroids, such as methylprednisolone, is appropriate. Long-term immunosuppression is unnecessary.
  - Maintenance therapy
    - Methotrexate, azathioprine, and rituximab are used for maintenance therapy.[46]

CASE 7. THE ATAXIC, DYSPNEIC PATIENT

An 84-year-old woman developed numbness in her hands and feet simultaneously 2 years earlier. She then developed dyspnea. A computed tomography scan of the chest demonstrated pulmonary fibrosis. Serologic testing revealed a positive anti–Sjögren's syndrome-related antigen A antibody. She established care with a rheumatologist who initiated hydroxychloroquine. Her numbness progressed and within 6 months of symptom onset she was using a rolling walker. At the time of presentation to the neurologist, she reported numbness affecting her entire body but sparing her face. She could not walk because her feet "do what they want."

On examination, she had absent vibratory sensation in the toes, ankles, and knees. In the fingers, vibratory sensation was diminished by 15 seconds. Proprioception was absent at the toes and ankles and diminished at the fingertips. She had absent pinprick sensation in the distal lower extremities. She was areflexic and had profound sensory ataxia. With her eyes closed, she demonstrated abnormal writhing movements of her fingers (ie, pseudoathetosis).

Clinical Questions

What is the most likely localization for this patient's neuropathy?

1. Dorsal columns
2. Small nerve fibers
3. Dorsal root ganglia
4. Large nerve fibers

The patient was suspected to have Sjögren's syndrome-associated sensory neuronopathy. What is the other major cause of acquired sensory neuronopathies?

1. Systemic lupus erythematosus
2. Paraneoplastic syndrome
3. Autoimmune hepatitis
4. Epstein-Barr virus

Discussion

- Sensory neuronopathies (or dorsal root ganglionopathies) result from damage to the dorsal root ganglia, which contain the sensory nerve cell bodies.
- The etiologies of these unique neuropathies are diverse and include autoimmune, degenerative, inherited, and toxic causes.[47]
- Given the rarity of these conditions, the incidence and prevalence remains unknown.
- The autoimmune causes of sensory neuronopathies include:
  - Paraneoplastic sensory neuronopathy
    - These are most often associated with anti-Hu and rarely anti-CV2/CRMP-5 antibodies.
    - Small cell lung cancer is the most common malignancy. Others include gynecologic, bladder, and prostate cancers.
    - Autonomic features (gastroparesis, tonic pupils) have been reported.
  - Sjögren's syndrome
    - It is less common than other Sjögren's syndrome-associated neurologic manifestations but is likely the most disabling.
    - Autonomic dysfunction often occurs.
  - Other autoimmune diseases
    - Case reports of autoimmune hepatitis, systemic lupus erythematosus, and celiac disease
    - Possible association with anti–fibroblast growth factor receptor 3 antibodies[48]

Clinical Presentation

- Typical clinical features of sensory neuronopathies include early ataxia, positive sensory symptoms, and multifocal and asymmetric sensory loss.
- Strength is normal, although patients with profound sensory loss have significant motor dysfunction.
- Deep tendon reflexes are often absent.

Diagnostic Approach

- Laboratory studies for autoimmune sensory neuronopathies include anti-Hu and anti-CV2/CRMP-5 antibodies, antinuclear antibody, anti–Sjögren's syndrome-related antigen A/B and occasionally anti–double-stranded DNA for systemic lupus erythematosus.[47]
- Electrodiagnostic studies demonstrate a non–length-dependent sensory neuropathy with low amplitude or absent sensory responses in a multifocal or non–length-dependent pattern. If the upper extremity sensory responses are disproportionately affected compared with the lower extremity responses, this finding strongly supports sensory neuronopathy.[49]
- If paraneoplastic sensory neuronopathy is suspected, a computed tomography scan of the chest looking for the primary malignancy should be performed. If negative, then a PET scan with fluorodeoxyglucose will increase yield.[50,51] If

no malignancy is found, cancer screening should continue with imaging every 6 months for up to 4 years.[52]

- Additionally, T2-weighted signal is often increased in the posterior columns of the spinal cord in sensory neuronopathies.[53]
- Dorsal root ganglion biopsy is discouraged given its high morbidity.
- **Table 6** reviews the sensory neuronopathy diagnostic criteria incorporating the exam, electrodiagnostic studies, and imaging.[49]

Table 6
Diagnostic criteria of sensory neuronopathy by Camdessanché and colleagues

Step A	Points
In a patient with clinically pure sensory neuropathy a diagnosis of sensory neuronopathy is considered as *possible* if total score is >6.5 points	
a. Ataxia in the lower or upper limbs at onset or full development of the neuropathy	+3.1
b. Asymmetrical distribution of sensory loss at onset or full development of the neuropathy	+1.7
c. Sensory loss not restricted to the lower limbs at full development	+2.0
d. At ≥SNAP absent or 3 SNAPs <30% of the LLN in the upper limbs, not explained by entrapment neuropathy	+2.8
e. <2 nerves with abnormal motor NCS in the lower limbs (abnormal if CMAP or MCV is <95% of LLN, distal latencies >110% of LLN or F waves latency>110% of LLN)	+3.1
Step B	
A diagnosis of sensory neuronopathy is *probable* if the patient's score is >6.5 points and if the initial workup does not show biological perturbations or electromyogram findings (such as conduction block or temporal dispersion) excluding sensory neuronopathy, Or if the patient has one of the following disorders: Onconeural antibodies (including anti-Hu and CRMP-5) or cancer within 5 y Cisplatin treatment Sjögren's syndrome Or MRI shows high signal in the posterior columns of the spinal cord	
Step C	
A diagnosis of sensory neuronopathy is *definite* if DRG degeneration is pathologically demonstrated although DRG biopsy is not recommended	

Abbreviations: CMAP, compound motor action potential; DRG, dorsal root ganglion; LLN, lower limit of normal; MCV, motor nerve conduction velocity; MRI, magnetic resonance imaging; NCS, nerve conduction studies; SNAP, sensory nerve action potential.

From Camdessanché J-P, Jousserand G, Ferraud K, et al. The pattern and diagnostic criteria of sensory neuronopathy: a case-control study. *Brain*. 2009;132(Pt 7):1723-1733; with permission. *Reproduced and slightly modified with permissions from the author and publisher.*

Treatment

- No randomized, controlled trials of autoimmune sensory neuronopathies exist.

Many treatments have been tried with variable success including IVIg, rituximab, plasma exchange, corticosteroids, and cyclophosphamide.[47] Poor response is common.

ACKNOWLEDGMENTS

The authors would like to acknowledge Dr Hope Richard, Dr Julia Nunley, and Dr Yang Tang for their assistance with the figures.

DISCLOSURE

Dr K.G. Gwathmey serves as a consultant to Alexion pharmaceuticals. Dr A.G. Smith serves as a consultant to Alexion, Argenx, Disarm, and Regenesis, and receives research funding from NINDS and NIDDK.

SUPPLEMENTARY DATA

Supplementary data related to this article can be found online at https://doi.org/10.1016/j.ncl.2020.03.008.

REFERENCES

1. Mesrati F, Vecchierini MF. F-waves: neurophysiology and clinical value. Neurophysiol Clin 2004;34(5):217–43.
2. Rees JH, Soudain SE, Gregson NA, et al. Campylobacter jejuni infection and Guillain-Barré syndrome. N Engl J Med 1995;333(21):1374–9.
3. Jacobs BC, Rothbarth PH, van der Meché FG, et al. The spectrum of antecedent infections in Guillain-Barré syndrome: a case-control study. Neurology 1998; 51(4):1110–5. Available at: http://www.ncbi.nlm.nih.gov/pubmed/9781538. Accessed August 2, 2013.
4. Willison HJ, Jacobs BC, van Doorn PA. Guillain-Barré syndrome. Lancet 2016; 388(10045):717–27.
5. Zheng X, Yu L, Xu Q, et al. Guillain-Barre syndrome caused by hepatitis E infection: case report and literature review. BMC Infect Dis 2018;18(1):50.
6. Nascimento OJM, da Silva IRF. Guillain-Barré syndrome and Zika virus outbreaks. Curr Opin Neurol 2017;30(5):500–7.
7. Vellozzi C, Iqbal S, Broder K. Guillain-Barre syndrome, influenza, and influenza vaccination: the epidemiologic evidence. Clin Infect Dis 2014;58(8):1149–55.
8. Ropper AH. The Guillain-Barré syndrome. N Engl J Med 1992;326(17):1130–6.
9. Fokke C, van den Berg B, Drenthen J, et al. Diagnosis of Guillain-Barré syndrome and validation of Brighton criteria. Brain 2014;137(Pt 1):33–43.
10. Wong AHY, Umapathi T, Nishimoto Y, et al. Cytoalbuminologic dissociation in Asian patients with Guillain-Barré and Miller Fisher syndromes. J Peripher Nerv Syst 2015;20(1):47–51.
11. Byun WM, Park WK, Park BH, et al. Guillain-Barré syndrome: MR imaging findings of the spine in eight patients. Radiology 1998;208(1):137–41.
12. Grimm A, Décard BF, Schramm A, et al. Ultrasound and electrophysiologic findings in patients with Guillain-Barré syndrome at disease onset and over a period of six months. Clin Neurophysiol 2016;127(2):1657–63.
13. Chevret S, Hughes RA, Annane D. Plasma exchange for Guillain-Barré syndrome. Cochrane Database Syst Rev 2017;(2):CD001798.
14. Hughes RAC, Swan AV, van Doorn PA. Intravenous immunoglobulin for Guillain-Barré syndrome. Cochrane Database Syst Rev 2014;(9):CD002063.
15. Ortiz-Salas P, Velez-Van-Meerbeke A, Galvis-Gomez CA, et al. Human immunoglobulin versus plasmapheresis in Guillain-Barre syndrome and myasthenia gravis: a meta-analysis. J Clin Neuromuscul Dis 2016;18(1):1–11.
16. van den Berg B, Walgaard C, Drenthen J, et al. Guillain-Barré syndrome: pathogenesis, diagnosis, treatment and prognosis. Nat Rev Neurol 2014;10(8):469–82.
17. Mori M, Kuwabara S, Fukutake T, et al. Clinical features and prognosis of Miller Fisher syndrome. Neurology 2001;56(8):1104–6. Available at: http://www.ncbi.nlm.nih.gov/pubmed/11320188.

18. Lo YL. Clinical and immunological spectrum of the Miller Fisher syndrome. Muscle Nerve 2007;36(5):615–27.
19. Koike H, Watanabe H, Sobue G. The spectrum of immune-mediated autonomic neuropathies: insights from the clinicopathological features. J Neurol Neurosurg Psychiatry 2013;84(1):98–106.
20. Kuwabara S, Sekiguchi Y, Misawa S. Electrophysiology in Fisher syndrome. Clin Neurophysiol 2017;128(1):215–9.
21. Broers MC, Bunschoten C, Nieboer D, et al. Incidence and prevalence of chronic inflammatory demyelinating polyradiculoneuropathy: a systematic review and meta-analysis. Neuroepidemiology 2019;52(3–4):161–72.
22. Köller H, Kieseier BC, Jander S, et al. Chronic inflammatory demyelinating polyneuropathy. N Engl J Med 2005;352(13):1343–56.
23. Lozeron P, Lacour M-C, Vandendries C, et al. Contribution of plexus MRI in the diagnosis of atypical chronic inflammatory demyelinating polyneuropathies. J Neurol Sci 2016;360:170–5.
24. Lichtenstein T, Sprenger A, Weiss K, et al. MRI biomarkers of proximal nerve injury in CIDP. Ann Clin Transl Neurol 2018;5(1):19–28.
25. Breiner A, Brannagan TH. Comparison of sensitivity and specificity among 15 criteria for chronic inflammatory demyelinating polyneuropathy. Muscle Nerve 2014;50(1):40–6.
26. Magda P, Latov N, Brannagan TH, et al. Comparison of electrodiagnostic abnormalities and criteria in a cohort of patients with chronic inflammatory demyelinating polyneuropathy. Arch Neurol 2003;60(12):1755–9.
27. Hughes RAC, Bouche P, Cornblath DR, et al. European Federation of Neurological Societies/Peripheral Nerve Society guideline on management of chronic inflammatory demyelinating polyradiculoneuropathy: report of a joint task force of the European Federation of Neurological Societies and the Peripher. Eur J Neurol 2006;13(4):326–32.
28. van Schaik IN, Bril V, van Geloven N, et al. Subcutaneous immunoglobulin for maintenance treatment in chronic inflammatory demyelinating polyneuropathy (PATH): a randomised, double-blind, placebo-controlled, phase 3 trial. Lancet Neurol 2018;17(1):35–46.
29. Mahdi-Rogers M, Brassington R, Gunn AA, et al. Immunomodulatory treatment other than corticosteroids, immunoglobulin and plasma exchange for chronic inflammatory demyelinating polyradiculoneuropathy. Cochrane Database Syst Rev 2017;(5):CD003280.
30. Gorson KC, Amato AA, Ropper AH. Efficacy of mycophenolate mofetil in patients with chronic immune demyelinating polyneuropathy. Neurology 2004;63(4):715–7.
31. Kaplan A, Brannagan TH. Evaluation of patients with refractory chronic inflammatory demyelinating polyneuropathy. Muscle Nerve 2017;55(4):476–82.
32. Cocito D, Paolasso I, Antonini G, et al. A nationwide retrospective analysis on the effect of immune therapies in patients with chronic inflammatory demyelinating polyradiculoneuropathy. Eur J Neurol 2010;17(2):289–94.
33. Uncini A, Susuki K, Yuki N. Nodo-paranodopathy: beyond the demyelinating and axonal classification in anti-ganglioside antibody-mediated neuropathies. Clin Neurophysiol 2013;124(10):1928–34.
34. Yeh WZ, Dyck PJ, van den Berg LH, et al. Multifocal motor neuropathy: controversies and priorities. J Neurol Neurosurg Psychiatry 2019. https://doi.org/10.1136/jnnp-2019-321532.

35. Beadon K, Guimarães-Costa R, Léger J-M. Multifocal motor neuropathy. Curr Opin Neurol 2018;31(5):559–64.
36. Meuth SG, Kleinschnitz C. Multifocal motor neuropathy: update on clinical characteristics, pathophysiological concepts and therapeutic options. Eur Neurol 2010;63(4):193–204.
37. Racosta JM, Sposato LA, Kimpinski K. Subcutaneous versus intravenous immunoglobulin for chronic autoimmune neuropathies: a meta-analysis. Muscle Nerve 2017;55(6):802–9.
38. Harbo T, Andersen H, Hess A, et al. Subcutaneous versus intravenous immunoglobulin in multifocal motor neuropathy: a randomized, single-blinded cross-over trial. Eur J Neurol 2009;16(5):631–8.
39. Bunschoten C, Jacobs BC, Van den Bergh PYK, et al. Progress in diagnosis and treatment of chronic inflammatory demyelinating polyradiculoneuropathy. Lancet Neurol 2019;18(8):784–94.
40. Querol L, Devaux J, Rojas-Garcia R, et al. Autoantibodies in chronic inflammatory neuropathies: diagnostic and therapeutic implications. Nat Rev Neurol 2017;13(9):533–47.
41. Vital C, Vital A, Canron M-H, et al. Combined nerve and muscle biopsy in the diagnosis of vasculitic neuropathy. A 16-year retrospective study of 202 cases. J Peripher Nerv Syst 2006;11(1):20–9.
42. Collins MP, Dyck PJB, Gronseth GS, et al. Peripheral Nerve Society Guideline on the classification, diagnosis, investigation, and immunosuppressive therapy of non-systemic vasculitic neuropathy: executive summary. J Peripher Nerv Syst 2010;15(3):176–84.
43. Jones RB, Tervaert JWC, Hauser T, et al. Rituximab versus cyclophosphamide in ANCA-associated renal vasculitis. N Engl J Med 2010;363(3):211–20.
44. Stone JH, Merkel PA, Spiera R, et al. Rituximab versus cyclophosphamide for ANCA-associated vasculitis. N Engl J Med 2010;363(3):221–32.
45. Collins MP, Hadden RD. The nonsystemic vasculitic neuropathies. Nat Rev Neurol 2017;13(5):302–16.
46. Gwathmey KG, Tracy JA, Dyck PJB. Peripheral nerve vasculitis: classification and disease associations. Neurol Clin 2019;37(2):303–33.
47. Gwathmey KG. Sensory neuronopathies. Muscle Nerve 2016;53(1):8–19.
48. Antoine J-C, Boutahar N, Lassablière F, et al. Antifibroblast growth factor receptor 3 antibodies identify a subgroup of patients with sensory neuropathy. J Neurol Neurosurg Psychiatry 2015;86(12):1347–55.
49. Camdessanché J-P, Jousserand G, Ferraud K, et al. The pattern and diagnostic criteria of sensory neuronopathy: a case-control study. Brain 2009;132(Pt 7):1723–33.
50. Titulaer MJ, Soffietti R, Dalmau J, et al. Screening for tumours in paraneoplastic syndromes: report of an EFNS task force. Eur J Neurol 2011;18(1):19-e3.
51. Rees JH, Hain SF, Johnson MR, et al. The role of [18F]fluoro-2-deoxyglucose-PET scanning in the diagnosis of paraneoplastic neurological disorders. Brain 2001;124(Pt 11):2223–31. Available at: http://www.ncbi.nlm.nih.gov/pubmed/11673324. Accessed November 5, 2014.
52. Rosenfeld MR, Dalmau J. Paraneoplastic neurologic syndromes. Neurol Clin 2018;36(3):675–85.
53. Bao Y-F, Tang W-J, Zhu D-Q, et al. Sensory neuronopathy involves the spinal cord and brachial plexus: a quantitative study employing multiple-echo data image combination (MEDIC) and turbo inversion recovery magnitude (TIRM). Neuroradiology 2013;55(1):41–8.

Printed and bound by CPI Group (UK) Ltd, Croydon, CR0 4YY
03/10/2024
01040478-0007